Orthogeriatrics: Surgical Procedures and Therapy

Orthogeriatrics: Surgical Procedures and Therapy

Editor: Hugo Hiddleston

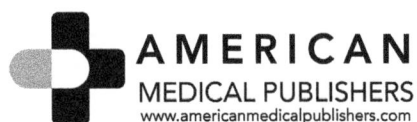

AMERICAN
MEDICAL PUBLISHERS
www.americanmedicalpublishers.com

AMERICAN
MEDICAL PUBLISHERS
www.americanmedicalpublishers.com

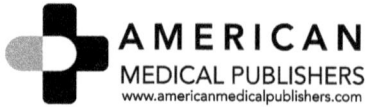

Cataloging-in-Publication Data

Orthogeriatrics: surgical procedures and therapy / edited by Hugo Hiddleston.
    p. cm.
Includes bibliographical references and index.
ISBN 978-1-63927-774-2
1. Geriatric orthopedics. 2. Orthopedic surgery. 3. Musculoskeletal diseases in old age.
4. Older people--Surgery. 5. Orthopedics. I. Hiddleston, Hugo.
RD732.3.A44 O78 2023
617.308 46--dc23

American Medical Publishers,
41 Flatbush Avenue,
1st Floor, New York,
NY 11217, USA

ISBN 978-1-63927-774-2 (Hardback)

Contents

Preface

I am honored to present to you this unique book which encompasses the most up-to-date data in the field. I was extremely pleased to get this opportunity of editing the work of experts from across the globe. I have also written papers in this field and researched the various aspects revolving around the progress of the discipline. I have tried to unify my knowledge along with that of stalwarts from every corner of the world, to produce a text which not only benefits the readers but also facilitates the growth of the field.

Orthogeriatrics refers to a subspecialty that was created in response to social, clinical and financial requirements for managing patients with fragility fractures. It is a multidisciplinary and integrated approach for the treatment of fracture patients who require surgical intervention. In patients who are unable to walk, hip fracture surgery can be seen as a palliative process with the aim of pain control. The evidence base for hip fracture care is strongest in orthogeriatrics. A mutual understanding, regard and trust of the roles among orthopedic surgery and geriatric medicine are necessary for the delivery of effective orthogeriatric care. It increases the standard of patient care and achieves a suitable level of clinical optimization throughout the perioperative period. It also reduces the length of hospital stays as well as hospital mortality, while achieving significant cost savings in the management of this medical condition. This book covers in detail some existent theories and innovative concepts revolving around the surgical procedures related to orthogeriatrics. Medical professionals and students actively engaged in this field will find it full of crucial and unexplored concepts.

Finally, I would like to thank all the contributing authors for their valuable time and contributions. This book would not have been possible without their efforts. I would also like to thank my friends and family for their constant support.

Editor

Missing Diagnosis, Pain and Loss of Function in Older Adults with Rheumatoid Arthritis and Insufficiency Fractures

Pia Simonsen Lentz [1], Anna Havelund Rasmussen [1], Aysun Yurtsever [2] and Dorte Melgaard [3,4,*]

[1] Department of Physiotherapy and Occupational Therapy North Denmark Regional Hospital, Bispensgade 37, DK-9800 Hjoerring, Denmark; psl@rn.dk (P.S.L.); annahavelundrasmussen@gmail.com (A.H.R.)

[2] Department of Rheumatology, North Denmark Regional Hospital, Bispensgade 37, DK-9800 Hjørring, Denmark; ayyu@rn.dk

[3] Centre for Clinical Research, North Denmark Regional Hospital, DK-9800 Hjoerring, Denmark

[4] Department of Clinical Medicine, Aalborg University, DK-9000 Aalborg, Denmark

* Correspondence: dmk@rn.dk

Abstract: Rheumatoid arthritis (RA) is characterised by a chronic, progressive inflammation in the joints and leads to substantial pain, disability, and other morbidities. Few studies document the occurrence of insufficiency fractures, but no studies document the patient's perspective on incurring an insufficiency fracture. The aim of this qualitative study was to explore the patients' perspective on how insufficiency fractures influence their level of activity and to detect their need for rehabilitation. Two focus-group interviews were performed with 10 patients diagnosed with RA and insufficiency fractures. The data from the focus-group interviews were subjected to thematic analysis to provide a sense of the important themes. The 10 patients were all females, aged 57–88 years. Magnetic resonance imaging were performed at a mean of six months and seven days. All patients identified the delayed diagnosis of fracture as a significant burden. They experienced pain but did not receive a diagnosis. When the patients were immobilised, some of them were offered aids such as crutches, which they were unable to use due to their RA. The patients needed a focus on diagnosis and individually customised rehabilitation, taking into account RA and including guidance concerning daily activities, aids, and the regain of physical function.

Keywords: rheumatoid arthritis; insufficiency fracture; stress fracture; rehabilitation; pain; delayed diagnosis; qualitative research

1. Introduction

Rheumatoid arthritis (RA) is the most common form of inflammatory arthritis [1], and the disease is characterised by chronic, progressive, systematic inflammation. This inflammation leads to substantial pain, disability, and other morbidities [2]. Patients with RA have an increased risk of osteoporosis and osteoporotic fractures [3], and other studies document that women with RA have an increased risk of fractures compared to women without RA [4–8]. Osteoporotic fracture is associated with the risk of falling [9,10]. An increased risk of osteoporosis and osteoporotic fractures is well reported, and the higher risk is related to inactivity or corticosteroid therapy [11].

Only occasionally has the medical literature reported the occurrence of insufficiency extremity fractures in rheumatoid arthritis [12,13]. An insufficiency fracture occurs when the mechanical strength of a bone is reduced to the point that physiological stress, which would not fracture a healthy bone, breaks a weak one. The condition that causes reduced bone strength typically does so throughout the skeleton (e.g., osteoporosis, osteomalacia, or osteogenesis imperfecta) but may be more localised (e.g., demineralisation in a limb due to disuse) [14].

Rheumatologists in the North Denmark Regional Hospital noticed some cases in which new-onset knee or ankle pain was misinterpreted as arthritis activity by the clinicians but was later shown to be insufficiency fractures [15]. X-ray examination did not show the insufficiency fractures, but MRI examination did reveal them. The fractures are at risk of being overlooked, and this fact may lead to a delay in diagnosis and the risk of ineffective treatment with, for example, steroid injections [12,13,15,16]. The included patients' RA status was well known, and they often experienced symptoms such as pain, reduced functionality, and loss of quality of life (QOL). The insufficiency fractures were treated conservatively, and the patients were immobilised for several weeks [15]. Due to their RA, the patients had difficulty using crutches and wheelchairs, and they often became care-dependent [17].

The complexity of the course of diseases due to RA and the immobilisation of the patients while the bone heals makes it relevant to involve the patient's experiences and perspective. This qualitative study aimed to explore what patients diagnosed with RA and insufficiency fractures experienced relevant during and after immobilisation.

2. Materials and Methods

2.1. Study Design

Two focus-group interviews were conducted to gather information about rehabilitation needs in patients with RA and insufficiency fractures during and after immobilisation. A loose model was used to structure the moderator guide with five starting questions in order to create an exploratory data production [18].

- "Did you experience pain?—if yes, how did the pain influence your life?"
- "How did you manage your daily activities?"
- "Were you challenged with physical activity when you were immobilized?"
- "Was your mood, sleep or social life influenced by the time you had the fracture?"
- "Is there anything you find important to tell about the time you had the fracture?"

This method was furthermore chosen to open the possibility of interaction among the group members and allow them to explore and clarify individual and common perspectives [19].

2.2. Participants

The rheumatologists identified a total of 15 patients with insufficiency fractures in the period from 2010 to 2015. They were all women aged 57–89. They had an average RA disease duration of 14.2 years, and all patients had a diagnosis delay of insufficiency fracture from about one month to more than one year and nine months. Two patients died, and the remaining 13 patients were invited for the interview, but three declined the invitation. A drop out analysis was not constructed.

The study was conducted in the physio- and occupational therapy unit in North Denmark Regional Hospital, Hjørring, in 2015. All the participating patients in this study were affiliated with the rheumatology department, North Denmark Regional Hospital. Initially, the patients were sent a letter to inform them about the aim of the study, and later they were contacted by telephone. Ten patients, aged 57–88 years and fulfilling the classification criteria for RA and insufficiency fractures, participated. The participants had an average RA disease duration of 14.2 years, and a magnetic resonance imaging (MRI) had been performed at a mean of six months and seven days after pain onset, as illustrated in Table 1.

Table 1. Patient characteristics.

	Pseudonym	Gender	Age	RA Duration	Diagnosis Delay
57–69 years (group 1)	1	F	61	38.5 y	1 m 24 d
	2	F	66	12 y	1 m 7 d
	3	F	57	19 y	1 y 9 m 14 d
	4	F	64	12 y	7 m 3 d
	5	F	62	11y	2 m 8 d
	6	F	66	12 y	5 m
71–88 years (group 2)	7	F	77	24 y	6 m 14 d
	8	F	69	32 y	3 m 12 d
	9	F	88	4 y	7 m 3 d
	10	F	69	10 y	6 m 20 d

RA: Rheumatoid arthritis; F: female; y: years; m: months; d: days.

The participating patients were divided into two focus groups. Each of the two groups was constructed based on age ranges, 57–69 years and 71–88 years. The groups were based on age due to the presumption that the groups then would be more homogenous to level of function and similar experiences. The purpose was furthermore to make a clear sense of the participants' reactions during the discussions and observe similarities and differences in their opinions and experiences [19].

2.3. Data Collection and Analysis

The focus-group interviews were carried out in an informal clinical setting, each lasting between 45 min and one hour. The interviews were conducted by P.S.L. and A.H.R. as moderators, one moderator for each group. If the patients responded individually to the moderator's questions, they were encouraged to talk and interact with each other [20]. The moderator guide consisted of questions of the following wide issues concerning difficulties in performing activities of daily living, difficulties in physical activity and exercise, modified function level, and delay of diagnosis.

Both focus-group interviews were audiotaped and afterwards transcribed by P.S.L. All patients were initially given a pseudonym from the numbers 1–10, later used in the processing of patients' statements. The analysis was conducted by coding in which meaningfully related data items were assigned to a unique theme [18,19].

The thematic analysis of the focus groups' data provided a sense of important themes. The authors discussed and studied in detail the statements of different patients, leading to the identification of key candidate themes. Subthemes and overarching themes were developed further and refined by discussion between the authors. Finally, the main themes were agreed upon and named.

2.4. Ethical Considerations

According to Danish legislation, the registration and publication of data from clinical registries do not require patient consent or approval by ethics committees, but all patients nevertheless signed informed written consent to ensure a high level of information. The Danish Data Protection Agency approved the study (No. 2015-41-4158).

3. Results

3.1. The Thematic Analysis Identified Two Main Themes: Delayed Diagnosis and Loss of Functionality
Delayed Diagnosis

All patients identified the missing diagnosis as a significant burden. They were feeling an unknown pain and did not get an explanation or diagnosis. Conventional X-ray examination may not identify the insufficiency fractures, and some of the patients waited months before an MRI detected the fracture: "*I was sent for a scan, and then they realised what it was*" (patient 3). The missing diagnosis and explanation for the pain led to frustrations: *"No, it's just that feeling that nobody really believes you"* (patient 1). Some of the patients had a delay of months before the diagnosis was made: *"Sometimes after I've been up here, I've sat and cried when I got home because I'd got absolutely nothing out of it. After about two weeks, I'd ring up and explain that it hadn't got any better, and then I'd get called in for the same treatment again"* (patient 8). Most of the patients were treated with intra-articular steroid injection in the fractured joint before the diagnosis was made: *"Then I got an adrenalin injection and it didn't help really as usual, so I got another one in November and that one didn't help either"* (patient 3). The diagnoses and explanation of the pain were very important for the patients: *"I've never been as happy as when I was told my leg was broken"* (patient 7).

3.2. Loss of Functionality

After the diagnosis, the patients were immobilised for several weeks: *"I wasn't allowed to do anything for two months. I wasn't even allowed to put any weight on my leg"* (patient 2). Some of the patients were still immobilised during the interview, and they were concerned about whether the fracture would heal as expected: *"I have to wear this boot for the next three months, and if I'm lucky, it'll be healed after the three months"* (patient 3).

All patients noticed a significant loss of function before the diagnosis was made and during immobilisation: *"I was so unhappy about not being able to do anything … even just getting up at night to go to the toilet"* (patient 7). The patients experienced challenges in performing daily activities: *"I can't even get to the toilet before I've wet myself"* (patient 7). Another patient who was still working said, *"I wasn't able to work there anymore; I had so much pain. I couldn't do anything"* (patient 1). Regarding daily activities, the patients mention as their main problem that they were immobilised: *"There were times when I couldn't even walk!"* (patient 2). Other patients were limited compared to their earlier walking distance: *"Even just being at home, you start thinking, 'How am I going to get to the other end of the house and back?'"* (patient 4). Most of the patients were very active in their daily life before the fracture, and the reduction in walking distance influenced their lives: *"Well, I've not been able to do the gardening"* (patient 4). The fear of falling and the fact that the patients experienced a higher risk of falling was also mentioned as another significant burden: *"It's still the same today … if I don't look where I'm going, suddenly, whoops, and I am lying on the ground. Just a small twig is enough to make me fall over"* (patient 1). Some of the other patients confirmed this: *"Suddenly, you fall, and you can't even see any reason for it afterwards"* (patient 5).

These patients face a challenge in having RA and a fracture. During the immobilisation, they were offered crutches, but they were not able to use standard crutches due to their RA: *"I have a problem with using crutches because I don't have enough strength in my arms to lift myself"* (patient 1). Due to a lack of power in the arms, some of the patients were provided a wheelchair even though it is not optimal due to the physiological consequences of being immobilised: *"I didn't have enough strength in my hands, so, after the operation, I was in a wheelchair for a while"* (patient 5). A patient asked whether it was possible to get axial crutches. The patients developed ways to solve their problems: *"So, now I use the office chair in the kitchen when I am cooking"* (patient 4). Another said, *"I couldn't really do the shopping. I went along sometimes and used the shopping trolley as a walking frame"* (patient 7).

Depending on other people was another psychological factor the patients mentioned: *"I'm lucky enough to have a husband that can cook a little and a grandchild that comes and does the cleaning"* (patient 1). The combination of dependence and the inability of performing daily activities was an issue: *"I used to be able to do the gardening, but now my husband has taken over, it really pains me that I can't do it"* (patient 4).

Most of the patients who were highly motivated for motion mentioned the importance of being active combined with the challenges of reduced walking distance: *"I wasn't allowed to do my exercises for my veins and my ankles … When I was in bed, I didn't have to wear the boot, so I would've been able to lift my legs and then do this to stretch them out, but I wasn't allowed to use my foot"* (patient 9). Another challenge is co-morbidity: *"But then I started getting out of breath and … then they found out that I also have heart*

fibrillations" (patient 4). Only one patient was offered rehabilitation: *"The rehabilitation was great ...
afterwards, I was able to walk properly again"* (patient 3).

Fatigue influenced most of the patients: *"But it was mostly the arthritis and not so much the fracture"*
(patient 5), and the other patients confirmed her statement. Mood was also affected for a couple of the
patients during the time they were waiting for a diagnosis and during the time they were immobilised:
"Yes, I also get upset and sad about it" (patient 9). Another patient said, *"I'm the type that tries to hide it and
finds it embarrassing"* (patient 10).

Most of the patients experienced more pain than usual with their RA: *"You suddenly have a lot more
pain, but you just don't know the reason"* (patient 5). After treatment with immobilisation, most of the
patients had less pain: *"I wasn't operated (on), and I was allowed to put weight on it. Having the plaster cast
on did help with the pain though"* (patient 6).

4. Discussion

The present study revealed that patients waited weeks or months to receive a diagnosis, and the
patients reported that the waiting time led to uncertainty among them; this reaction is also known
among other groups of patients who are misdiagnosed or where the diagnosis is delayed [21–23].

Delay in diagnosis is defined as a non-optimal interval of time between onset of symptoms,
identification, and initiation of treatment. A delayed diagnosis occurs when the correct diagnosis is
delayed due to failure in or untimely ordering of tests (e.g., lab work, colonoscopies, or breast imaging
studies) [24]. Patients with RA are accustomed to pain and coping with it, and this is common for
patients with RA [25]. This is confirmed in this study where patients do not focus on their pain in
general, but on the fact that they experienced a new and inexplicable pain that was more difficult to
cope with and which caused uncertainty and worries.

This study confirms that immobilised patients with insufficiency fractures experience functional
disability, a decrease in muscle strength, and fatigue [26]. Most of the patients in the present study had
an ankle fracture, and a study demonstrated that supervised physical therapy after the immobilisation
can reverse the decrease in muscle performance, functional ability, and fatigue [26]. Only the youngest
patient was offered rehabilitation, and she was very positive about the effect of the training. It seems
very relevant to offer supervised physiotherapy to this group of patients in future practice. This study
documents that it is not common practice to offer physiotherapy to this group of patients.

Women with RA demonstrate a twofold increase in osteoporosis [5]. The fact that most of the
women in the project were incorrectly treated with glucocorticoids, and afterwards immobilised,
further increased the risk of developing osteoporosis [27].

Most patients talked about their risk of falling. It is well known that patients with RA are at
increased risk of falling, and when they have fallen once they are more likely to fall again [28–31]. It is
relevant to offer supervised physiotherapy and the aids necessary to prevent falling [28].

RA has an impact on loss of functionality and social life, but the women in this study take pride in
their role as a housewife and so forth. More of the women explain that their dependency on other
people was very difficult for them to handle. The aids they obtained from the hospital made them
more independent, but often the aids were not useful due to their RA. There is a need for special aids
for patients with RA. The insufficiency fracture and the immobilisation influenced them negatively,
both psychologically and socially. Due to this, it is very important to offer the patients aids that are
useful with decreased muscle strength, also documented by Gold et al. [32].

Limitations and Strengths

A limitation of this study is that therapists conducted the interviews, and this may have influenced
the answers, due to the patients' dependency on the staff of the hospital and thus the unequal balance
of power, although there was no ongoing therapist–patient relationship when the interviews were
conducted. The interviews took place in the hospital, and, while the particular location was a conference
room, this venue may have had an impact on the patients and may have created a medical agenda for

the discussion. A limitation of a focus-group interview is that a social control in the group may lead the informants in one direction [33]. Also, several of the patients had fractures years ago, and this led to a risk-of-recall bias [34]. Accordingly, during the interviews, some of the patients were challenged to distinguish between their experiences with the insufficient fracture and other former fractures. Information about comorbidity was not obtained; however, it would have been relevant, as comorbidity can affect the participants' quality of life.

A strength of this study is that the informants are widely represented in relation to age and activity level. A second strength is the qualitative approach and the use of focus-group interviews to gain an understanding of these patients with RA experiencing an insufficiency fracture, which gives insight into the patients' universe in relation to their experience of diagnosis, pain, limitations in relation to activities, and offers of rehabilitation and aids. The interactions between participants with diverse characteristics allowed the identification of multiple meanings. Interaction between group participants is considered the distinct advantage of focus-group research, because the group dynamics, agreements, disagreements, and the way people account for their opinions are essential for the content of the data [35].

The knowledge about insufficiency fractures in patients with RA is limited, and there is a need for more focus on this problem to diagnose the insufficiency fracture early by pain onset and to offer the needed rehabilitation and aids.

5. Conclusions

In conclusion, the present study documents that patients with RA and insufficiency fractures experience the delayed diagnosis as a burden, and it is stressful for them to wait for an explanation of their pain. Due to the patients' inability to use crutches or a wheelchair, it is important to find other aids that patients with RA and insufficiency fractures can use. When the patients were immobilised, they experienced the loss of function, but were not offered supervised physical therapy. This points to the need to focus on the diagnosis and guidance of these patients in relation to daily activities, training, and aids.

Author Contributions: Conceptualization, A.H.R., P.S.L., A.Y. and D.M.; methodology, P.S.L., A.H.R. and D.M.; formal analysis, A.H.R., P.S.L. and D.M.; data curation, D.M.; writing—original draft preparation, D.M., A.H.R., P.S.L. and A.Y.; writing—review and editing, D.M., A.H.R., P.S.L. and A.Y. All authors have read and agreed to the published version of the manuscript.

Acknowledgments: The authors thank the participating patients for their involvement in the interviews.

References

1.   Rasch, E.K.; Hirsch, R.; Paulose-Ram, R.; Hochberg, M.C. Prevalence of rheumatoid arthritis in persons 60 years of age and older in the United States: Effect of different methods of case classification. *Arthritis Rheum.* **2003**, *48*, 917–926. [CrossRef]

2.   Mikuls, T.R. Co-morbidity in rheumatoid arthritis. *Best Pract. Res. Clin. Rheumatol.* **2003**, *17*, 729–752. [CrossRef]

3.   Hooyman, J.R.; Melton, L.J.; Nelson, A.M.; O'Fallon, W.M.; Riggs, B.L. Fractures after rheumatoid arthritis a population-based study. *Arthritis Rheum.* **1984**, *27*, 1353–1361. [CrossRef]

4.   Lane, N.E.; Pressman, A.R.; Star, V.L.; Cummings, S.R.; Nevitt, M.C. Rheumatoid arthritis and bone mineral density in elderly women. *J. Bone Miner. Res.* **2009**, *10*, 257–263. [CrossRef]

5.   Haugeberg, G.; Uhlig, T.; Falch, J.A.; Halse, J.I.; Kvien, T.K. Bone mineral density and frequency of osteoporosis in female patients with rheumatoid arthritis: Results from 394 patients in the Oslo County rheumatoid arthritis register. *Arthritis Rheum.* **2000**, *43*, 522–530. [CrossRef]

6.   Kroger, H.; Honkanen, R.; Saarikoski, S.; Alhava, E. Decreased axial bone mineral density in perimenopausal women with rheumatoid arthritis–a population based study. *Ann. Rheum. Dis.* **1994**, *53*, 18–23. [CrossRef]

7. Kinjo, M.; Setoguchi, S.; Solomon, D.H. Bone mineral density in older adult patients with rheumatoid arthritis: An analysis of NHANES III. *J. Rheumatol.* **2007**, *34*, 1971–1975.

8. Sinigaglia, L.; Nervetti, A.; Mela, Q.; Bianchi, G.; Del Puente, A.; Di Munno, O.; Frediani, B.; Cantatore, F.; Pellerito, R.; Bartolone, S.; et al. A multicenter cross sectional study on bone mineral density in rheumatoid arthritis. Italian Study Group on Bone Mass in Rheumatoid Arthritis. *J. Rheumatol.* **2000**, *27*, 2582–2589. [PubMed]

9. Leveille, S.G.; Jones, R.N.; Kiely, D.K.; Hausdorff, J.M.; Shmerling, R.H.; Guralnik, J.M.; Kiel, D.P.; Lipsitz, L.A.; Bean, J.F. Chronic Musculoskeletal Pain and the Occurrence of Falls in an Older Population. *JAMA* **2009**, *302*, 2214–2221. [CrossRef] [PubMed]

10. Durward, G.; Pugh, C.N.; Ogunremi, L.; Wills, R.; Cottee, M.; Patel, S. Detection of risk of falling and hip fracture in women referred for bone densitometry. *Lancet* **1999**, *354*, 220–221. [CrossRef]

11. Arnett, F.C.; Edworthy, S.M.; Bloch, D.A.; McShane, D.J.; Fries, J.F.; Cooper, N.S.; Healey, L.A.; Kaplan, S.R.; Liang, M.H.; Luthra, H.S.; et al. The american rheumatism association 1987 revised criteria for the classification of rheumatoid arthritis. *Arthritis Rheum.* **1988**, *31*, 315–324. [CrossRef] [PubMed]

12. Elkayam, O.; Paran, D.; Flusser, G.; Wigler, I.; Yaron, M.; Caspi, D. Insufficiency fractures in rheumatic patients: Misdiagnosis and underlying characteristics. *Clin. Exp. Rheumatol.* **2000**, *18*, 369–374. [PubMed]

13. Kay, L.J.; Holland, T.M.; Platt, P.N. Stress fractures in rheumatoid arthritis: A case series and case-control study. *Ann. Rheum. Dis.* **2004**, *63*, 1690–1692. [CrossRef] [PubMed]

14. Pentecost, R.L.; Murray, R.A.; Brindley, H.H. Fatigue, Insufficiency, and Pathologic Fractures. *JAMA* **1964**, *187*, 1001–1004. [CrossRef] [PubMed]

15. Yurtsever, A.; Fagerberg, S.K.; Rasmussen, C. Insufficiency fractures of the knee, ankle, and foot in rheumatoid arthritis: A case series and case-control study. *Eur. J. Rheumatol.* **2020**, *7*, 124–129. [CrossRef]

16. Yurtsever, A.; Rasmussen, C. AB0308 Spontaneous Ankle and Knee Fractures in Rheumatoid Arthritis: A CASE Report Study. *Ann. Rheum. Dis.* **2014**, *73*, 906. [CrossRef]

17. Herrera-Saray, P.; Pelaez-Ballestas, I.; Ramos-Lira, L.; Sanchez-Monroy, D.; Burgos-Vargas, R. Usage problems and social barriers faced by persons with a wheelchair and other aids. Qualitative study from the ergonomics perspective in persons disabled by rheumatoid arthritis and other conditions. *Reumatol. Clin.* **2013**, *9*, 24–30. [CrossRef]

18. Halkier, B. Focus groups as social enactments: Integrating interaction and content in the analysis of focus group data. *Qual. Res.* **2010**, *10*, 71–89. [CrossRef]

19. Morgan, D.L. *Qualitative Research Methods: Focus Groups as Qualitative Research*; SAGE Publications: Thousand Oaks, CA, USA, 1997.

20. Krueger, R.A. *Focus Groups: A Practical Guide for Applied Research*; SAGE Publications: Thousand Oaks, CA, USA, 2000.

21. Stockl, A. Complex syndromes, ambivalent diagnosis, and existential uncertainty: The case of Systemic Lupus Erythematosus (SLE). *Soc. Sci. Med.* **2007**, *65*, 1549–1559. [CrossRef]

22. Dubayova, T.; Van Dijk, J.P.; Nagyova, I.; Rosenberger, J.; Havlikova, E.; Gdovinova, Z.; Middel, B.; Groothoff, J.W. The impact of the intensity of fear on patient's delay regarding health care seeking behavior: A systematic review. *Int. J. Public Health* **2010**, *55*, 459–468. [CrossRef]

23. Van Der Linden, M.P.M.; Le Cessie, S.; Raza, K.; Van Der Woude, D.; Knevel, R.; Huizinga, T.W.; van der Helm-van Mil, A.H. Long-term impact of delay in assessment of patients with early arthritis. *Arthritis Rheum.* **2010**, *62*, 3537–3546. [CrossRef] [PubMed]

24. Definiciont of Delayed Diagnosis. Published 2020. Available online: http://www.reference.md/files/D057/mD057210.html (accessed on 18 October 2020).

25. Keefe, F.J.; Caldwell, D.S.; Martinez, S.; Nunley, J.; Beckham, J.; Williams, D.A. Analyzing pain in rheumatoid arthritis patients. Pain coping strategies in patients who have had knee replacement surgery. *Pain* **1991**, *46*, 153–160. [CrossRef]

26. Shaffer, M.A.; Okereke, E.; Esterhai, J.J.L.; Elliott, M.A.; Walter, G.A.; Yim, S.H.; Vandenborne, K. Effects of Immobilization on Plantar-Flexion Torque, Fatigue Resistance, and Functional Ability Following an Ankle Fracture. *Phys. Ther.* **2000**, *80*, 769–780. [CrossRef] [PubMed]

27. Abud-Mendoza, C. Considerations on treatment recommendations for rheumatoid arthritis. *Reumatol Clin.* **2015**, *11*, 193–195. [CrossRef]

28. Stanmore, E.K. Recommendations for assessing and preventing falls in adults of all ages with rheumatoid arthritis. *Br. J. Community Nurs.* **2015**, *20*, 529–533. [CrossRef]

29. Hayashibara, M.; Hagino, H.; Katagiri, H.; Okano, T.; Okada, J.; Teshima, R. Incidence and risk factors of falling in ambulatory patients with rheumatoid arthritis: A prospective 1-year study. *Osteoporos. Int.* **2010**, *21*, 1825–1833. [CrossRef]

30. Smulders, E.; Van Lankveld, W.; Eggermont, F.; Duysens, J.; Weerdesteyn, V. Step Performance in Persons With Rheumatoid Arthritis: A Case-Control Study. *Arch. Phys. Med. Rehabil.* **2011**, *92*, 1669–1674. [CrossRef]

31. Brenton-Rule, A.; Dalbeth, N.; Bassett, S.; Menz, H.B.; Rome, K. The incidence and risk factors for falls in adults with rheumatoid arthritis: A systematic review. *Semin. Arthritis Rheum.* **2015**, *44*, 389–398. [CrossRef]

32. Gold, D. The clinical impact of vertebral fractures: Quality of life in women with osteoporosis. *Bone* **1996**, *18*, S185–S189. [CrossRef]

33. Halkier, B. *Fokusgrupper.* 2; Roskilde Universitetsforlag: Roskilde, Denmark, 2008.

34. Coughlin, S.S. Recall bias in epidemiologic studies. *J. Clin. Epidemiol.* **1990**, *43*, 87–91. [CrossRef]

35. Grønkjær, M.; Curtis, T.; De Crespigny, C.; Delmar, C. Analysing group interaction in focus group research: Impact on content and the role of the moderator. *Qual. Stud.* **2011**, *2*, 16–30. [CrossRef]

Social Image Impacting Attitudes of Middle-Aged and Elderly People toward the Usage of Walking Aids: An Empirical Investigation in Taiwan

Shao-Wei Huang [1] and **Tsen-Yao Chang** [2,*]

1   Graduate School of Design, National Yunlin University of Science and Technology, Yunlin 640, Taiwan; d10530017@gemail.yuntech.edu.tw
2   Department of Creative Design, National Yunlin University of Science and Technology, Yunlin 640, Taiwan
*   Correspondence: changty@gemail.yuntech.edu.tw

Abstract: The elderly need the assistance of walking aids due to deterioration of their physical functions. However, they are often less willing to use these aids because of their worries about how others may think of them. Not using professional walking aids often makes elderly people fall easily when walking. This study explores the behavioral intention factors of middle-aged people (45–64 years old) and elderly people (65 years and older) that affect the use of walking aids. Based on the Theory of Reasoned Action (TRA), subjective norms, attitude toward usage, behavior intention, safety, and usefulness were combined with social image to establish the research framework. This study used questionnaire surveys both in paper form assisted by volunteers and in online electronic form. A total of 457 questionnaires were collected. Data analysis was carried out in three stages: descriptive analysis, measurement model verification, and structural equation model analysis. The results showed that social image had a significant impact on the attitude toward using walking aids. Factors such as attitude toward usage, subjective norms, and safety of walking aids also had a significant positive impact on behavioral intention. Finally, through the research results, some suggestions are proposed for stakeholders to improve the elderly's concerns about the social image of using walking aids.

Keywords: walking aids; social image; Theory of Reasoned Action (TRA)

1. Introduction

The world is currently facing a serious aging trend, and the speed of aging is rapidly accelerating. For example, it took 150 years for the population over 60 years old in France to go from 10% to 20%. However, it took only around 20 years for countries such as Brazil, China, and India to reach the same level [1]. The "2019 Revision of World Population Prospects" launched by the United Nations pointed out that the world is facing three major trends: a decrease in the new population, a rapid increase in the elderly population, and a decline in population in many countries [2]. According to data from the World Health Organization, in the period from 2015 to 2050, the proportion of the world's population over 60 will be almost double, from 12% to 22%. The aging population structure has become a major challenge for the entire world. In 2016, the World Health Organization and its members formulated the Global Aging and Health Strategy and Action Plan in the World Health Assembly (Document A69/17) [3]. In addition to focusing on healthy aging, providing a good supportive environment so that the elderly can walk easily is also one of the key points of continuous promotion, which include providing a barrier-free environment or the use of assistive devices. At the same time, the elderly can perform regular exercises to improve their physical and mental functions. It can help the elderly to delay aging [1].

According to the report, "Taiwan Population Estimates (2018–2065)" [4], released by the National Development Council, Taiwan is currently facing three major trends. First, the total population will turn to negative growth in 3–10 years. Second, if the total fertility rate remains the same, the number of births in 2065 will be halved. Third, Taiwan will become an overaged society in the next eight years. The rate of aging has surpassed developed countries such as European nations, America, and Japan. Moreover, once the number of births in the future decreases and the average age of the population increases, this means that the dependency ratio will continue to increase. In addition to major changes in the demographic structure, the social burden will also increase. Moreover, the report pointed out that in the future, the proportion of people over 65 in the total population will rise from 14.5% in 2018 to 41.2% in 2065. This means that four out of 10 people will be elderly [5]. Therefore, in order to deal with the aging social structure, Taiwan is currently actively improving the friendly environment for the elderly, including elderly-friendly workplaces, long-term care programs, and the economic security of the elderly.

The National Health Interview Survey, conducted by Taiwan's National Health Administration [6], interviewed 3280 elderly people in 2017. It stated that one out of six elderly people fell in the past year (495 people, 15.5%). As the physical functions of the elderly, including muscle strength and balance ability, etc., decline, they are gradually going downhill. Moreover, the survey also mentioned that the most common places to fall at home are the bedroom, living room, and bathroom. Among the top 10 causes of death among the elderly in Taiwan in 2019, accidents ranked sixth [7], even higher than kidney disease or high blood pressure. In addition to deaths in traffic accidents, the most common accidents are caused by falls.

Because of the deterioration of the body, many abilities of the elderly are not as good as when they were young, including vision, hearing, balance, reaction time, muscle strength, or endurance. Yang et al. conducted a study on elderly people with mild to moderate difficulties living in institutions [8]. The survey found that the functions affected by the activities of daily living (ADLs) of these elderly people included climbing stairs (62.9%), bathing (47.2%), and walking (40.4%). At the same time, it was also found that functional movements such as knee extension muscle strength, 3-m timed up and go, 30-s sitting and standing, and 2-min stance stepping were worse than in other normal elderly people.

Therefore, with age the performance of the elderly in ADLs is most often affected by the ability to walk. Suwannarat et al. conducted interviews and surveys on 343 elderly people over 65 years old in rural Thailand in 2015 [9]. The types of walking aids used by these elderly people and their mobile functions were discussed. The elders who participated in the survey had a significant correlation with the need for walking aids, especially the elderly over 75. The ability of daily living can be obviously improved through walking aids.

Some studies have mentioned that the elderly encounter several major obstacles when using assistive technologies, including privacy violations, insufficient trust in technical assistance tools, lack of value-added features, consideration of purchase costs, and lack of training or embarrassment [10]. Related researches tend to focus on high-tech assistive technologies, and rarely mention low-tech walking aids such as canes or walkers. On the topic of preventing the elderly from falling, researchers found out that many elderly people do not want to be associated with health problems. They think that the problem is "not for me" or they are afraid to feel stigmatized after using assistive devices [11]. The elderly do not want to use assistive devices because of their worry about dependence [12].

Simpson and Richardson [13] suggested that when a patient needs to use walking aids, medical staff should actively check the walking aids used by the patient and his or her health promotion needs. At the same time, the elderly are encouraged to seek professional advice before using walking aids. However, it can be observed in Taiwan that there are still many elders who have difficulty in moving and are reluctant to use walking aids such as canes or walkers, whether or not they need disability care services or are provided assistive device purchase subsidies. They are concerned about their social image and are afraid of being laughed at by others or being labeled as "disabled." They would rather struggle to walk or use umbrellas to assist themselves in walking. There is still a lack of relevant empirical research on the phenomenon of elderly people resisting the use of walking aids from the perspective of social image.

In 2014, the Technology Acceptance Model (TAM) was used to study the technology acceptance of the elderly in Hong Kong [14]. The results of the study pointed out that because Chinese people are more introverted and afraid of being laughed at for poor performance, it is easy to influence the intention of the elderly to use technology. In addition, Tural, Lu, and Cole [15] also discussed the attitudes and intentions of elderly people who use staircase-assisted design at home. Among them, if the appearance or aesthetics of the related equipment is well-designed, the elderly will still regard it as a continuous stigma of disability due to the association of negative images. For example, poor social acceptance or loss of independence [16] will affect their willingness to use related equipment. It can be seen that the elderly want to look like ordinary elderly people but do not want to be regarded as dependent or disabled, which will affect their behavioral intentions and attitudes when using assistive devices.

Therefore, this research will focus on the factors that influence the behavior of middle-aged (45–64 years old) and elderly (65 years and older) people toward using walking aids in Taiwan. The subjects of the study were not people with severe walking disabilities, but people with mild walking disabilities or those who needed walking supporters because of old age. As Asians live in a closely connected social environment, middle-aged and elderly people are more concerned with social image. Based on the rational behavior theory, the relationship between "social image", "attitude toward usage", "subjective norm", "safety level", "usefulness", and "behavior intention" will be verified by a survey investigation. According to the results of this study, it can provide a reference for government agencies and private manufactories to promote walking aids for middle-aged and elderly people.

2. Background and Hypotheses Development

2.1. Middle-Aged and Elderly People

Middle-aged citizens are considered to be those aged 45 to 65 years old, and the elderly those over 65 years old by the Middle-aged and Elderly Employment Promotion Act of the Ministry of Labor [17] in Taiwan. The Executive Yuan stated the purpose of formulating the regulations: "This middle-aged and senior citizens are mainly faced with age discrimination, decreased physical endurance, and social stereotypes" [18]. It can also be seen that the physical functions of middle-aged and elderly people gradually decline, which also leads to the decline of their social image, that is, the outside world tends to look down on their abilities. As of the end of last year (2019), the total population of middle-aged and older (45 years and older) was 10,681,705, accounting for 45.26% of the total population of the country (23,631,121). The phenomena bring the reality that many countries have to deal with them.

As the aging population increases, the proportion of people with reduced mobility is also increasing. Koon et al. [19] pointed out that decreased mobility is the most common disability condition among the elderly. Fifteen percent of the population over 65 years old (65–74 years old) have mobility problems and the population over 85 years old is as high as 48%. In addition, elderly people are prone to lower limb function weakness and poor balance due to illness or physical degradation, which may lead to falls [20]. Furthermore, the elderly rely on assistive devices to enhance their walking ability and improve the quality of life [21]. Therefore, even middle-aged people (45–64 years old), due to degeneration or disease, already face mobility problems. At the same time, the number of people with mobility impairments is increasing with age, and those with severe disabilities may even require assistance from others.

2.2. Design and Development of Walking Aids

In the Assistive Technology Act of the United States, assistive technology is divided into assistive technology equipment (devices) and assistive technology service (service) [17]. According to regulations in Taiwan, assistive technology equipment is the so-called assistive device, which refers to any product (including devices, equipment, instruments, technology, and software) [18]. The Bureau of Standards, Metrology, Inspection, and Quarantine of the Ministry of Economic Affairs in Taiwan formulated the classification standard CNS15390 for assistive devices in reference to the ISO 9999 specifications, which are divided into 11 categories such as personal medical assistive devices and personal mobility assistive devices. Wheelchairs, crutches, and walking aids are also personal mobility aids [20]. Others include one-arm operation walking aids, such as single crutches and four-legged crutches, and double-arm operation walking aids, such as axillary crutches, walkers, etc., as shown in Figure 1.

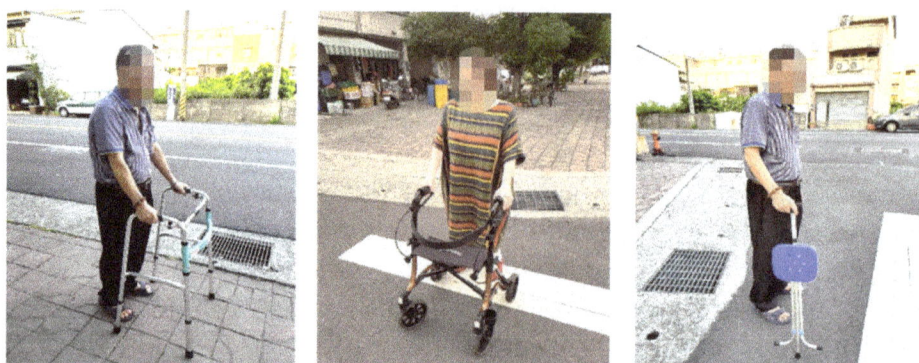

Figure 1. Walking aids (the images were shot by the authors).

At present, in the design and research of walking aids, most of them are developed based on the consideration of biomechanics, functional aspect, or appearance [21–24]. In addition, Juan, Wang, and Sie [25] and others used the Situational Story Method or the Quality Function Deployment Method to explore the usage scenario and user's needs. However, the psychological aspects of users or their attitudes toward the use of assistive devices are still rarely explored. It is also very important to understand the user's willingness and use of the walking aids.

2.3. Social Image

Social image usually plays the role of motivation and cognition. It is a perception that will arouse and imitate real experience in the heart; the feedback obtained after a certain content is disseminated to the public [26]; and also a subjective cognition of the external objective world [27]. Cepeda Zorrilla, Hodgson, and Jopson [28] pointed out that social image results when people put forward different tastes or prestige views as a reaction to public opinion. Guo et al. believed that social image is an evaluation of the image of a certain behavior participant [29]. For walking aids users, social image is how people see them while using walking aids, which is different from seeing people who do not use them.

In addition, social image is a topic of concern in care-services-related research fields. Li and Wu [30] discussed the working environment and social image of care attendants by dividing social image into two aspects: "social status" and "professional license." Moreover, Tsen [31] explored the benefits of promoting the social image of the mentally handicapped community, including social recognition, educational learning, and social care. Then, Hui-Fen [32] described some users' reactions in the research of the elderly using assistive devices. Many elderly people think that the use of assistive devices will make them become disabled people and expressed other reactions, such as "I am not a patient, and why do I use these assistive devices?" The common thought among elderly people is that using assistive devices reveals a negative social image. Therefore, the elderly are unwilling to use assistive devices.

Salifu Yusif et al. reviewed academic journals from 1976 to 2015 and searched 39 articles from Google and Google scholar from 2000 to 2015 [10]. They found that among the barriers to the use of assistive technology by the elderly, the "Privacy" factor was most frequently mentioned (15 articles). "Stigma", "Loss of Dignity", "Lack of accessibility and social inclusion" and other factors were also related to the social image of the elderly as being unwilling to use assistive technology. From exploring the research and application of disadvantaged groups, it was found that social images are obviously related to the user's attitude and intention of using assistive devices.

Since 2012, Dr. Chang has released conceptual designs of assistive devices that are based on a culturally creative and farsighted technology perspective, thinking about food, clothing, housing, transportation, education, and entertainment (shown in Figure 2) [33]. The design project emphasizes the need to provide basic health care and truly humane ways of responding to the needs of the elderly by considering their psychological aspects and providing aesthetic and practical designs, so that they can continue to live a decent and joyful life even in their twilight years. One of the works of the project, named "Puzzle for life" received the best work of the year. The concepts of the designs respond from the viewpoint of social image.

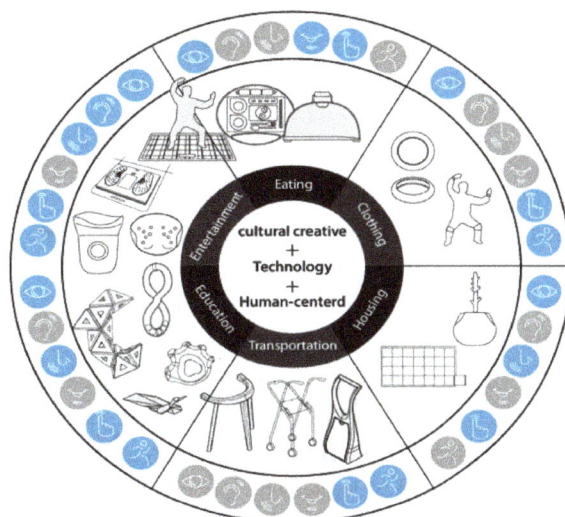

Figure 2. Conceptual design of assistive devices.

2.4. Theory of Reasoned Action

Theory of Reasoned Action (TRA) was proposed by Fishbein and Ajzen [34] to analyze how people change their behavior patterns through personal will. Human behavior is the result of rational thinking. The variables include attitudes, subjective norms, and behavioral intentions to explain and predict personal behavior. Attitude refers to the perception and evaluation of the implementation of specific behavior and also includes consideration of the subsequent results [35]. Subjective norms are the views and opinions held toward social pressure when engaging in specific behaviors. If other people hold opinions for (or against) something, the easier (or harder) it is to execute the act [36]. Furthermore, behavioral intention is the willingness to engage in a specific behavior, and it is a prerequisite for actual execution [37]. It will be affected by two elements: attitude and subjective norms.

Concerning health care and medicine-related fields, for example, the study of organ donation after death [38] explored the attitude and intention of organ donation through rational behavior theory and explained the rational decision-making process of this behavior. Moreover, in the study of the condom use behavior of people living with HIV [39] it was found that the subjective norms of condom use in individual cases can significantly predict the possibility of condom use in future sex. TRA is also used to explain how to improve health and develop good habits by increasing healthy behaviors and reducing habitual behaviors [40], for example, teachers' use of interventions to develop student habits to reduce the sitting time in the classroom [41] or related research on pregnant women's exercise behavior [42]. Rational behavior theory is also widely used in the study of the behavioral intentions of healthy people, patients, and middle-aged and elderly people.

Regarding empirical research on social image and usage attitude, Lin and Bhattacherjee [43] discussed the use of online entertainment systems. The research result showed that perceived entertainment and social image positively affect usage attitude. Therefore, social image will have a positive impact on the user's attitude.

In short, for middle-aged and elderly people, the perception of the social image of using a walker will have a positive impact on their attitude toward usage. Similarly, changes in attitudes and subjective norms will also affect the behavioral intention of using walking aids. Therefore, this research proposes the following hypotheses:

Hypothesis 1. *Social image will have a positive and significant influence on the attitude toward using walking aids.*

Hypothesis 2. *The attitude toward using walking aids will have a positive and significant influence on behavioral intention.*

Hypothesis 3. *Subjective norms will have a positive and significant influence on the behavioral intention of using walking aids.*

2.5. Safety

The safety aspect refers to safety awareness, which means whether people can be aware of their own safety [44]. The higher the awareness of safety, the more care and attention is paid to health or life [45]. In addition, the user's perception of safety is a cognitive process that affects emotions and behavioral intentions. It is expressed through the interaction between cognition, emotion, and behavioral intention. The need for safety means the importance of and attitude to safety, which are also proportional to the intention of use [46,47]. The safety level of walking aids refers to the stability and support of the walking aids [22,24], that they will not cause falls and secondary injuries [21].

In addition, safety needs to be considered in the research on intelligent nursing aids. For example, Kwee-Meier, Bützler, and Schlick [48] found in the study of wearable positioning systems that perceptual safety performance has a positive and significant impact on behavioral intentions. Consideration of the potential safety risks of smart home devices also is an important factor in whether consumers are willing to use smart devices [49]. In addition, research on intelligent nursing services for the elderly found that due to uncertain factors, especially perceived safety, the elderly are reluctant to use the intelligent call system. If the elderly can feel the degree of safety, the intention of use will be more obvious [50].

All in all, the perceived security level has a positive effect on behavioral intentions. For the elderly, the higher the perceived safety, the higher their intention to use walking aids. Therefore, this research infers that the perception of the middle-aged and elderly of the safety level has a positive and significant impact on behavioral intentions. The proposed hypothesis is:

Hypothesis 4. *The perceived safety level of walking aids will positively and significantly affect the behavioral intention of using walking aids.*

2.6. Usefulness

Fred Davis [51] proposed the Technology Acceptance Model (TAM), which pointed out that through perceived usefulness and perceived ease of use, as well as other variables, it is possible to predict whether users can accept a particular technology. Perceived usefulness means that when a certain technology can improve work performance, the willingness to use it will be greatly increased, and the work performance will also be improved accordingly. In addition, if users believe that related services are beneficial to their daily life or work, they will increase their intentions; if they find them easy to use, they will also increase their overall willingness to use them [52].

There are many related studies. For example, Lin and Chang [53] studied the factors that affect the willingness of the elderly to use, such as production and sales systems. It was found that subjective norms, the visibility of pictures and labels all have a significant impact on perceived usefulness. In addition, when discussing the opinions of the elderly on the practicality and their attitudes toward autonomous vehicles, the acceptance was very high [53]. Therefore, it can be stated that usefulness has a significant positive impact on usage intention and attitude.

In summary, usefulness has a positive effect on behavioral intentions. For users of walking aids, the higher the perceived usefulness, the higher will be their behavioral intention to use the aids. Therefore, the proposed hypothesis is:

Hypothesis 5.   *The usefulness of walking aids will positively and significantly affect the user's behavioral intentions.*

2.7. Mediation Effect

In the applied research on social image and usage attitude, Lin and Schlick [44] verified the positive correlation between social image and usage attitude. Attitudes positively influence behavioral intentions. Moreover, researches on the behavior of the different genders on the recycling of resources on campus and the behavioral research on information acceptance by the elderly have found that there is a direct correlation between use attitude and behavioral intention [54,55].

Based on the above research, social image has a positive influence on usage attitude, and usage attitude has a positive influence on behavior intention. For the user of walking aids, the more positive the social image of using walking aids is, the more positive the attitude toward using aids will be. Therefore, this study infers that middle-aged and elderly people's social image perception of using walking aids will have a positive and significant impact on behavioral intentions through their attitudes. The proposed hypothesis is:

Hypothesis 6. *The attitude toward the usage of walking aids has a mediation effect between social image and behavioral intention.*

This research explores the behavioral intentions of the middle-aged and the elderly toward the use of walking aids and studies the influencing factors. This study took social image, usage attitude, subjective norms, safety level, and usefulness as independent variables. Among them, usage attitude also played the role of a mediating variable. Behavioral intention was the dependent variable. Through the literature review, the research model is drawn as shown in Figure 3.

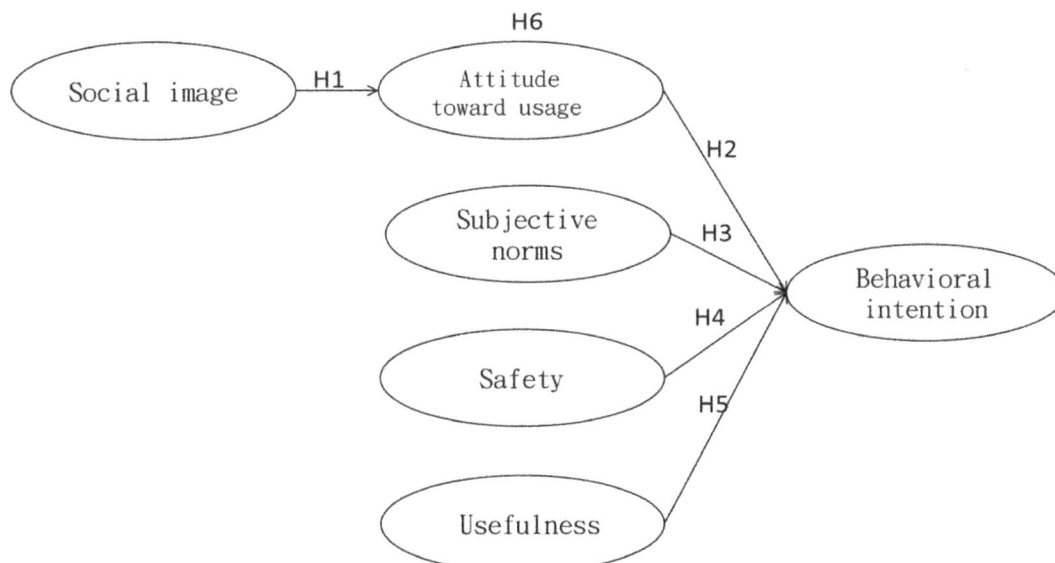

Figure 3. Research Model.

3. Materials and Methods

3.1. Data Collection

This study explored the intention of middle-aged and elderly people to use walking aids, so the research subjects were people over 45 years old. This research used questionnaires, which were conducted online and in the form of paper, which was assisted by volunteers. In the north, middle, south, and east of Taiwan, we collected research data through community elderly associations, religious groups, civil organizations, and assistive device manufacturers. The questionnaire collection period of time was from 1 May 2020 to 30 June 2020. After deleting invalid questionnaires, there were a total of 406 valid questionnaires. According to the sample size requirement formula from the survey system website [56], when the statistical confidence was 95% and the confidence interval was 5%, the sample size of the total population of Taiwan was 384 copies. Therefore, the sample size of this research was sufficient.

3.2. Measurement Instrument

The research questionnaire included the investigation of the basic participants' background information and their opinions of the research constructs. The background information, including gender, age, education, marital status, occupation, family environment, and residential area, was investigated in the first part of the questionnaire. Then, in the second part of the questionnaire the six latent variables were measured by a Likert seven-point scale ranging from "strongly disagree" (1) to "strongly agree" (7). The measurement items were mainly adapted from the previous studies. All items were originally written in Chinese and modified to the suitable walking aids usage scenario for the survey participants. First, there were five items related to users' attitudes toward using walking aids. Three items were adapted from Wu and Lin's study [57], one item was from Chen and Zheng's study [58], and the other one item was from Zhu, Huang, and Weng's work [59]. Then, for the subjective norm construct, all five items were adapted and modified from Zhang and Sink's study [60], which concerned people's walking activities in Taipei. The research target and scenario were similar to the present study. It contained encouragement from several aspects, such as families, friends, the elderly, the government, and environmental groups. After that, there were also five items about safety consideration. One item came from Lai's research [61] in the safety design of a public bicycle. Two items were adapted from Zhou and Lee's study [62] about the safety level of club members. The other two items were modified from Zhuang and Huang's study [63] about the well-being of native elementary students while walking on the community roads. Then, usefulness was also evaluated by five items. The first two items were adapted from Zeng, Hong, and Lin's research [64]. Their research concerned using technology to solve problems. The other three items were from Xu et al.'s study, which concerned how a blog can provide useful information [65]. Moreover, three items about social image measurement were taken from Yang et al.'s research providing social image evaluation items for wearable devices [66]. The other two items came from Lin and Bhattacherjee's study [43], which was originally designed for online video game users about their perceived social image. Then, for the behavioral intention of using walking aids, the first two items were adapted from Lee and Gu's research [67] about the behavioral intention of purchasing souvenirs abroad. The other two items came from Chen et al.'s study, which explored the purchasing information and recommendation effects on purchasing intention [68]. The last item was adapted from Zhang et al.'s study about the usage of the voice message board [69].

3.3. Data Analysis

The results were processed in three sections: descriptive statistical analysis, measurement model verification, and structural equation modeling analysis. In this study, the structural equation model (SEM) was used to obtain the relevant conclusions. The Likert seven-point scale used in the questionnaire was a continuous scale, which is statistically consistent with a normal distribution and obtains relatively accurate results. However, some of the research variables in this study were nominal scales, such as gender, marriage, or occupation. These variables could not be analyzed using structural equations, which limit the results of the research [70–72]. Descriptive statistical analysis by SPSS contained two parts: one was the frequency distribution calculation of demographic data for a basic understanding of the sample set; and the other one was the mean value and standard deviation of the items of each construct. Then, according to Anderson and Gerbing [73], the study provided verification of the measurement model by confirmatory reliability analysis, convergent validity, and discriminant validity. After that, based on the research model, the structural equation model was analyzed, including path analysis and mediation effect analysis by statistic software AMOS (SPSS Inc., Chicago, IL, USA).

4. Results

4.1. Descriptive Statistical Analysis

4.1.1. Frequency Distribution

The categorical data elements of the 406 valid questionnaires included gender, age, education, marital status, occupation, family environment, and residential area. The respondents were 70.2% female. Most of respondents were aged 45–64, which was the definition of middle-aged people. A total of 45.32% of the respondents were aged between 45 and 54, and 39.66% of respondents were aged between 55 and 64. Regarding the education level, the largest group was college and university, which was 47.04%. A total of 361 respondents were married, which was 88.92%. The data are shown in Table 1.

Table 1. Frequency distribution table.

Variable	Value Label	Frequency	Percent	Accumulated Percent
Gender	Male	121	29.80	29.80
	Female	285	70.20	100.00
	Total	406	100.0	
Age	45–54 years old	184	45.32	45.32
	55–64 years old	161	39.66	84.98
	65 years or above	61	15.02	100.00
	Total	406	100.0	
Education	Elementary	4	0.99	0.99
	Junior school	6	1.48	2.46
	High school/vocational school	94	23.15	25.62
	College/University	191	47.04	72.66
	Master or above	111	27.34	100.00
	Total	406	100.0	
Marital status	Married	361	88.92	88.92
	Unmarried	45	11.08	100.00
	Total	406	100.0	
Occupation (Background)	Medical	32	7.88	7.88
	Agriculture, Forestry and Fisheries	10	2.46	10.34
	Military service/civil servants/teachers	96	23.65	33.99
	Service industry	93	22.91	56.90
	Manufacture/business	61	15.02	71.92
	Freelance	41	10.10	82.02
	Housekeeping	54	13.30	95.32
	Others	19	4.68	100.00
	Total	406	100.0	

Table 1. *Cont.*

Variable	Value Label	Frequency	Percent	Accumulated Percent
	Bungalow	13	3.20	3.20
	Townhouse	236	58.13	61.33
Family environment	Apartment (no elevator)	40	9.85	71.18
	Building (with elevator)	117	28.82	100.00
	Total	406	100.0	
	Suburbs	45	11.08	11.08
	Urban area	229	56.40	67.49
Residential area	Countryside	42	10.34	77.83
	Small town	75	18.47	96.31
	Medium-sized city	15	3.69	100.00
	Total	406	100.0	

4.1.2. Item Statistical Analysis

Table 2 shows the mean values and standard deviation values of items of each construct. The lowest average score of all items was 4.57, which was for "I can get the envy of my friends by using advanced walking aids" of the social image construct. The highest average score was 6.37, for "If I use walking aids well, I will convey positive news to others" of the behavioral intention. This time also had the highest standard deviation value of all items. There were two tied lowest standard deviation values in the behavioral intention construct.

Table 2. Mean and standard deviation of items.

Construct	Item	Mean	SD [1]
	1. I use walking aids to make a good impression.	4.98	1.31
	2. Using walking aids can enhance my image among community residents.	4.85	1.32
Social image	3. I feel that using walking aids brings me recognition from others.	5.01	1.36
	4. I will get more respect from others when I walk with walking aids.	4.97	1.40
	5. I can get the envy of my friends by using advanced walking aids.	4.57	1.50
Total		4.876	
	1. I think the use of walking aids will meet my requirements.	5.83	1.12
	2. I think using walking aids will be a pleasant experience.	5.37	1.30
Attitude toward usage	3. Overall, my evaluation of the use of walking aids is positive.	6.10	0.91
	4. I think using walking aids is a good choice.	6.07	0.93
	5. I think the use of walking aids is really needed by the elderly.	6.10	1.18
Total		5.894	
	1. I will use it because my family members (including my spouse) persuaded the use of walking aids to be healthy.	6.17	0.81
	2. I will try to use it because my friends agree with the use of walking aids.	5.96	1.00
Subjective norm	3. I will try to use it because my neighbors persuaded the advantage of walking aids.	5.78	1.09
	4. I will use walking aids as much as possible because of government policies.	5.77	1.10
	5. I will try to use it because the professional recommended the benefits of walking aids.	6.36	0.77
Total		6.008	
	1. The design of the walking aid itself is extremely safe.	6.00	0.85
	2. I think walking aids are trustworthy.	5.94	0.85
Safety	3. Using walking aids always makes people feel safe.	5.93	0.90
	4. I think it is safe to walk on the street with a walking aid alone.	5.50	1.18
	5. I think it is safe to use walking aids to walk in the community.	5.82	1.00

Table 2. *Cont.*

Construct	Item	Mean	SD [1]
Total		5.838	
Usefulness	1. I think using walking aids can help achieve the goal of independent walking.	6.10	0.80
	2. Using walking aids will solve my walking problems.	5.97	0.90
	3. Using walking aids will help me walk more safely.	6.11	0.83
	4. Using walking aids will increase my walking speed.	5.71	1.07
	5. Using walking aids will help me effectively prevent falls.	6.16	0.85
Total		6.010	
Behavioral intention	1. If I have difficulty walking, I plan to use a walker.	6.28	0.76
	2. If I have difficulty walking, I will be willing to use walking aids.	6.32	0.72
	3. If I use walking aids well, I would recommend them to others.	6.34	0.76
	4. If I use walking aids well, I will convey positive news to others.	6.37	0.72
	5. If I have difficulty walking, I will often use walking aids.	6.31	0.73
Total		6.324	

[1] SD = Standard Deviation.

The F-test of different ages in the social image construct reached a significant level (F = 10.676, $p < 0.05$). It meant that age made a significant difference in the social image construct. After comparing with the Scheffe method, it was found that subjects 55–64 years old had a significantly higher opinion in the social image construct than those 45–54 years old, and subjects 65 years or above had a significantly higher opinion in social image than those 45–54 years old. The testing results are shown in Table 3.

Table 3. Age vs. Social image research construct analysis of variance table.

Construct	Age	N	Mean	Std. Deviation	F-Test	*p*-Value Sig.	Scheffe
Social image	1. 45–54 years old	184	4.834	1.163	10.676	$p < 0.001$	2 > 1, 3 > 1
	2. 55–64 years old	161	5.201	1.061			
	3. 65 years or above	61	5.525	0.958			
	Total	406	5.083	1.120			

N = Number; Std. = Standard; Sig. = Significant.

4.2. Measurement Model Verification

4.2.1. Convergent Validity

A complete structural equation model should be implemented by two phases; the first phase is to verify the measurement model and then the second phase is the structure mode analysis [73]. Confirmatory factor analysis provides standardized factor loading, composite reliability, and average variance extracted to test the convergent validity. After the acceptance of convergent validity verification, the next phase of structure model can be processed [74]. The standardized factor loading should be larger than 0.6. It is better that the value is larger than 0.7 [75]. If the loading value is less than 0.45, the item should be deleted [76]. Then, the suggested value for composite reliability should be larger than 0.6, and the average variance extracted value should be larger than 0.5 [77–79].

Table 4 shows the results of the confirmatory factor analysis. All standardized factor loadings were between 0.634 and 0.956, larger than 0.6, which meant all items had acceptable reliability. All composite reliability values were between 0.875 and 0.964, larger than 0.7, which meant all constructs had acceptable reliability. Finally, all average variance extracted values were between 0.589 and 0.843, larger than 0.5, which meant all constructs had acceptable convergence validity.

Table 4. Confirmatory factor analysis.

Construct	Ite	Significance of Estimated Parameters				Item Reliability		Composite Reliability	Convergence Validity
		Unstd. [1]	S.E.	Unstd./S.E.	p-Value	Std. [2]	SMC [3]	CR [4]	AVE [5]
Social image	SOCI1	1.000				0.900	0.810		
	SOCI2	1.046	0.033	31.284	0.000	0.930	0.865		
	SOCI3	1.041	0.035	29.774	0.000	0.917	0.841	0.951	0.796
	SOCI4	1.060	0.036	29.508	0.000	0.917	0.841		
	SOCI5	1.003	0.047	21.455	0.000	0.791	0.626		
Attitude toward usage	ATTU1	1.000				0.634	0.402		
	ATTU2	1.255	0.105	11.999	0.000	0.672	0.452		
	ATTU3	1.105	0.077	14.394	0.000	0.898	0.806	0.875	0.589
	ATTU4	1.130	0.077	14.595	0.000	0.918	0.843		
	ATTU5	0.918	0.079	11.586	0.000	0.666	0.444		
Subjective norm	SUBN1	1.000				0.841	0.707		
	SUBN2	1.259	0.051	24.590	0.000	0.921	0.848		
	SUBN3	1.300	0.059	21.940	0.000	0.870	0.757	0.922	0.705
	SUBN4	1.259	0.063	20.024	0.000	0.820	0.672		
	SUBN5	0.843	0.048	17.414	0.000	0.735	0.540		
Safety	SAFE1	1.000				0.874	0.764		
	SAFE2	1.001	0.037	26.713	0.000	0.905	0.819		
	SAFE3	1.014	0.038	26.346	0.000	0.903	0.815	0.931	0.730
	SAFE4	1.147	0.059	19.471	0.000	0.777	0.604		
	SAFE5	1.009	0.049	20.670	0.000	0.805	0.648		
Usefulness	USEF1	1.000				0.793	0.629		
	USEF2	1.268	0.061	20.920	0.000	0.892	0.796		
	USEF3	1.201	0.056	21.459	0.000	0.913	0.834	0.918	0.694
	USEF4	1.268	0.079	15.975	0.000	0.730	0.533		
	USEF5	1.128	0.061	18.592	0.000	0.823	0.677		
Behavioral intention	BEHI1	1.000				0.934	0.872		
	BEHI2	0.991	0.024	40.596	0.000	0.956	0.914		
	BEHI3	0.926	0.032	28.941	0.000	0.881	0.776	0.964	0.843
	BEHI4	0.898	0.030	30.339	0.000	0.897	0.805		
	BEHI5	0.954	0.028	34.019	0.000	0.921	0.848		

[1] Unstd. = Unstandardized factor loading, [2] Std. = Standardized factor loading, [3] SMC = Squared Multiple Correlations, [4] CR = Composite reliability, [5] AVE = Average Variance Extracted.

4.2.2. Discriminant Validity

This study used average variance extracted as the criteria for testing the discriminant validity of research constructs. According to Fornell and Larcker [77], the square root of the average variance extracted (AVE) value (the bold figures in Table 5) should be larger than the Pearson correlative coefficients with other constructs (the figures under the diagonal) in order to be discriminant with each other. Table 5 shows the discriminant validity test of the measurement model. The values under the diagonal are the Pearson correlation coefficients between constructs, which were smaller than the square root of average variance extracted values on the diagonal. Therefore, all the discriminant validity of research constructs were acceptable.

Table 5. The result of discriminant validity analysis.

	AVE	SOCI	ATTU	SUBN	SAFE	USEF	BEHI
SOCI [1]	0.796	**0.892**					
ATTU [2]	0.589	0.454	**0.767**				
SUBN [3]	0.705	0.515	0.234	**0.84**			
SAFE [4]	0.730	0.590	0.268	0.740	**0.854**		
USEF [5]	0.694	0.571	0.259	0.630	0.693	**0.833**	
BEHI [6]	0.843	0.481	0.399	0.587	0.632	0.557	**0.918**

[1] SOCI = Social Image, [2] ATTU = Attitude toward Usage, [3] SUBN = Subjective Norm, [4] SAFE = Safety, [5] USEF = Usefulness, [6] BEHI = Behavioral Intention.

4.3. Structural Equation Model

4.3.1. Structural Model Analysis

Schumacker and Lomax [80] and Kline [74] pointed out that, since the big sample analysis would cause a p-value smaller than 0.05, the model fit would be affected as a bad result. Therefore, the quantitative research should adapt several different methods to test the model fit. The present study implemented eight common models of fit verification methods proposed by Jackson, Gillaspy, and Purc-Stephenson [81]. Moreover, if the sample size was big, larger than 200, the Chi-square value easily got a bad result. The bootstrap method provides an alternative way to get a better result [82]. By using Chi-square divided by degree of freedom (DF), the ideal result should be less than three. Moreover, other criteria provide a more rigorous standard for model fit verification, as Table 6 shows. For example, the Root Mean Square Error of Approximation (RMSEA) value should be smaller than 0.08 [83]. Comparative Fit Index (CFI) criteria should be larger than 0.9. The tested results are shown in Table 6. All the model fit criteria tested fitted the suggested standards [80].

Table 6. Model fit verification.

Model Fit	Criteria	Model Fit of Research Model
χ^2 [1]	The smaller the better	522.511
DF [2]	The larger the better	394.000
Normed Chi-square (χ^2/DF)	$1 < \chi^2/DF < 3$	1.326
RMSEA [3]	<0.08	0.028
TLI (NNFI) [4]	>0.9	0.989
CFI [5]	>0.9	0.990
GFI [6]	>0.9	0.960
AGFI [7]	>0.9	0.952

[1] χ^2 = Chi-square, [2] DF = Degree of Freedom, [3] RMSEA = Root Mean Square Error of Approximation, [4] TLI (NNFI) = Tucker-Lewis Index (Non Normed Fit Index), [5] CFI = Comparative Fit Index, [6] GFI = Goodness of Fit Index, [7] AGFI = Adjusted Goodness of Fit Index.

4.3.2. Path Analysis

Table 7 shows the path coefficient analysis for verification of the causal relationship between variables. As the results show, social image positively impacted the attitude toward usage of walking aids significantly. The unstandardized regression coefficient from social image to attitude toward usage was 0.243. The p-value was less than 0.001, which meant social image impacted attitude toward usage significantly. The explainable variation was 0.206. The coefficients from attitude toward usage, subjective norm, safety, and usefulness to behavioral intention, were 0.246, 0.208, 0.283, and 0.178, respectively. Their p-values also were less than 0.001, except usefulness. The explainable variation was 0.495. Figure 4 shows the regression coefficients of the structural equation model.

Table 7. Path analysis.

DV [7]	IV [8]	Unstd. [9]	S.E. [10]	Unstd./S.E.	p-Value	Std. [11]	R2 [12]
ATTU	SOCI [1]	0.243	0.031	7.889	$p < 0.001$	0.454	0.206
	ATTU [2]	0.246	0.068	3.616	$p < 0.001$	0.228	0.495
BEHI [6]	SUBN [3]	0.208	0.069	2.992	0.003	0.206	
	SAFE [4]	0.283	0.062	4.535	$p < 0.001$	0.315	
	USEF [5]	0.178	0.073	2.426	0.015	0.151	

[1] SOCI = Social Image, [2] ATTU = Attitude toward Usage, [3] SUBN = Subjective Norm, [4] SAFE = Safety, [5] USEF = Usefulness, [6] BEHI = Behavioral Intention, [7] DV = Dependent Variable, [8] IV = Independent Variable, [9] Unstd. = Unstandardized regression coefficients, [10] S.E. = Standard Error, [11] Std. = Standardized regression coefficients, [12] R2 = Explainable variations.

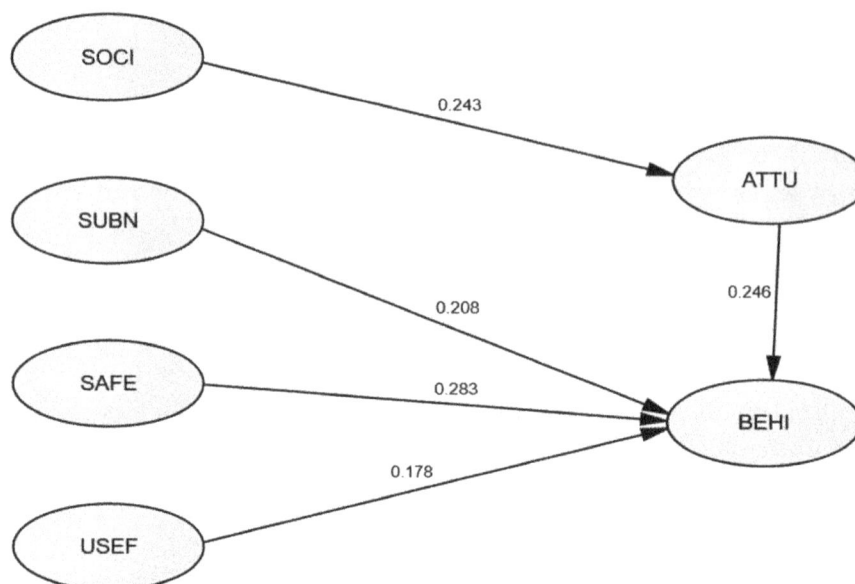

Figure 4. SEM statistic model.

4.3.3. Mediation Effect Analysis

This study used bootstrapping as the repeated sampling method to produce statistical confidence intervals for indirect effects. Table 8 shows the results of social image impacting behavioral intention through attitude toward usage. The confidence intervals were 0.003 to 0.113, and the p-value was less than 0.05. The value of lower bound and upper bound was not across 0, which meant the indirect effect existed.

Table 8. Indirect effect analysis.

Indirect Effect	Point Estimate	Product of Coefficients			Bootstrap 1000 Times Bias-Corrected 95%	
		S.E.	Z-Value	p-Value	Lower Bound	UPPER BOUND
SOCI [1]→ATTU [2]→BEHI [3]	0.060	0.027	2.215	0.027	0.003	0.113

[1] SOCI = Social Image, [2] ATTU = Attitude toward Usage, [3] BEHI = Behavioral Intention.

5. Discussion

This research was mainly to investigate the behavioral intention of middle-aged and elderly people to use walking aids and to explore its influencing factors. Based on the Theory of Reasoned Action (TRA), combined with the social image and attitude toward usage as mediating variables, the research framework and related hypotheses were proposed. After collecting data through a questionnaire survey, the structural equation model was used to test the model and verify related hypotheses. Based on the Theory of Reasoned Action (TRA), this research attempted to explore the factors affecting the behavior of middle-aged and elderly users from the perspective of social image. Therefore, integrating factors such as safety, usefulness, and social image dimensions were used to discuss the influence on middle-aged and elderly people's intention to use walking aids. The research results are as follows.

5.1. The Influence of Social Image on the Attitude toward Using Walking Aids

The results of the study showed that social image has a significant positive impact on attitudes toward using walking aids. This result was consistent with the previous research [43]. The average score of social image measurement was 4.876, which was the lowest score of all constructs. It could be that the middle-aged and elderly people think that the use of walking aids cannot be socially recognized. They are obviously worried about the external image of using a walker, so they have reservations about using a walker, and even have a sense of resistance. At the same time, the standard deviation of the social image item "I use walking aids to make a good impression" was greater than 1.3, indicating that users' opinions varied greatly. Moreover, the item "I can get the envy of my friends by using advanced walking aids" had the lowest mean score, 4.57, and the highest standard deviation, 1.5. The low score may show that on the issue of the use of walking aids, the users thought that even choosing high-end-style walking aids would not necessarily reverse the social image. Therefore, they could not gain support and recognition for using walking aids. At the same time, the high standard deviation may indicate that users had greatly inconsistent opinions, and it also may show that the public has unequal attitudes and opinions toward people who use walking aids.

In the path analysis of the influence of social image on use attitude, the non-standardized regression coefficient reached 0.243, indicating that social image factors had a high proportion of influence on use attitude. It also confirms the hypothesis of this study that social image has a significant influence on the attitude toward using walking aids. Therefore, it is also proved that middle-aged and elderly users are obviously concerned about the social impression of disability, aging, and the dependence caused by the use of walking aids. This differs from ordinary people, so it affects their attitude toward using mobility aids. At the same time, if they were to choose a more advanced walker, whether it was for a change in function or appearance, it would not enhance the attitude toward using a walker.

5.2. The Influence of Attitude and Subjective Norms on the Behavioral Intention of Walking Aids

The results of this study showed that the attitude toward using walking aids has a significant positive effect on behavioral intentions. This result was similar to the results of previous studies [55]. In addition, subjective norms have a significant positive effect on the behavioral intention of using walking aids. This result was also consistent with the results of previous studies [39,84], and all fit into the framework of the TRA.

In the attitude toward usage construct, a positive view appeared, which meant that users agree that if their walking function was affected in the future, they would be open and willing to accept using walkers. The behavioral intention construct reached the highest average score of 6.324, indicating that if having difficulty walking in the future, the participants would use walking aids to assist walking, and even to convey positive messages or to recommend it to others. The subjective norm item "I will try to use it because the professional recommended the benefits of walking aids" gained the highest average score, 6.36, and its standard deviation value was 0.77. That means not only high agreement among the participants on this question, but also that as long as the use of walking aids is recommended by professionals, the user's willingness to use it will be greatly increased.

5.3. The Impact of Safety and Usefulness on the Behavioral Intention of Using Walking Aids

The intensity of the perception of safety has a significant impact on the behavioral intention of using walking aids. This result was similar to the results of previous studies [46,47]. In addition, the usefulness of walking aids also has a significant positive impact on behavioral intentions. This result was also similar to the results of previous studies [19,85].

For users, the average score of the safety aspect was 5.838, which meant that they are less worried about the safety of walking aids. At the same time, in the safety construct, the non-standardized regression coefficient of behavioral intention reached 0.283. In addition to being an important influencing factor on the behavioral intention of using walking aids, it also meant that after users feel that safety is guaranteed, their willingness to use walking aids will increase significantly. In addition, the score of related items in usefulness also reached 6.01, and standard deviation was 0.85, indicating that users agree that walking aids are useful. However, since the regression coefficient was 0.178, the lowest of all factors, the degree it affected the behavioral intention of using walking aids was not so obvious.

5.4. Social Image Influences Behavioral Intention through Attitude toward Usage

Social image affects the attitude toward usage, and the attitude toward usage significantly positively affects the behavior intention, that is, the social image of using walking aids indirectly affects the behavioral intention. The attitude toward usage had a mediating effect, and this result was similar to the previous studies [19,42]. It can be seen that if middle-aged and elderly people are more concerned about their social image, it will affect their attitudes to using walking aids, which, in turn, will affect their behavioral intention to use walking aids.

6. Conclusions

The World Health Organization (WHO) proposed the Global Aging and Health Strategy and Action Plan in 2016 [3], which mentioned that the physical and mental functions of the elderly are rapidly decreasing. The impact of the elderly on the whole of society is very important. If the elderly can maintain their functional capacity through their interaction with the environment, and be provided with adequate support for improving their health, then the life span of the elderly can be extended. The elderly can participate in society and improve their own health and well-being. Therefore, the use of assistive equipment and a barrier-free environment are the best supports for maintaining the functions of the elderly.

Taiwan began to implement National Ten-year Long-term Care Plan in 2008, providing assistive equipment and barrier-free environment improvement subsidies, including crutches, walking aids, or walkers. In 2018, the National Ten-year Long-term Care Plan 2.0 was promoted [86], and the "Reablement" service was updated. Professional medical staff provide daily life function training, physical function training and maintenance, assistive devices use training, and other services. The goals of the program include improving the individual's ability to live independently, achieving ability recovery, and increasing the ability to act independently.

As many elderly people get older, the function of their lower limbs deteriorates, which affects their walking function. However, they are afraid of being laughed at, their external image becoming morbid or weak. This may be why the middle-aged and elderly are reluctant to use walking aids. Instead, they will walk with umbrellas or bamboo poles, which is not only very laborious but also prone to danger. Therefore, it is very important to understand the influence of "social image" on users for the research on the use of walking aids by middle-aged and elderly people. In the past, research on assistive devices mostly focused on the design of the mechanics, functional aspects, and appearance of walking assistive devices. The behavior of assistive devices from the perspective of the user's mentality and the relationship between related influencing variables were rarely studied.

Therefore, improving life functions through assistive devices is very important in an aging society. According to the present study, for these middle-aged or elderly people who are facing gradual degradation of functions, if the use of assistive devices cannot overcome the existing poor social image, no matter how sophisticated the assistive device is, it still cannot increase the willingness to use it. The group between the ages of 45–55, especially, was more concerned with social image than other elderly groups. It also becomes impossible to use assistive devices to achieve social participation, thereby delaying aging and increasing physical and mental health.

This study mainly sampled the middle-aged and elderly people in the urban area. The results of the study indicated that the sampled subjects had relatively high academic qualifications; a college degree or above accounted for 74.4%. However, the higher the level of education, the higher the ability to absorb information about assistive devices, and the higher the proportion of self-help ability in understanding the use of assistive devices. This study may not be able to fully present the attitudes and intentions of other people with lower academic qualifications. In addition, the majority of the subjects were under 65 years old (85%), and the elderly group sample (65 years old or above) was relatively small. Future research can improve in the sampling process. In addition, this research focuses on walking aids. In the future, research can focus on the intention of using other types of assistive devices, such as wheelchairs, hearing aids, or visual-impairment-related assistive devices, providing more about the use of various assistive devices.

Author Contributions: Conceptualization, S.-W.H. and T.-Y.C.; writing—original draft preparation, S.-W.H.; writing—review and editing, T.-Y.C.; visualization, T.-Y.C. All authors have read and agreed to the published version of the manuscript.

References

1. W.H.O. Ageing and Health. Available online: https://www.who.int/zh/news-room/fact-sheets/detail/ageing-and-health (accessed on 20 July 2020).

2. United Nations. World Population Prospects 2019. Available online: https://population.un.org/wpp2019/ (accessed on 20 July 2020).

3. W.H.O. The Global Strategy and Action Plan on Ageing and Health. Available online: https://www.who.int/ageing/global-strategy/en/ (accessed on 20 July 2020).

4. National Development Council. *Report of Population Projections for the R.O.C. (Taiwan) (2018-2065)*; National Development Council: Taipei, Taiwan, 2018.

5. National Development Council. National Development Council Population Projections for the R.O.C. (Taiwan). Available online: https://pop-proj.ndc.gov.tw/ (accessed on 11 July 2020).

6. Health Promotion Administration, Ministry of Health and Welfare. 5 Points to Prevent Falls at Home for the Elderly. Available online: https://www.hpa.gov.tw/Pages/Detail.aspx?nodeid=4141&pid=12132 (accessed on 21 July 2020).

7. Department of Statistics, Ministry of Health and Welfare. *2019 Statistical Results on Causes of Death in Taiwan*; Ministry of Health and Welfare: Taipei, Taiwan, 2019.

8. Yang, Y.-A.; Chen, Y.-S.; Lin, C.-F.; Lee, H.-C.; Tsai, Y.-J.; Tsauo, J.-Y.; Wang, C.-Y. An investigation of ADL disability status and associated physical performances in mobile but unstable institutionalized older adults. *Formos. J. Phys. Ther.* **2017**, *42*, 135–136. [CrossRef]

9. Suwannarat, P.; Thaweewannakij, T.; Kaewsanmung, S.; Mato, L.; Amatachaya, S. Walking devices used by community-dwelling elderly: Proportion, types, and associated factors. *Hong Kong Physiother. J.* **2015**, *33*, 34–41. [CrossRef]

10. Yusif, S.; Soar, J.; Hafeez-Baig, A. Older people, assistive technologies, and the barriers to adoption: A systematic review. *Int. J. Med. Inform.* **2016**, *94*, 112–116. [CrossRef] [PubMed]

11. Nam, C.S.; Bahn, S.; Lee, R. Acceptance of assistive technology by special education teachers: A structural equation model approach. *Int. J. Hum.-Comput. Interact.* **2013**, *29*, 365–377. [CrossRef]

12. Aidemark, J.; Askenäs, L. Fall Prevention as Personal Learning and Changing Behaviors: Systems and Technologies. *Procedia Comput. Sci.* **2019**, *164*, 498–507. [CrossRef]

13. Simpson, J.; Richardson, B. Why Do Elderly People Use Walking Aids? *Physiotherapy* **2002**, *88*, 174–175. [CrossRef]

14. Chen, K.; Chan, A.H.S. Predictors of gerontechnology acceptance by older Hong Kong Chinese. *Technovation* **2014**, *34*, 126–135. [CrossRef]

15. Tural, E.; Lu, D.; Cole, D.A. Factors predicting older Adults' attitudes toward and intentions to use stair mobility assistive designs at home. *Prev. Med. Rep.* **2020**, *18*. [CrossRef]

16. Bailey, C.; Hodgson, P.; Aitken, D.; Wilson, G. Primary research with practitioners and people with lived experience—To understand the role of home adaptations in improving later life. *Cent. Ageing Better* **2018**, 1–152. [CrossRef]

17. United States Federal Legislation. *Assistive Technology Act (AT Act)*; United States Federal Legislation: Washington, DC, USA, 1988.

18. CNS 15390 Assistive Technology Classification Technical Manual. Available online: https://newrepat.sfaa. gov.tw/home/download-file/2c90e4c7638695fc01638aed2beb004d (accessed on 25 November 2020).

19. Koon, L.M.; Remillard, E.T.; Mitzner, T.L.; Rogers, W.A. Aging Concerns, Challenges, and Everyday Solution Strategies (ACCESS) for Adults Aging with a Long-Term Mobility Disability. *Disabil. Health J.* **2020**, *13*. [CrossRef]

20. Popularization, C.F.A.T.R.A. CNS 15390. Available online: https://newrepat.sfaa.gov.tw/home/cns15390 (accessed on 11 July 2020).

21. Jian, L.; Li, F.L.; Hui, L. Biomechanical study on axillary crutches. *J. Med. Biomech.* **2014**, *29*, 93–98.

22. Chen, J.-C.; Liang, C.-C.; Huang, P.; Hung, D.; Wu, Y.-Z. Design and functional analysis of a convenient household stair-climbing device. *Formos. J. Phys. Ther.* **2010**, *35*, 263–267.

23. You, J.-S. Motion experiment and effect assessment for assisting elderly to stand up from toilet seat. *J. Gerontechnol. Serv. Manag.* **2018**, *6*, 435–442. [CrossRef]

24. Cai, Z.-M.; Chen, H.-D.; Chen, J.-Y.; Chen, B.-W.; Yang, C.-L. Design of assistive device: A telescopic cane for one-hand operation. *J. Gerontechnol. Serv. Manag.* **2015**, *3*, 277–278. [CrossRef]

25. Juan, Y.-C.; Wang, M.W.; Sie, M.-J. Applying scenario approach and quality function deployment to custom design of elder cane. *J. Gerontechnol. Serv. Manag.* **2013**, *1*, 1–12. [CrossRef]

26. Cooke, L.; Munroe Chandler, K.; Hall, C.; Tobin, D.; Guerrero, M. Development of the children's active play imagery questionnaire. *J. Sports Sci.* **2014**, *32*, 860–869. [CrossRef] [PubMed]

27. Lin, C.-H.; He, Y.-Z. A study on the social image of librarians in Taiwan. *J. Infolib. Arch.* **2016**, 1–24. [CrossRef]

28. Cepeda Zorrilla, M.; Hodgson, F.; Jopson, A. Exploring the influence of attitudes, social comparison and image and prestige among non-cyclists to predict intention to cycle in Mexico City. *Transp. Res. Part F Traffic Psychol. Behav.* **2019**, *60*, 327–342. [CrossRef]

29. Guo, B.W.; Hu, J.P.; Zhang, Q.Y.; Zhang, W. Sensation seeking and adolescents' online game addiction: The intermediary effect of social impression and emotional connection. *J. South. China Norm. Univ. (Soc. Sci. Ed.)* **2014**, *3*, 84–89.

30. Tu, Y.-J.L.; Cheng, S.M.-W. A study of the care servicers on the working environment and social image: According to the Pingtung County. *J. Taiwan Health Care Assoc.* **2011**, *11*, 1–21. [CrossRef]

31. Tsen, J.-M. Social Imagery of the developmentally disabled in Taiwanese media. *J. Des.* **2014**, *19*, 23–40.

32. Mao, H.-F. Assistive devices, a good helper for the elderly to make life more colorful. *Health World* **2010**, 20–28. [CrossRef]

33. Chang, T.-Y. *Enjoy Aging: Blending Cultural Creativity with Technology into Eldercare. The Project Report of NSC 101 Interdisciplinary Collaboration for Creative Value-Added Planning on Forward-looking Concept Development*; National Science Council: Taipei, Taiwan, 2012.

34. Fishbein, M.; Ajzen, I. *Belief, Attitude, Intention and Behaviour: An Introduction to Theory and Research*; Addison-Wesley: Boston, MA, USA, 1975.

35. Verma, P.; Sinha, N. Integrating perceived economic wellbeing to technology acceptance model: The case of mobile based agricultural extension service. *Technol. Forecast. Soc. Chang.* **2018**, *126*, 207–216. [CrossRef]

36. Procter, L.; Angus, D.J.; Blaszczynski, A.; Gainsbury, S.M. Understanding use of consumer protection tools among Internet gambling customers: Utility of the Theory of Planned Behavior and Theory of Reasoned Action. *Addict. Behav.* **2019**, *99*. [CrossRef] [PubMed]

37. Papa, A.; Mital, M.; Pisano, P.; Del Giudice, M. E-health and wellbeing monitoring using smart healthcare devices: An empirical investigation. *Technol. Forecast. Soc. Chang.* **2020**, *153*. [CrossRef]

38. Alsalem, A.; Fry, M.-L.; Thaichon, P. To donate or to waste it: Understanding posthumous organ donation attitude. *Australas. Mark. J. (AMJ)* **2020**, *28*, 87–97. [CrossRef]

39. Chuang, H.-L.; Kuo, C.-P.; Jiu, E.-C.; Yeh, C.-H. Investigation of condom use intention among people at high risk for HIV infection by the Theory of Reasoned Action. *Formos. J. Med.* **2006**, *10*, 10–19. [CrossRef]

40. Sheeran, P.; Conner, M. Degree of reasoned action predicts increased intentional control and reduced habitual control over health behaviors. *Soc. Sci. Med.* **2019**, *228*, 68–74. [CrossRef]
41. Köykkä, K.; Absetz, P.; Araújo-Soares, V.; Knittle, K.; Sniehotta, F.F.; Hankonen, N. Combining the reasoned action approach and habit formation to reduce sitting time in classrooms: Outcome and process evaluation of the Let's Move It teacher intervention. *J. Exp. Soc. Psychol.* **2019**, *81*, 27–38. [CrossRef]
42. Huang, P.; Peng, W.-T.; Luo, B.-R. A survey and analysis of exercise among pregnant women conducted using the Theory of Reasoned Action. *J. Nurs.* **2016**, *63*, 50–59. [CrossRef]
43. Lin, C.P.; Bhattacherjee, A. Extending technology usage models to interactive hedonic technologies: A theoretical model and empirical test. *Inf. Syst. J.* **2010**, *20*, 163–181. [CrossRef]
44. Barling, J.; Loughlin, C.; Kelloway, E.K. Development and test of a model linking safety-specific transformational leadership and occupational safety. *J. Appl. Psychol.* **2002**, *87*, 488–496. [CrossRef] [PubMed]
45. Wang, E.S.-T.; Chu, Y.-H. Influence of Consumer's Long-term Orientation and Safety Consciousness on Intention to Repurchase Certified Functional Foods. *J. Food Prod. Mark.* **2020**, *26*, 247–261. [CrossRef]
46. Bhattacherjee, A. Understanding Information Systems Continuance: An Expectation-Confirmation Model. *MIS Q.* **2001**, *25*, 351–370. [CrossRef]
47. Lim, S.; Kim, D.; Hur, Y.; Park, K. An Empirical Study of the Impacts of Perceived Security and Knowledge on Continuous Intention to Use Mobile Fintech Payment Services. *Int. J. Hum.-Comput. Interact.* **2019**, *35*, 886–898. [CrossRef]
48. Kwee-Meier, S.T.; Bützler, J.E.; Schlick, C. Development and validation of a technology acceptance model for safety-enhancing, wearable locating systems. *Behav. Inf. Technol.* **2016**, *35*, 394–409. [CrossRef]
49. Klobas, J.E.; McGill, T.; Wang, X. How perceived security risk affects intention to use smart home devices: A reasoned action explanation. *Comput. Secur.* **2019**, *87*. [CrossRef]
50. Lee, Y.-H.; Yang, C.-C.; Chen, T.-T. Barriers to incident-reporting behavior among nursing staff: A study based on the theory of planned behavior. *J. Manag. Organ.* **2015**, *22*, 1–18. [CrossRef]
51. Davis, F.D. A Technology Acceptance Model for Empirically Testing New End-User Information Systems: Theory and Results. Ph.D. Thesis, MIT Sloan School of Management, Cambridge, MA, USA, 1986.
52. Xu, X.-D.; He, D.-D. An empirical study on the influencing factors of the willingness to use library mobile services—TAM based on information security perception and mobility. *Library* **2019**, *293*, 83–89. [CrossRef]
53. Lin, H.-C.; Chang, T.-Y.; Kuo, S.-H. Effects of social influence and system characteristics on traceable agriculture product reuse intention of elderly people: Integrating trust and attitude using the Technology Acceptance Model. *J. Res. Educ. Sci.* **2018**, *63*, 291–319. [CrossRef]
54. Oztekin, C.; Teksöz, G.; Pamuk, S.; Sahin, E.; Kilic, D.S. Gender perspective on the factors predicting recycling behavior: Implications from the theory of planned behavior. *Waste Manag.* **2017**, *62*, 290–302. [CrossRef] [PubMed]
55. Menéndez Álvarez-Dardet, S.; Lorence Lara, B.; Pérez-Padilla, J. Older adults and ICT adoption: Analysis of the use and attitudes toward computers in elderly Spanish people. *Comput. Hum. Behav.* **2020**, *110*. [CrossRef]
56. The Survey System. Available online: https://www.surveysystem.com/sscalc.htm (accessed on 22 June 2020).
57. Wu, M.-Y.; Lin, I.-C. A study of Taiwan universities' intention and behavior to use library 2.0. *Libr. Inf. Sci. Res.* **2011**, *6*, 139–180.
58. Chen, Y.-L.; Zheng, S.H. Digital learning and virtual community in adult education: A study of behavioral intention in blended learning. *J. Inf. Manag.* **2010**, *17*, 177–196. [CrossRef]
59. Xu, J.; Huang, F.; Zhang, X.; Wang, S.; Li, C.; Li, Z.; He, Y. Sentiment analysis of social images via hierarchical deep fusion of content and links. *Appl. Soft Comput.* **2019**, *80*, 387–399. [CrossRef]
60. Chang, H.-L.; Shen, Y.-C. People's intention to walk-A case study for Taipei citizens. *J. Chin. Inst. Transp.* **2005**, *17*, 233–260. [CrossRef]
61. Lai, S.-F. An acceptance and satisfaction study on public bike system—A case study on Taipei U-bike system. *J. Chin. Inst. Transp.* **2012**, *24*, 379–405. [CrossRef]
62. Qiang, Z.; Xiang, -K.L. Empirical study of relationships among perceived service quality, user satisfaction and behavioral intentions among fitness club members. *J. Wuhan Inst. Phys. Educ.* **2011**, *45*, 45–51.
63. Chuang, L.-H.; Hwang, Y.-S. An empirical study on happiness of indigenous people in Taiwan: Implications for indigenous social policy and social work. *NTU Soc. Work Rev.* **2019**, *39*, 105–151. [CrossRef]

64. Tseng, C.-H.; Hung, P.-H.; Lin, I.-H. The development of a literacy-based technology application scale. *Int. J. Digit. Learning Technol.* **2011**, *3*, 81–98.

65. Hsu, L.-L.; Hsu, T.-H.; Tang, J.-W.; Liang, C.-Y. An empirical study of user's experiential value impact user's continuance intention in blog context. *J. Inf. Manag.* **2010**, *17*, 89–117. [CrossRef]

66. Yang, H.; Yu, J.; Zo, H.; Choi, M. User acceptance of wearable devices: An extended perspective of perceived value. *Telemat. Inform.* **2016**, *33*, 256–269. [CrossRef]

67. Lee, S.-H.; Goo, Y.-J. Exploring the factors in outbound gift purchase behavior. *J. Leis. Res.* **2019**, *25*, 197–224. [CrossRef]

68. Chen, K.-Y.; Chen, P.-Y.; Dai, Y.-D.; Wu, L.-Y. Perceived quality, perceived value, and behavior intention from the perspective of transaction cost. *NTU Manag. Rev.* **2016**, *27*, 191–224. [CrossRef]

69. Chang, C.-T.; Su, P.-C.; Ho, H.-P.; Su, P.-S. Extending the TAM for the voice message board interactive function of website. *J. e-Business* **2009**, *11*, 469–487. [CrossRef]

70. Carayon, P.; Kianfar, S.; Li, Y.; Xie, A.; Alyousef, B.; Wooldridge, A. A systematic review of mixed methods research on human factors and ergonomics in health care. *Appl. Ergon.* **2015**, *51*, 291–321. [CrossRef]

71. Stefanini, A.; Aloini, D.; Gloor, P. Silence is golden: The role of team coordination in health operations. *Int. J. Oper. Prod. Manag.* **2020**. [CrossRef]

72. Stefanini, A.; Aloini, D.; Gloor, P.; Pochiero, F. Patient satisfaction in emergency department: Unveiling complex interactions by wearable sensors. *J. Bus. Res.* **2020**. [CrossRef]

73. Anderson, J.C.; Gerbing, D.W. Structural equation modeling in practice: A review and recommended two-step approach. *Psychol. Bull.* **1988**, *103*. [CrossRef]

74. Kline, R.B. *Principles and Practice of Structural Equation Modeling*; Guilford Publications: New York, NY, USA, 2015.

75. Chin, W.W. Commentary: Issues and Opinion on Structural Equation Modeling. *MIS Q.* **1998**, *22*, 7–16.

76. Hooper, D.; Coughlan, J.; Mullen, M. Structural equation modelling: Guidelines for determining model fit. *Electron. J. Bus. Res. Methods* **2008**, *6*, 53–60.

77. Fornell, C.; Larcker, D.F. Evaluating structural equation models with unobservable variables and measurement error. *J. Mark. Res.* **1981**, *18*, 39–50. [CrossRef]

78. Hair, J.F.; Black, W.C.; Babin, B.J.; Anderson, R.E.; Tatham, R.L. *Multivariate Data Analysis*, 5th ed.; Prentice hall Upper Saddle River: Jersey City, NJ, USA, 1998.

79. Nunnally, J.C. *Psychometric Theory 3E*; Tata McGraw-hill Education: New York, NY, USA, 1994.

80. Schumacker, R.E.; Lomax, R.G. *A Beginner's Guide to Structural Equation Modeling*, 3rd ed.; Routledge Taylor & Francis Group: New York, NY, USA, 2010.

81. Jackson, D.L.; Gillaspy, J.A., Jr.; Purc-Stephenson, R. Reporting practices in confirmatory factor analysis: An overview and some recommendations. *Psychol. Methods* **2009**, *14*, 6–23. [CrossRef] [PubMed]

82. Bollen, K.A.; Stine, R.A. Bootstrapping goodness-of-fit measures in structural equation models. *Sociol. Methods Res.* **1992**, *21*, 205–229. [CrossRef]

83. Hu, L.T.; Bentler, P.M. Cutoff criteria for fit indexes in covariance structure analysis: Conventional criteria versus new alternatives. *Struct. Equ. Modeling Multidiscip. J.* **1999**, *6*, 1–55. [CrossRef]

84. Grimes, M.; Marquardson, J. Quality matters: Evoking subjective norms and coping appraisals by system design to increase security intentions. *Decis. Support. Syst.* **2019**, *119*, 23–34. [CrossRef]

85. Hamidi, H.; Chavoshi, A. Analysis of the essential factors for the adoption of mobile learning in higher education: A case study of students of the University of Technology. *Telemat. Inform.* **2018**, *35*, 1053–1070. [CrossRef]

86. Ministry of Health and Welfare. *National Ten-Year Long-Term Care Plan 2.0*; Ministry of Health and Welfare: Taipei, Taiwan, 2016.

3

Immediate Effects of Aquatic Therapy on Balance in Older Adults with Upper Limb Dysfunction

Maria Graça [1,2,3,*], José Alvarelhão [2], Rui Costa [2], Ricardo J. Fernandes [3,4], Andrea Ribeiro [3,5], Daniel Daly [6] and João Paulo Vilas-Boas [3,4]

1 Research Centre for Physical Activity, Health and Leisure, Faculty of Sport, University of Porto, 4200-450 Porto, Portugal
2 School of Health Sciences, University of Aveiro, 3810-193 Aveiro, Portugal; jalvarelhao@ua.pt (J.A.); rcosta@ua.pt (R.C.)
3 Porto Biomechanics Laboratory (LABIOMEP-UP), University of Porto, 4200-450 Porto, Portugal; ricfer@fade.up.pt (R.J.F.); andrear@ufp.edu.pt (A.R.); jpvb@fade.up.pt (J.P.V.-B.)
4 Centre of Research, Education, Innovation and Intervention in Sport, Faculty of Sport, University of Porto, 4200-450 Porto, Portugal
5 School of Health, Fernando Pessoa University, 4200-253 Porto, Portugal
6 Department of Movement Sciences, KU Leuven, 3001 Leuven, Belgium; daniel.daly@kuleuven.be
* Correspondence: maria.graca@ua.pt

Abstract: Background: Aquatic physiotherapy has been shown to be effective in developing balance, strength, and functional reach over time. When dealing with immediate effects, the literature has concentrated more on the body's physiological response to the physical and mechanical properties of water during passive immersion. The purpose of this study was to evaluate the effects of a single 45-min active aquatic physiotherapy session on standing balance and strength, and its relationship with functional reach in persons 55 years and older with upper limb dysfunction. Methods: The intervention group ($n = 12$) was assessed before and after a single aquatic physiotherapy session, while the control group ($n = 10$) was evaluated before and after 45 min of sitting rest. Functional assessment was made using the visual analogue pain scale (points), step test (repetitions), functional reach test (cm), and global balance-standing test on a force platform (% time). A two-way repeated-measures ANOVA was applied ($p < 0.05$). Results: The intervention group showed non-significant improvements between measurement before and after the intervention: Pain: 6.2 ± 1.9 vs. 5.2 ± 2.3 cm, steps: 7.0 ± 2.0 vs. 7.4 ± 1.8 repetitions, reach: 9.1 ± 2.8 vs. 10.4 ± 3.8 cm, and balance: 61.7 ± 5.9 vs. $71.3 \pm 18.2\%$ time in balance on the platform. The control group showed fewer changes but had better baseline values. A comparison between groups with time showed no significant differences in these changes. Conclusions: No significant immediate effects were found for one session of aquatic physiotherapy applied to patients older than 55 years with upper limb dysfunction.

Keywords: single aquatic intervention; outcomes; functional performance

1. Introduction

Recent research has studied the benefits of exercise on the enhancement of functional capacity and reduction in risk and rate of falling in older adults [1]. Exercise interventions should focus on increasing the muscle strength, muscle mass, improving balance, and increasing gait ability [2,3]. Exercise programs that stimulate several physical capacities, such as muscle strength and endurance, cardiorespiratory fitness, balance and coordination, appear to result in greater improvements in aging adults' ability to perform activities of daily living [3–5].

Aquatic therapy has been proposed as an effective therapeutic approach to maintain performance, improve balance, and reduce the risk of falls in older adults over the long-term [6,7]. It has several advantages compared to non-aquatic exercise, due to the physical properties of water [8–10]. Buoyancy acts on the body to reduce the vertical load on the joints [11] and this antigravity effect may reduce the perception of fatigue and aid energy conservation [12]. Furthermore, the viscosity of water and the associated resistive hydrodynamic force requires the individual to exert more force when performing immersed movements [11]. In other words, aquatic therapy allows high-intensity exercise, while ensuring both low joint impact and greater comfort for the individual.

The thermal properties of water afford a higher capacity to dissipate heat, which helps maintain a constant body temperature and thus better controlling oedema and inflammation, diminishing fatigue and pain, and promoting recovery in one single immersion [13]. Another important property of water is hydrostatic pressure, which leads to the improved conduction of fluids from the extremities towards the central cavity of the human body [13]. The decrease in perception of fatigue may also be due to reduced neuromuscular responses during water immersion [12,14]. Other advantages include low risk of injury from falling and the consequent lack of fear of falling during water exercise with a moderate and high intensity load [15,16].

Although several studies show the efficacy of aquatic therapy on balance gain, pain relief, and functionality in longer term interventions for older adults [17,18], the sustainable effects [19] or the immediate effects, e.g., of a single aquatic therapy session remain unclear for functional tests. In a study of immediate effects, Waller et al. (2017) looked at the walking speed in persons with mild knee osteoarthritis after a 4-month intervention. They found increased walking speed and decreased fat mass. However, in a 12-month follow up, fat mass returned to the base line while walking speed maintained its improvement. These authors did not examine at what point in the 4-month intervention (3× week) the actual improvements were reached. They also found regression in outcome measures with the exception of walking speed in a long-term follow up. Increased leisure time activity did hinder this regression. With an eye on determining the optimal frequency of intervention, which achieves clinically relevant results and promotes lifelong adherence, it might be of interest to examine if any improvements could be obtained after only a single session of aquatic therapy.

Therefore, the aim of this exploratory study was to measure the immediate effects of a single session of aquatic therapy on balance, strength, and functional reach in persons with chronic osteoarthritis, older than 55 years of age. This cut-off age is based on the European Innovation Partnership on Active and Healthy Ageing (EIP-AHA), who consider persons from 55 years and older in their studies of fall risk. Martins et al. (2015) [20] showed this relation. On the other hand, Linaker and Walker-Bone (2015) presented an overview of upper limb dysfunction related with occupation and daily life activities and also found this age group to be of increased risk [21]. Our hypothesis was that functional test results should show an effective significant change after one aquatic therapy session.

2. Materials and Methods

2.1. Study Design and Setting

A quasi-experimental trial was carried out, with participants recruited from the Hospital after ethical approval. First, the volunteers filled in a sociodemographic data and health condition questionnaire, the disability arm shoulder and hand (DASH) scale and signed the informed consent. An expert physiotherapist performed a fixed protocol of aquatic therapeutic exercises each session. Three physiotherapists performed the measures: Stadiometer scale, balance weighing scale, visual analogic scale for pain (VAS_Pain), step test (ST), functional reach test (FRT), and the global balance standing test (GBST), before and no more than 2 min after the intervention. The control group without aquatic therapy intervention followed the same procedure, with measurements taken before and after 45 min of a rest period in a chair. The study design and reporting follow the CONSORT recommendations for conduction and reporting. This was not a randomized controlled trial [22].

2.2. Subjects

From the hospital falls risk assessment program, all potential subjects 55 years and older were invited to participate. A sample of 48 subjects was available for eligibility assessment. Twenty-two participants met the inclusion criteria and agreed to participate in the study. All participants provided informed consent according to the Helsinki Declaration and Oviedo Convention. All 22 participants experienced one or more of the following: Disability of upper limb, problems with balance and/or lower limb weakness. The stratified allocation resulted in an experimental group with poorer health. In practice, those persons had an indication for aquatic physiotherapy to decrease body impact. The control group was of better health and took part in land activities during therapy and had less body impact problems. The intervention group ($n = 12$) included those with several health problems on the waiting list to start an aquatic therapy program. These persons had some previous experience in this type of therapy but were coming from a wash-out period during the 2 months summer vacation break prior to the study. The remaining sample with upper limb dysfunction, fewer health problems, and little or no experience with aquatic therapy were waiting for a fall risk assessment as part of a general functional health screening. These were included in the control group ($n = 10$), as healthier older persons but with upper limb disability and balance problems (Figure 1). It was essential that the experimental group have at least some experience in aquatic therapy to assure that the single session could be organised efficiently. The inclusion criteria were: (a) No severe mobility deficits, (b) be able to walk and stand independently, and (c) do not present mental disorders or deficits in communication and understanding instructions. Individuals with severe mobility deficits ($n = 14$), inability to walk or stand independently ($n = 6$), and individuals unable to communicate or understand commands ($n = 6$) to perform the proposed activities were excluded.

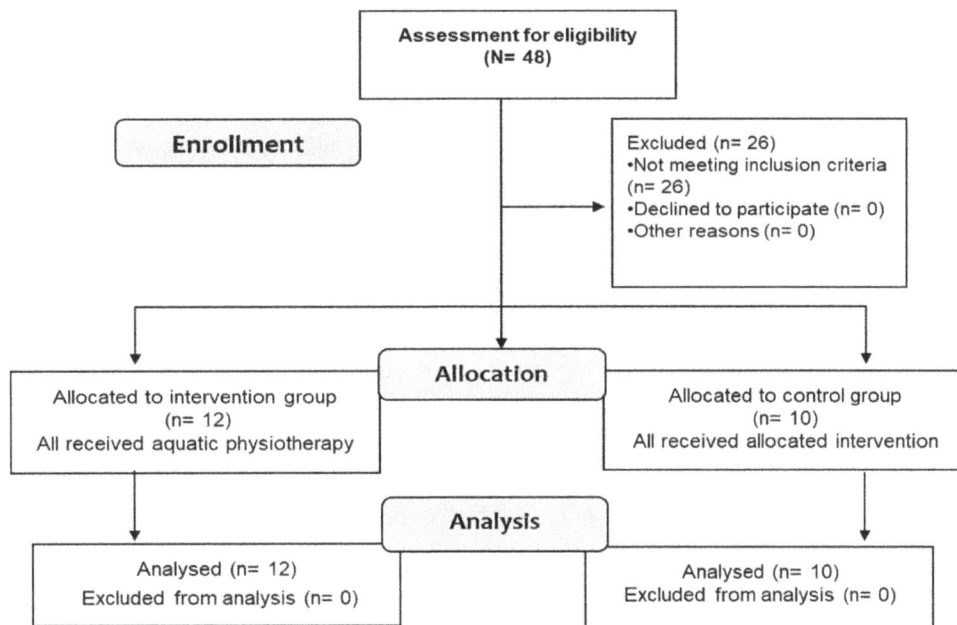

Figure 1. Study design (CONSORT 2010).

2.3. Procedures for Data Collection

Initially, when volunteers agreed to participate in the study, they completed a written questionnaire for sociodemographic data, health conditions, informed consent, and DASH scale. The data for the intervention group were collected in the pool building in a quiet room, temperature 25 °C, with the participants wearing comfortable clothes (t-shirt and swim suit). We started by measuring the height and body mass using a stadiometer and body weighting scales. The outcomes measurements (VAS_Pain, ST, FRT, GBST) were then made immediately before and after the 45 min aquatic therapy program (not more than 2 min after the session of aquatic exercises). To decrease the bias, researchers used the same protocol [23] in three sessions to collect data of four participants in each session. The data collection of the control group took part in the hospital sport hall. First, all participants completed the written questionnaire for sociodemographic data, health conditions, and DASH scale, and signed the informed consent. After this, the outcome measurements (VAS_Pain, ST, FRT, and GBST) were taken before and after sitting quietly for 45 min without the activity.

2.4. Intervention

The aquatic therapy intervention used a protocol with upright exercises (walking in different patterns and directions, lower limbs movements, sitting and standing) [24] and active relaxation exercises from the Halliwick and Clinical Ai chi methods [18,25]. Each session lasted 45 min and included a warm-up, conditioning, and cooling down period. The warm-up included gait exercises in all directions, with a change of pace, gait with dissociation of the waist, and walking on toes and heels [7,23]. The main objective of conditioning was to improve balance. Exercises such as bicycling with legs, upper limb reach, pushing the water, and slips with a noodle float support were included. Balancing exercises were also performed in the sitting and standing positions with floating plates [8,26,27] and Ai-chi movements with exercises in unipodal or bipodal support according to the participant's tolerance [18,28]. Cooling down included gait exercises with waist dissociation, standing-balancing with Ai-chi upper limb movements (first five movements), followed by relaxing cervical movements, shoulder rotations, and slow stretches [29–34].

2.5. Outcomes for Data Collection

The DASH is a scale that assesses the perception of upper limb functionality. It consists of 21 questions related to pain or other symptoms, activities of daily living, leisure activities, and professional activities. A lower score indicates a musculoskeletal upper limb problem and disability [35]. VAS_Pain is a 10 cm scale where the users quantified their pain from 0 to 10 in real time in a sheet of paper with the scale printed. Zero is no pain and 10 is considered the worst pain imaginable. The score is categorized as follows: Less than 3 cm—little pain, between 3 and 6.9 cm—moderate pain, equal to or more than 7 cm—severe pain [36], with a minimal clinically important difference found for adults with musculoskeletal as 1.4 cm change [36–38].

The ST is a test of dynamic balance. The users were instructed to stand in front of a step 7.5 cm high without support while simulating the ascent and descent of stairs alternately on the right and left foot (Figure 2). Complete repetitions were counted during 15 s [39]. The mean values of three trials were recorded. The speed of performance in the step movement provided a significant prediction of non-fallers with a success rate of 70%. Seven or less steps in 15 s suggested high instability [15].

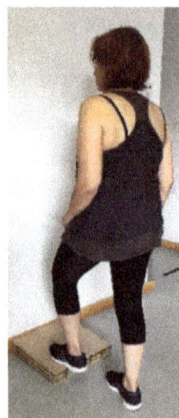

Figure 2. Step test example.

The FRT is a test that evaluates the frontal dynamic balance. The patient must be able to stand independently for at least 30 s without support and also be able to flex the shoulder to at least 90° (Figure 3). The participant was instructed to stand next to a wall so that he can reach forward along the length of the metric stick as far as possible. The movement is repeated three times and the evaluator measures the distance achieved in centimeters [40]. The mean of the second and third attempt is recorded. The performance in FRT should be between 15 and 25 cm to be considered as a safe frontal dynamic balance [41].

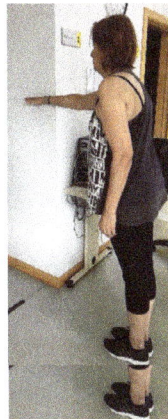

Figure 3. Functional reach test example [41].

The GBST on the force platform (Hercules model from Sensing Future, 60 × 48 × 45 cm), used Wi-Fi to monitor communication, acquisition frequency until 100 Hz, and software (from Sensing Future) to evaluate the static balance with biofeedback in the computer monitor, using a red and green cross as an indicator of bad or good equilibrium, respectively [42]. The equation for calculating the percentage in equilibrium is as follows:

$$\%balance = \left(\frac{equilibrium\ time(in\ seconds)}{total\ time\ (in\ seconds)} \right) \times 100 \qquad (1)$$

Equation (1)—Calculating percent values of equilibrium time on the force platform.

The equilibrium time is the time inside the green indicator. In other words, when the weight difference between the left and right side and the difference of weight between the front and back are within the defined tolerance. Tolerance (5%) is the allowable weight margin for the indicator to remain green (Figure 4). Each user was asked to stand up straight and completely still, with eyes open, during 1 min and repeat it three times. The best score is recorded, in trials for which at least 70% of the time in the equilibrium zone was achieved with biofeedback to have safe equilibrium reactions [20,43].

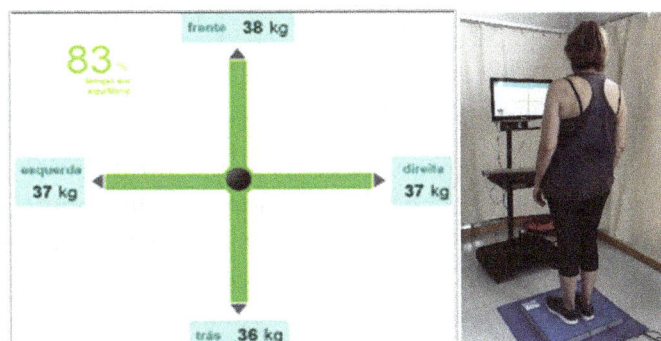

Figure 4. Monitor picture of physio sensing platform for feedback on balance.

2.6. Ethical Procedures

Researchers received permission from the local hospital Ethics Committee (07/12/2017-CE) and National Data Protection Commission (number 7103/2017) to treat the data and publish the results.

2.7. Statistical Analysis

The analysis was conducted with the statistic software SPSS version 24.0 (SPSS Inc., Chicago, IL, USA). Twelve participants were allotted to the intervention group as recommended by Julious et al. (2005) for a pilot study [44]. The normality of all outcome variables was assessed using the Shapiro-Wilk test and homogeneity of variances were verified using the Levene test. Two-way repeated-measures ANOVA allowed comparing data before and after the intervention and between groups (experimental and control) for VAS_Pain, ST, FRT, and GBST. For all ANOVAs, Mauchly's sphericity test was performed, and where this assumption was violated, Greenhouse Geisser adjustments were used [45,46].

3. Results

After the baseline assessment, all participants were included in the data analysis. Subsequently, 22 participants, 12 in the intervention group and 10 controls took part. No outcome measures showed any significant deviation from the normal distribution. No differences were found regarding age, height, weight, and BMI between groups, but there are differences for gender, health conditions, medication, osteoarthritis status, and DASH. The proportion of subjects with health conditions, medication, and osteoarthritis was higher in the intervention group. Although all participants had experienced some upper limb disability, at the time of data collection the control group had a lower DASH score (Table 1).

Table 1. Baseline characteristics of the participants (mean/standard deviation (SD)).

Characteristics	Intervention		Control	
	Female	Male	Female	Male
Gender/n	11	1	7	3
Age (years)/mean (SD)	62.9 (5.9)	58	61.9 (5.6)	75 (8.7)
Height (m)/mean (SD)	1.6 (0.1)	1.7	1.7 (0.8)	1.7 (0.7)
Weight (Kg)/mean (SD)	70.6 (12.4)	100	65.9 (11.2)	72.0 (11.8)
BMI (kg/m^2)/mean (SD)	27.8 (4.1)	35	27.0 (4)	25.0 (2)
Health condition * (yes/no)/n	11/0	1/0	4/3	1/2
Medication (yes/no)/n	7/4	0/1	1/6	0/3
Osteoarthritis (yes/no)/n	10/1	1/0	1/6	0/3
DASH Score/mean (SD)	54 (13.8)	67	28.7 (21.8)	6.11 (5.9)

* (High blood pressure or high cholesterol or diabetes mellitus 2).

Results showed better values after the aquatic intervention for the VAS_pain (6.2 (1.9) vs. 5.2 (2.3)) and for the GSBT (61.7 (5.9) vs. 71.3 (18.2). The analysis showed a time effect but no significant changes in the intervention group. There are no differences between groups in the post-test (ANOVA $p < 0.05$) results but the control group was better in the pre-test ($p < 0.01$). Actually, immediately after the intervention, the scores of all tests increased in the intervention group but remained almost unchanged in the control group (Table 2).

Table 2. Changes due to the immediate effects on pain and balance performance after the aquatic therapy, two-way repeated measures ANOVA.

Outcomes		Before Mean (SD)	After Mean (SD)		
VAS_Pain (cm)	Intervention ($n = 12$)	6.2 (1.9)	5.2 (2.3)	Time: F (1.20) = 4.31 Time*group: F (1.20) = 3.86	$p < 0.05$ $p = 0.06$
	Control ($n = 10$)	0.9 (1.9)	0.9 (1.9)	Group*inter subjects: F (1.20) = 97.60	$p < 0.01$
ST (n)	Intervention ($n = 12$)	7.0 (2.0)	7.4 (1.8)	Time: F (1.20) = 11.20 Time*group: F (1.20) = 0.39	$p < 0.01$ $p = 0.54$
	Control ($n = 10$)	11.23 (3.1)	11.80 (3.3)	Group*inter subjects: F (1.20) = 297.04	$p < 0.01$
FRT (cm)	Intervention ($n = 12$)	9.1 (2.8)	10.4 (3.8)	Time: F (1.20) = 4.67 Time*group: F (1.20) = 1.31	$p < 0.05$ $p = 0.27$
	Control ($n = 10$)	20.41 (5.9)	20.91 (5.5)	Group*inter subjects: F (1.20) = 270.43	$p < 0.01$
GBST (% T in balance)	Intervention ($n = 12$)	61.7 (5.9)	71.3 (18.2)	Time: F (1.20) = 2.24 Time*group: F (1.20) = 3.34	$p = 0.15$ $p = 0.08$
	Control ($n = 10$)	73.24 (24.3)	72.24 (22.9)	Group*inter subjects: F (1.20) = 237.80	$p < 0.01$

4. Discussion

The purpose of this exploratory study was to evaluate the immediate effects of one aquatic therapy session in a patient's group older than 55 years, following a wash-out period of no aquatic therapy after the summer vacation. Many studies look for improvements due to longer interventions [6,8,25,30,33,36,37], but in this study, the key point was to find what changes occur immediately after a single training session. The literature showed significant benefits in several patient groups [47], however, the outcome measures used in previous studies were not consistent. Due to the limited time for assessment, researchers chose measures relevant to the health problems of the participants, as well as valid, reliable, and sensitive to training [6,17,38–40].

In the current study for pain evaluation, the VAS_Pain showed a 1 cm improvement in the intervention group, while the control group showed no change after 45 min of sitting rest. No minimal clinically differences were shown in accordance with Salaffi et al. (2004), who proposed 1.4 cm as the minimal clinically important change [38]. On the other hand, Simmerman et al. (2011) found efficacy in two sessions of aquatic vertical traction in patients with persistent low back symptoms with changes in spinal length and pain, 2.7 (2.1) cm. As in our study of one session, pain deceased [48]. For the step test, the intervention group showed a score of about seven steps both before vs. after the intervention. These results might be affected by poor one-foot standing balance in the intervention group. The control group had better baseline results of about 11 steps, with no change before vs. after [40,49].

The literature suggests functional reach test values between 25.5 and 28.9 cm as an indication of good functional reach test performance in community-dwelling older adults [4,41]. Our intervention group results were more than 15 cm under this level and did not change with a single session of aquatic therapy. The control group showed better scores (≈20 cm) suggesting a moderate balance control. There were no minimum important changes, which suggested no improvement with the aquatic physiotherapy, but also no effect on the test learning process in the control group [50].

Finally, for the global balance standing test [5,18,40] based on the predictive study of Martins et al. (2015), a person should be more than 60% of the time within balance in the test to predict a low risk of falling. The results showed improved performance in the GBST for the intervention group, whereas this change was not observed in the control group. However, there was no significant interaction as the intervention group had a significantly lower baseline performance than the control group. The improvement, although not significant, did bring the intervention group up to the level of the control group. This suggested some influence of aquatic therapy in the standing balance for older adults with upper limb disability and that they do not loose balance even shortly after an aquatic session.

On the other hand, the control group showed better baseline results compared to the intervention group. Our control group were a non-active sample to study the influence of the repetition (learning effect) on the functional measurements. However, even with a better baseline, we expected some effect of learning and/or resting [51]. In addition, as the control group had lower values on BMI, with higher height, lower weight, and less additional health problems, we might have expected more and greater baseline differences.

The intervention group showed a tendency toward greater improvements in the outcomes used particularly in the global balance test, although no significance was found. The immediate changes of aquatic therapy observed in this sample, reinforces the importance of patients with upper limb dysfunction repeating a series of aquatic therapy sessions annually although the immediate improvement was not significant. As function decreases with age, we recommend aquatic therapy programs for maintenance of function as age increases [52,53]. Furthermore, the study of Cronin et al. [54] suggested that water immersion may offer promise as a low-risk, non-invasive, and non-pharmaceutical method of decreasing peripherally reflex excitability in persons with hemiplegia. Therefore, relaxation can be related with a decrease of peripheral reflex excitability.

The limitations of this study are related to the non-randomization, the different baseline level of the groups, and the study of only a single aquatic therapy session. However, this exploratory study pointed out no differences. On the other hand, the results of the experimental group showed a slight decrease in pain and an increase in balance with one single aquatic therapy session. Importantly, there were no decrements in performance. Moreover, the current study suggests that this population with fragile health (11 vs. 1) and osteoarthritis (10 vs. 2) needs to remain active (in aquatic therapy) and our immediate effect results re-enforce this goal.

Further studies should measure one single session several times to understand the evolution of the participants in a long-term program. Further, the monitoring of physiological and kinematic parameters, related to the clinically relevant expectations, can be important to better understand why returning patients are attracted to aquatic therapy in long-term programs. The establishment of the minimal important clinical changes could provide important goals and motivation for patients and physiotherapists in the practice performance.

5. Conclusions

This study had no immediate functional effects. No decrements in performance on balance or pain were found. Findings showed that participants in the intervention group experienced immediate positive changes in one single session, which enforces the motivation to continue the aquatic therapy program. The outcomes suggest that people older than 55 years have a disability in the balance test and risk. For future studies, the measurement of one single session several times is needed to understand the participant's evolution in the long-term program. Additionally, an important goal will be to establish a minimal observable difference for one single session of an aquatic therapy program for persons older than 55 years with upper limb dysfunction and other related problems of this age group.

Author Contributions: Conceptualization, M.G., D.D., and J.P.V.-B.; methodology, M.G.; validation, R.C. and D.D.; formal analysis, J.A.; investigation, M.G.; resources, R.C.; data curation, M.G.; writing—original draft preparation, M.G.; writing—review and editing, R.J.F., D.D., A.R., and J.P.V.-B.; supervision, J.P.V.-B. All authors have read and agreed to the published version of the manuscript.

Acknowledgments: The present study did not receive the financial supports.

References

1. Turpela, M.; Häkkinen, K.; Haff, G.G.; Walker, S. Effects of different strength training frequencies on maximum strength, body composition and functional capacity in healthy older individuals. *Exp. Gerontol.* **2017**, *98*, 13–21. [CrossRef]

2. Sherrington, C.; Tiedemann, A.; Fairhall, N.; Close, J.C.; Lord, S.R. Exercise to prevent falls in older adults: An updated meta-analysis and best practice recommendations. *N. S. W. Pub. Health Bull.* **2011**, *22*, 78–83. [CrossRef]

3. Cadore, E.L.; Rodríguez-Mañas, L.; Sinclair, A.; Izquierdo, M. Effects of different exercise interventions on risk of falls, gait ability, and balance in physically frail older adults: A systematic review. *Rejuvenation Res.* **2013**, *16*, 105–114. [CrossRef]

4. Freiberger, E.; Haberle, L.; Spirduso, W.W.; Zijlstra, G.A. Long-term effects of three multicomponent exercise interventions on physical performance and fall-related psychological outcomes in community-dwelling older adults: A randomized controlled trial. *J. Am. Geriatr. Soc.* **2012**, *60*, 437–446. [CrossRef]

5. Hagedorn, D.K.; Holm, E. Effects of traditional physical training and visual computer feedback training in frail elderly patients. A randomized intervention study. *Eur. J. Phys. Rehabil. Med.* **2010**, *46*, 159–168. [PubMed]

6. Kars Fertelli, T.; Mollaoglu, M.; Sahin, O. Aquatic exercise program for individuals with osteoarthritis: Pain, stiffness, physical function, self-efficacy. *Rehabil. Nurs. J.* **2018**, *44*, 290–299. [CrossRef]

7. Adsett, J.; Morris, N.; Kuys, S.; Hwang, R.; Mullins, R.; Khatun, M.; Paratz, J.; Mudge, A. Aquatic exercise training is effective in maintaining exercise performance in trained heart failure patients: A randomised crossover pilot trial. *Heart Lung Circ.* **2017**, *26*, 572–579. [CrossRef] [PubMed]

8. Alikhajeh, Y.; Hosseini, S.R.A.; Moghaddam, A. Effects of hydrotherapy in static and dynamic balance among elderly men. *Procedia Soc. Behav. Sci.* **2012**, *46*, 2220–2224. [CrossRef]

9. Kaneda, K.; Sato, D.; Wakabayashi, H.; Hanai, A.; Nomura, T. A comparison of the effects of different water exercise programs on balance ability in elderly people. *J. Aging Phys. Act.* **2008**, *16*, 381–392. [CrossRef]

10. Avelar, N.C.P.; Bastone, A.C.; Alcântara, M.A.; Gomes, W.F. Efetividade do treinamento de resistência à fadiga dos músculos dos membros inferiores dentro e fora d'água no equilíbrio estático e dinâmico de idosos. *Braz. J. Phys. Ther.* **2010**, *14*, 229–236. [CrossRef]

11. Miyoshi, T.; Shirota, T.; Yamamoto, S.; Nakazawa, K.; Akai, M. Effect of the walking speed to the lower limb joint angular displacements, joint moments and ground reaction forces during walking in water. *Disabil. Rehabil.* **2004**, *26*, 724–732. [CrossRef]

12. Wilcock, I.M.; Cronin, J.B.; Hing, W.A. Physiological response to water immersion: A method for sport recovery? *Sports Med.* **2006**, *36*, 747–765. [CrossRef]

13. Torres-Ronda, L.; Del Alcazar, X.S. The properties of water and their applications for training. *J. Hum. Kinet.* **2014**, *44*, 237–248. [CrossRef] [PubMed]

14. Verhagen, A.P.; Cardoso, J.R.; Bierma-Zeinstra, S.M. Aquatic exercise & balneotherapy in musculoskeletal conditions. *Best Pract. Res. Clin. Rheumatol.* **2012**, *26*, 335–343. [PubMed]

15. Simmons, V.; Hansen, P.D. Effectiveness of water exercise on postural mobility in the well elderly: An experimental study on balance enhancement. *J. Gerontol. Ser. A Biol. Sci. Med. Sci.* **1996**, *51*, M233–M238. [CrossRef] [PubMed]

16. Waller, B.; Munukka, M.; Multanen, J.; Rantalainen, T.; Poyhonen, T.; Nieminen, M.T.; Kiviranta, I.; Kautiainen, H.; Selanne, H.; Dekker, J.; et al. Effects of a progressive aquatic resistance exercise program on the biochemical composition and morphology of cartilage in women with mild knee osteoarthritis: Protocol for a randomised controlled trial. *BMC Musculoskelet. Disord.* **2013**, *14*, 82. [CrossRef]

17. Waller, B.; Ogonowska-Slodownik, A.; Vitor, M.; Rodionova, K.; Lambeck, J.; Heinonen, A.; Daly, D. The effect of aquatic exercise on physical functioning in the older adult: A systematic review with meta-analysis. *Age Ageing* **2016**, *45*, 593–601. [CrossRef]

18. So, B.C.L.; Kong, I.S.Y.; Lee, R.K.L.; Man, R.W.F.; Tse, W.H.K.; Fong, A.K.W.; Tsang, W.W.N. The effect of Ai Chi aquatic therapy on individuals with knee osteoarthritis: A pilot study. *J. Phys. Ther. Sci.* **2017**, *29*, 884–890. [CrossRef]

19. Kim, Y.; Mehta, T.; Lai, B.; Motl, R.W. Immediate and sustained effects of interventions for changing physical activity in people with multiple sclerosis: Meta-analysis of randomized controlled trials. *Arch. Phys. Med. Rehabil.* **2020**, *101*, 1414–1436. [CrossRef]

20.   Martins, A.C.; Andrade, S.; Santos, D. Screening and assessment of the risk of fall: An initiative to prevent falls in community dwelling older adults. *Physiotherapy* **2015**, *101*, e958. [CrossRef]

21.   Linaker, C.H.; Walker-Bone, K. Shoulder disorders and occupation. *Best Pr. Res. Clin. Rheumatol.* **2015**, *29*, 405–423. [CrossRef]

22.   Moher, D.; Hopewell, S.; Schulz, K.F.; Montori, V.; Gøtzsche, P.C.; Devereaux, P.J.; Elbourne, D.; Egger, M.; Altman, D.G. CONSORT 2010 explanation and elaboration: Updated guidelines for reporting parallel group randomised trials. *BMJ* **2010**, *340*, c869. [CrossRef]

23.   Graça, M. Development of an aquatic therapy group's protocol program for older adults with upper limb disability. In Proceedings of the International Congress of Health and Well-Being Intervention (ICHWBI 2019), Viseu, Portugal, 31 May–1 June 2019; Desouzart, G., Ed.; Work Journal: Viseu, Portugal, 2019; p. 146.

24.   Meredith-Jones, K.; Waters, D.; Legge, M.; Jones, L. Upright water-based exercise to improve cardiovascular and metabolic health: A qualitative review. *Complementary Ther. Med.* **2011**, *19*, 93–103. [CrossRef]

25.   Lambeck, J.; Gamper, U. The Halliwick Concept. In *Comprehensive Aquatic Therapy*, 3rd ed.; Bruce, E., Becker, A.J.C., Eds.; Washington State University Press: Pullman, WA, USA, 2010.

26.   Lord, S.R.; Ward, J.A.; Williams, P.; Anstey, K.J. An epidemiological study of falls in older community-dwelling women: The Randwick falls and fractures study. *Aust. J. Public Health* **1993**, *17*, 240–245. [CrossRef]

27.   Methajarunon, P.; Eitivipart, C.; Diver, C.J.; Foongchomcheay, A. Systematic review of published studies on aquatic exercise for balance in patients with multiple sclerosis, Parkinson's disease, and hemiplegia. *Hong Kong Physiother. J.* **2016**, *35*, 12–20. [CrossRef]

28.   Pérez-de la Cruz, S.; García Luengo, A.V.; Lambeck, J. Effects of an Ai Chi fall prevention programme for patients with Parkinson's disease. *Neurología* **2016**, *31*, 176–182.

29.   Assis, M.R.; Silva, L.E.; Alves, A.M.; Pessanha, A.P.; Valim, V.; Feldman, D.; Neto, T.L.; Natour, J. A randomized controlled trial of deep water running: Clinical effectiveness of aquatic exercise to treat fibromyalgia. *Arthritis Rheum.* **2006**, *55*, 57–65. [CrossRef]

30.   Rewald, S.; Mesters, I.; Lenssen, A.F.; Emans, P.J.; Wijnen, W.; de Bie, R.A. Effect of aqua-cycling on pain and physical functioning compared with usual care in patients with knee osteoarthritis: Study protocol of a randomised controlled trial. *BMC Musculoskelet. Disord.* **2016**, *17*, 88. [CrossRef]

31.   Brady, B.; Redfern, J.; MacDougal, G.; Williams, J. The addition of aquatic therapy to rehabilitation following surgical rotator cuff repair: A feasibility study. *Physiother. Res. Int. J. Res. Clin. Phys. Ther.* **2008**, *13*, 153–161. [CrossRef]

32.   Burmaster, C.; Eckenrode, B.J.; Stiebel, M. Early incorporation of an evidence-based aquatic-assisted approach to arthroscopic rotator cuff repair rehabilitation: Prospective case study. *Phys. Ther.* **2016**, *96*, 53–61. [CrossRef]

33.   Bidonde, J.; Busch, A.J.; Webber, S.C.; Schachter, C.L.; Danyliw, A.; Overend, T.J.; Richards, R.S.; Rader, T. Aquatic exercise training for fibromyalgia. *Cochrane Database Syst. Rev.* **2014**, *10*, Cd011336. [CrossRef] [PubMed]

34.   Candeloro, J.; Caromano, F. Efeito de um programa de hidroterapia na flexibilidade e na força muscular de idosas. *Braz. J. Phys. Ther.* **2007**, *11*, 303–309. [CrossRef]

35.   Atroshi, I.; Gummesson, C.; Andersson, B.; Dahlgren, E.; Johansson, A. The disabilities of the arm, shoulder and hand (DASH) outcome questionnaire: Reliability and validity of the Swedish version evaluated in 176 patients. *Acta Orthop. Scand.* **2000**, *71*, 613–618. [CrossRef]

36.   Hawker, G.A.; Mian, S.; Kendzerska, T.; French, M. Measures of adult pain: Visual analog scale for pain (VAS Pain), numeric rating scale for pain (NRS Pain), McGill pain questionnaire (MPQ), short-form McGill pain questionnaire (SF-MPQ), chronic pain grade scale (CPGS), short form-36 bodily pain scale (SF-36 BPS), and measure of intermittent and constant osteoarthritis pain (ICOAP). *Arthritis Care Res.* **2011**, *63*, S240–S252.

37.   Tashjian, R.Z.; Deloach, J.; Porucznik, C.A.; Powell, A.P. Minimal clinically important differences (MCID) and patient acceptable symptomatic state (PASS) for visual analog scales (VAS) measuring pain in patients treated for rotator cuff disease. *J. Shoulder Elb. Surg.* **2009**, *18*, 927–932. [CrossRef] [PubMed]

38.   Salaffi, F.; Stancati, A.; Silvestri, C.A.; Ciapetti, A.; Grassi, W. Minimal clinically important changes in chronic musculoskeletal pain intensity measured on a numerical rating scale. *Eur. J. Pain* **2004**, *8*, 283–291. [CrossRef]

39.   Devereux, K.; Robertson, D.; Briffa, N.K. Effects of a water-based program on women 65 years and over: A rrandomised controlled trial. *Aust. J. Physiother.* **2005**, *51*, 102–108. [CrossRef]

40.   Brauer, S.G.; Burns, Y.R.; Galley, P. A prospective study of laboratory and clinical measures of postural stability to predict community-dwelling fallers. *J. Gerontol. Ser. A Biol. Sci. Med. Sci.* **2000**, *55*, M469–M476. [CrossRef]

41. Duncan, P.W.; Weiner, D.K.; Chandler, J.; Studenski, S. Functional reach: A new clinical measure of balance. *J. Gerontol.* **1990**, *45*, M192–M197. [CrossRef]
42. Martins, A.C.; Silva, J.; Baltazar, D.; Silva, A.J.; Santos, A.; Madureira, J.; Alcobia, C.; Ferreira, L.; Mendes, P.; Tonelo, C.; et al. Fatores ambientais e prevenção de quedas_o FallSensing como solução integradora. *Segurança Saúde Ocup. E Ambient.* **2016**. Available online: https://docplayer.com.br/51053574-Fatores-ambientais-e-prevencao-de-quedas-o-fallsensing-como-solucao-integradora.html (accessed on 15 December 2020).
43. Whyatt, C.; Merriman, N.A.; Young, W.R.; Newell, F.N.; Craig, C. A Wii bit of fun: A novel platform to deliver effective balance training to older adults. *Games Health J.* **2015**, *4*, 423–433. [CrossRef] [PubMed]
44. Julious, S.A. Sample size of 12 per group rule of thumb for a pilot study. *Pharm. Stat.* **2005**, *4*, 287–291. [CrossRef]
45. Blanca, M.J.; Alarcón, R.; Arnau, J.; Bono, R.; Bendayan, R. Non-normal data: Is ANOVA still a valid option? *Psicothema* **2017**, *29*, 552–557.
46. Field, A. *Discovering Statistics Using SPSS*, 5th ed.; SAGE Publishing: Newbury Park, CA, USA, 2013.
47. Dias, J.M.; Cisneros, L.; Dias, R.; Fritsch, C.; Gomes, W.; Pereira, L.; Santos, M.L.; Ferreira, P.H. Hydrotherapy improves pain and function in older women with knee osteoarthritis: A randomized controlled trial. *Braz. J. Phys. Ther.* **2017**, *21*, 449–456. [CrossRef]
48. Simmerman, S.M.; Sizer, P.S.; Dedrick, G.S.; Apte, G.G.; Brismée, J.M. Immediate changes in spinal height and pain after aquatic vertical traction in patients with persistent low back symptoms: A crossover clinical trial. *PM R J. Inj. Funct. Rehabil.* **2011**, *3*, 447–457. [CrossRef]
49. Moore, M.; Barker, K. The validity and reliability of the four square step test in different adult populations: A systematic review. *Syst. Rev.* **2017**, *6*, 187. [CrossRef]
50. Schmitt, J.S.; Di Fabio, R.P. Reliable change and minimum important difference (MID) proportions facilitated group responsiveness comparisons using individual threshold criteria. *J. Clin. Epidemiol.* **2004**, *57*, 1008–1018. [CrossRef]
51. Lord, S.; Mitchell, D.; Williams, P. Effect of water exercise on balance and related factors in older people. *Aust. J. Physiother.* **1993**, *39*, 217–222. [CrossRef]
52. Alcalde, G.E.; Fonseca, A.C.; Bôscoa, T.F.; Gonçalves, M.R.; Bernardo, G.C.; Pianna, B.; Carnavale, B.F.; Gimenes, C.; Barrile, S.R.; Arca, E.A. Effect of aquatic physical therapy on pain perception, functional capacity and quality of life in older people with knee osteoarthritis: Study protocol for a randomized controlled trial. *Trials* **2017**, *18*, 317. [CrossRef]
53. Bocalini, D.S.; Serra, A.J.; Rica, R.L.; Dos Santos, L. Repercussions of training and detraining by water-based exercise on functional fitness and quality of life: A short-term follow-up in healthy older women. *Clinics* **2010**, *65*, 1305–1309. [CrossRef]
54. Cronin, N.J.; Valtonen, A.M.; Waller, B.; Pöyhönen, T.; Avela, J. Effects of short term water immersion on peripheral reflex excitability in hemiplegic and healthy individuals: A preliminary study. *J. Musculoskelet. Neuronal. Interact.* **2016**, *16*, 58–62. [PubMed]

4

The Influence of Preoperative Physical Activity on Postoperative Outcomes of Knee and Hip Arthroplasty Surgery in the Elderly

Sebastiano Vasta [1]**, Rocco Papalia** [1]**, Guglielmo Torre** [1,*]**, Ferruccio Vorini** [1]**, Giuseppe Papalia** [1]**, Biagio Zampogna** [1]**, Chiara Fossati** [2]**, Marco Bravi** [3]**, Stefano Campi** [1] **and Vincenzo Denaro** [1]

[1]   Department of Orthopaedic and Trauma Surgery, Campus Bio-Medico University of Rome, 00128 Rome, Italy; s.vasta@unicampus.it (S.V.); r.papalia@unicampus.it (R.P.); f.vorini@unicampus.it (F.V.); g.papalia@unicampus.it (G.P.); b.zampogna@unicampus.it (B.Z.); s.campi@unicampus.it (S.C.); denaro@unicampus.it (V.D.)

[2]   Department of Movement, Human and Health Sciences, University of Rome "Foro Italico", 00100 Rome, Italy; chiara.fossati@uniroma4.it

[3]   Department of Physical Medicine and Rehabilitation, Campus Bio-Medico University of Rome, 00128 Rome, Italy; m.bravi@unicampus.it

*   Correspondence: g.torre@unicampus.it

Abstract: Total hip arthroplasty (THA) and total knee arthroplasty (TKA) represent two of the most common procedures in orthopedic surgery. The growing need to avoid physical impairment in elderly patients undergoing this kind of surgery puts the focus on the possibility to undertake a preoperative physical activity program to improve their fit and physical health at the time of surgery. A systematic review has been carried out with online databases including PubMed-Medline, Cochrane Central and Google Scholar. The aim was to retrieve available evidence concerning preoperative physical activity and exercise, before total knee or total hip arthroplasty in patients older than 65 years, and to clarify the role of this practice in improving postoperative outcomes. Results of the present systematic analysis showed that, for TKA, most of the studies demonstrated a comparable trend of postoperative improvement of Visual Analogue Scale (VAS), range of movement (ROM) and functional scores, and those of quality of life. There is insufficient evidence in the literature to draw final conclusions on the topic. Prehabilitation for patients undergoing TKA leads to shorter length of stay but not to an enhanced postoperative recovery. Concerning THA, although currently available data showed better outcomes in patients who underwent prehabilitation programs, there is a lack of robust evidence with appropriate methodology.

Keywords: knee; hip; arthroplasty; physical activity; elderly; prehabilitation

1. Introduction

The prevalence of osteoarthritis in the elderly population is relevant, especially for lower limb weight-bearing joints. Total knee arthroplasty (TKA) and total hip arthroplasty (THA) are the two major surgeries for end-stage osteoarthrosis, usually advocated when all conservative treatments are inefficient. The healthcare-related economic burden is extensive for these surgeries, especially concerning postoperative hospitalization, leading in recent years to the development of several fast-track strategies aimed to improve results and decrease hospital stay expenses [1,2].

Arthroplasty aims to restore the function of the joint and soothe the pain derived from bone-on-bone arthritic conditions. After hip and knee arthroplasty, a consistent rehabilitation program is usually undertaken in order to provide the patient with the adequate strength and mobility to bear the prosthetic implant and to guarantee a correct function [1]. Isometric strengthening of the muscle responsible for the index joint movement (gluteal muscles for the hip and quadriceps for the knee) is a key feature of postoperative rehabilitation, providing the limb with the appropriate muscular support for the mobilization of the hip or the knee. Furthermore, an antagonist stretching program is mandatory to achieve a full range of movement (ROM), avoiding postoperative stiffness and walking disabilities. In a consecutive phase, neuromuscular education to walking is advocated to eventually restore the locomotor function of the limb [3].

In recent years there has been growing interest in the possibility to prepare patients for surgery through a "prehabilitation" program, composed of strengthening and stretching exercises in the immediate preoperative period. The focus of several research projects at present is to understand whether a prehabilitation program of specific exercises or physical activities may influence and improve the postoperative outcomes of the patients. Physical exercise has been already reported to be beneficial in the knee and hip OA as a conservative treatment [4]. Activity improves function and decreases pain; thus, it is actually suggested for those patients affected, independently from the schedule of the surgery. However, it is not clear if specific exercise programs improve surgical outcomes and postoperative parameters of the patient, including the length of stay in the hospital and the quality of life. The aim of the present systematic review of the literature is to collect evidence concerning preoperative programs of activity and exercises for those patients scheduled for hip and knee arthroplasty. A specific focus of our research frame is the elderly, as there are major concerns about functional recovery and length of hospital stay in this sub-population. This intension was firstly determined from the examination of previous literature, where heterogeneity of population characteristics compromised the internal consistency of results of systematic reviews and meta-analyses [5]. The primary endpoint is to clarify the impact of specific training on subjective and objective surgical outcomes; the secondary endpoint focuses on the influence on postoperative parameters including the length of hospitalization and the quality of life of the patient.

2. Methods

The present systematic review was carried out in accordance with the Preferred Reporting Items for Systematic Review and Meta-analysis (PRISMA) guidelines and followed the Cochrane methodology for systematic reviews [6]. However, no protocol for systematic review has been registered. Furthermore, PICO (Poipulation, Intervention, Comparison, Outcome) methodology has been used to formulate the study hypothesis. According to PICO, the following elements have been used to frame the study question:

Population—patients who are candidates for TKA or THA;
Intervention—prehabilitation; preoperative physical activity program;
Comparison—no preoperative intervention;
Outcome of interest—postoperative functional outcomes and length of stay.

2.1. Criteria for Considering Studies for This Review

The studies considered for inclusion were randomized controlled trials (RCT), prospective cohort studies (PCS), case-control studies (CCS) and case series (CS). Case reports, reviews and meta-analyses were excluded. Furthermore, basic science and in-vitro studies, biomechanical and cadaver evaluations were excluded. Studies considered should concern the preoperative physical activity in elderly patients that were scheduled for TKA or THA. According to WHO's definition of the elderly, only studies where the average age of the cohorts was greater than 65 years were considered.

2.2. Primary Outcomes

Subjective and objective clinical measurements were considered as the primary outcome of the analysis, taking into account the clinical scores reported, which included Knee injury and Osteoarthritis Outcome Score (KOOS) Western Ontario McMaster University Osteoarthritis Index (WOMAC),

Knee Society Score (KSS) and range of motion (ROM) of the index joint. Furthermore, the outcomes of physical performance tests were considered, including the 6 min walking test (6-MWT), the time up and go test (TUG), and gait speed and distance.

2.3. Secondary Outcomes

Postoperative length of stay was the main secondary outcome considered. Furthermore, the quality of life of the patients after surgery was considered, measured through Short Form-36 (SF-36) and the quality of life section of the Knee injuries and Osteoarthritis Outcome Score (KOOS).

2.4. Search Methods for Identification of Studies

Online databases were searched for relevant articles, including PubMed-Medline, Cochrane Central and Google Scholar. The search was carried out between March and November 2019. Search strings used were the following: ("exercise" [MeSH Terms] OR "exercise" [All Fields] OR ("physical" [All Fields] AND "activity" [All Fields]) OR "physical activity" [All Fields]) AND ("aged" [MeSH Terms] OR "aged" [All Fields] OR "elderly" [All Fields]) AND ("arthroplasty" [MeSH Terms] OR "arthroplasty" [All Fields]); Prehabilitation [All Fields] AND ("aged" [MeSH Terms] OR "aged" [All Fields] OR "elderly" [All Fields]) AND ("arthroplasty" [MeSH Terms] OR "arthroplasty" [All Fields]).

No time interval was set for publication date. The studies retrieved were firstly screened by title, and where relevant, the whole abstract was read. After a first selection and exclusion of not-relevant papers, the full text of the potentially eligible articles was retrieved and read by two reviewers for eventual inclusion. Discordant opinions were solved through the consultation of a third reviewer. After the electronic search was completed, the bibliography of the relevant articles included was screened manually to identify further papers potentially missed in the electronic search. The search process is summarized in the flow diagram in Figure 1.

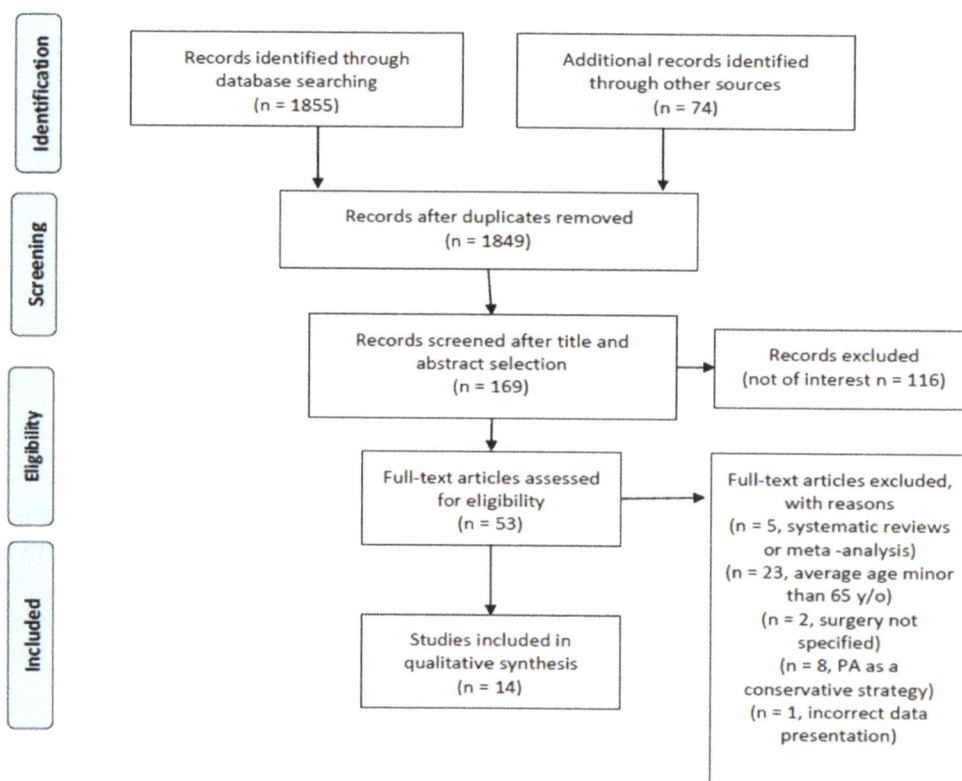

Figure 1. Preferred Reporting Items for Systematic Review and Meta-analysis (PRISMA) flow diagram. PA: Physical Activity

2.5. Data Collection and Analysis

Data were extracted from the included articles according to the primary and secondary outcomes considered for the aim of this review. After extraction, generic data concerning the paper and specific outcome data were reported in tables. The protocol of preoperative physical activity intervention was analyzed and reported in a specific table. For an appropriate presentation of data, the results were divided on the basis of the surgery (TKA or THA).

2.6. Risk of Bias Assessment

Given the heterogeneity of the included studies, two different critical appraisal tools were utilized. For randomized clinical trials, the Cochrane risk of bias assessment tool was used, providing a grade of risk (low or high risk) of bias for the index study in five elements of the study design (sequence generation, allocation concealment, blinding, incomplete data addressing and selective reporting). For non-randomized studies, the Methodological Index for Non-Randomized Studies (MINORS) score was used.

3. Results

3.1. Results of the Search

From the electronic search, a total of 1855 articles were retrieved. One of the authors (G.T.) screened the results by title and abstract and manually searched the bibliographies of the relevant papers, especially reviews and meta-analyses. Of the articles retrieved through electronic and manual search, 14 were finally included (Figure 1) [7–20].

3.2. Included Studies

Of the included studies, 12 were RCT of Level Of Evidence (LOE) I, 1 was a prospective case–control study of LOA II, and 1 was a CS of LOE IV [7]. Of these, 10 presented outcomes of TKA [7,11–19], 3 of THA and one evaluated both TKA and THA results [8–10].

3.3. Excluded Studies

Several studies retrieved were excluded for the following main reasons: average age of the cohort < 65 years [20,21], reviews or meta-analyses [22] and/or no surgery scheduled (assessment of physical activity as a conservative treatment).

3.4. Demographic Data

The included studies reported data on a total of 1175 patients, with an average age ranging from 66 to 76.9 years. A total of 1096 patients were scheduled for TKA, while 79 were scheduled for THA. Details on demographic data of the cohorts are shown in Tables 1 and 2.

Table 1. TKA.

Study	Type of Study	LOE	Number of Patients	Mean Age (y)	Type of Scheduled Surgery	Type of Intervention	Outcomes Summary
Evgeniadis et al., 2008	RCT	I	53	68.76	TKA	General strengthening exercise program 3 weeks before surgery vs. specific strengthening exercise program 8 weeks postoperatively	Preoperative SF-36 was slightly better in patients treated with preoperative strengthening. ILAS and active ROM resulted significantly improved at the termination of the program in the group treated with strengthening postoperatively
Gill et al., 2009	RCT	I	82	70.3	TKA, THA	Land-based vs. pool-based preoperative exercise programs, 6 preoperative weeks	Significant improvement in postoperative performance for both groups, although no difference occurred between groups in terms of WOMAC and SF-36
Gstoettner et al., 2011	RCT	I	38	72.8 (study group) 66.9 (control group)	TKA	Preoperative proprioceptive training	Stance stability improved significantly in the study group at 6 weeks after surgery (Biodex Stability System evaluation). No difference between study and control group occurred in postoperative (6 weeks) WOMAC and KSS
Huang et al., 2012	RCT	I	273	70	TKA	Home-based rehabilitation educational program (4 weeks before surgery)	Medical expenditure of hospital stay in the study group was significantly lower ($P = 0.001$). VAS and ROM was not significantly different in patients of both groups in the early day after surgery (5 days after admission)
Matassi et al., 2012	RCT	I	122	66 (study group), 67 (control group)	TKA	Home-based exercise program (6 weeks before surgery)	Exercise program improved the recovery of knee motion and yielded a shorter hospital stay. Differences were balanced in the long-term follow-up.
Skoffer et al., 2015	RCT	I	59	70.7 (study group), 70.1 (control group)	TKA	Progressive resistance training in the 4 preoperative weeks	Significant differences were found in the study group when compared to controls in terms of 30sCST, TUG, knee flexors strength. No difference was found in KOOS, VAS and a 100-points quality of life rating scale.
Twiggs et al., 2017	CS	IV	91	67.5	TKA	Fitbit wristband activity goals (step count)	Poor positive correlation (not statistically significant) between higher preoperative step count and hospital stay. KOOS QOL was significantly associated to step count 6-weeks postoperatively and KOOS Pain was significantly correlated to step count at preoperative and postoperative day 2–4 step count.
VanLeeuwen et al., 2014	RCT	I	22		TKA	Standard training with additional program of progressive strength training	No difference was found between groups in 6MWT and chair stand. Moreover, no difference was found in recovery time

Table 1. *Cont.*

Study	Type of Study	LOE	Number of Patients	Mean Age (y)	Type of Scheduled Surgery	Type of Intervention	Outcomes Summary
Williamson et al., 2007	RCT	I	181	72.4 (Acupuncture group) 70 (Physiotherapy group) 69.6 (Controls)	TKA	Supervised strengthening exercises 6 weeks before surgery	Shorter in-patient stay was observed in the physiotherapy group (1 day less than other groups)
Aytekin et al., 2018	CCS	II	44	67.8 (Prehabilitation) 69.7 (Controls)	TKA	Education and home-based exercise 12 weeks before surgery	No significant difference in VAS and KOOS occurred at 3 and 6 months between groups. Length of stay was higher for the control group. Of the intervention group, 4 subjects changed their operation decision.
Beaupre et al., 2004	RCT	I	131		TKA	Exercise and education program 4 weeks before surgery	No difference was observed in ROM and strength of the knee, pain and HRQOL

LOE: Level Of Evidence, RCT: Randomized Controlled Trial, WOMAC: Western Ontario McMaster universities Arthritis Index, CS: Case Series, CCS: Case-Control Study, ILAS: Iowa Level of Assistance Scale, THA: total hip arthroplasty, TKA: total knee arthroplasty, VAS: Visual Analogue Scale, ROM: range of motion, TUG: time up and go, 6MWT: 6-minute walking test, 30sCST: 30 s chair stand test, KOOS: Knee injury and Osteoarthritis Outcome Score, HRQOL: Health Related Quality of Life.

Table 2. THA.

Study	Type of Study	LOE	N.er of Patients	Mean Age (y)	Type of Scheduled Surgery	Type of Intervention	Outcomes Summary
Hoogeboom et al., 2010	RCT	I	21	76	THA	Preoperative strengthening exercises and tailor-made activity	No difference occurred between study and control groups in length of stay and functional recovery after surgery
Oosting et al., 2012	RCT	I	30	76.9 (study group), 75 (control group)	THA	Supervised walking and functional activities from 6 to 3 weeks preoperatively	Functional improvements were observed with better results in the study group in the postoperative TUG test and 6MWT (6 weeks after surgery)
Wang et al., 2002	RCT	I	28	68.3	THA	Preoperative customized exercise program	Exercise group showed greater stride length and gait speed at 3 weeks after surgery. Gait speed was also greater at 12 and 24 weeks, while 6MWT distance was greater at 12 and 24 weeks

ILAS: Iowa Level of Assistance Scale, THA: total hip arthroplasty, TKA: total knee arthroplasty, VAS: Visual Analogue Scale, ROM: range of motion, TUG: time up and go, 6MWT: 6-minute walking test, 30sCST: 30 s chair stand test, KOOS: Knee injury and Osteoarthritis Outcome Score, HRQOL: Health Related Quality of Life.

3.5. Total Knee Arthroplasty

3.5.1. Main intervention

Studies concerning knee arthroplasty focused on preoperative muscle strengthening or proprioceptive exercises. Timing of intervention ranged between 2 and 12 weeks before surgery. Specific training included strengthening with elastic resistance band [19], combined land-based and pool-based exercises [18], supervised proprioceptive training [17] and progressive resistance training [12,16]. Several papers intervened by instructing patients of the study group in a home-based exercise program [14,15], while several other administered supervised training sessions [13,16–19]. Some of the studies reported a continuation of the activity program in weeks 4 to 8, after surgery [16,19]. In Table 3 specific programs were summarized in comparison to control group activity.

Table 3. Protocols of intervention.

Study	Main Intervention	Control Group Intervention
Evgeniadis et al., 2008	Trunk and upper extremity elastic band (thera-band) strengthening for the 3 weeks before surgery.	No exercise before surgery, rehabilitation protocol for the 8 weeks after surgery.
Gill et al., 2009	Ingroups of 4 to 6 participants, under physiotherapist instructions: 1 h for 2 times a week for the 6 preoperative weeks. Exercises were completed at a moderate intensity between 12 and 14 on the BRPES. Home exercises were also encouraged 3 times a week. Specific program: "5 to 10 min of forward, sideways, and backward walking; 20 min pedaling a stationary exercise bike; resistance exercises; calf, hamstrings, and quadriceps stretches (2 sets of 30 s)."	Similar program schedule to land based group. Specific program: "walking and active range of movement Exercises; calf, hamstring, and quadriceps stretches (2 sets of 30 s)."
Gstoettner et al., 2011	Preoperative proprioceptive program in the 6 weeks preceding surgery: once a week, 45min training session supervised one-to-one by a physiotherapist. Daily home training instructions were given. Exercises include: slide step forward/backward, step forward/backward, single leg stance and squat.	No preoperative training
Hoogeboom et al., 2010	Supervised training twice a week for the 6 to 3 weeks preceding the index surgery. Four-phases training was administered: "First, patients started with a 5-min walk to warm up. Subsequently, they trained their lower extremity with the leg-press (sets of 10–20) through the full possible range of motion, both concentric and eccentric. Then, patients trained their aerobic capacity on a bicycle ergometer for 20–30 min. Finally, they followed a specific tailor-made training which integrates functional physical activities into the patient's daily living"	Usual preoperative and postoperative care
Huang et al., 2012	Experienced physiotherapist educated the subjects for a home-based program in a 40 min meeting 2 to 4 weeks before the index surgery. "Exercises included straight leg raising, knee setting, ankle pumping, and hip abduction with resistance"	No activity restrictions in the period before surgery. No specific training or educational, except routine.
Matassi et al., 2012	Patients were instructed for a home.-based program to undertake 5 days a week in the 6 weeks preceding surgery (without the help of a therapist). Exercises included: quadriceps and hamstring stretching, isometric and isotonic quadriceps strengthening, isotonic hamstring contractions, and dynamic stepping.	Regular activities until surgery
Oosting et al., 2012	Supervised 30-min sessions twice a week for the preoperative 6 to 3 weeks. Training was tailored to the patient and his/her environment with focus on walking ability and functional daily activities.	Single supervised session 3 weeks before surgery. The session provided education on postoperative course, walking with crutches and exercises.

Table 3. *Cont.*

Study	Main Intervention	Control Group Intervention
Skoffer et al., 2015	Progressive resistance training supervised sessions (60 min each) were undertook 3 times a week in the 4 preoperative weeks and continued the program in the 4 postoperative weeks. After warm-up, the exercise session included leg press, knee extension, knee flexion, hip extension, hip abduction, and hip adduction in strength training machines.	Regular activities until surgery and progressive resistance training program in the postoperative period (4 weeks, as the study group).
VanLeeuwen et al., 2014	Standard strengthening with the adjunction of progressive strength training, including: leg press, step-up, squat, leg extension.	Standard strengthening
Wang et al., 2002	Two supervised sessions and two home-based sessions were scheduled per week, in the 8 weeks before surgery. "All exercise programs were customized to the subject and his or her level of pain, age, and general physical ability". Supervised sessions included hydrotherapy, stationary bike riding, and resistive training for thigh abduction, thigh flexion and extension, leg flexion and extension, and ankle plantar flexion.	Standard advices on preoperative activities given by the physiotherapist of the hospital.
Williamson et al., 2007	Patients were divided in groups of 6–10 patients and attended 1 h session once a week for 6 weeks before surgery. Exercise circuits were either devised or supervised.	Acupuncture group (II arm) received lower limb acupuncture. Control group (III arm) received an informative leaflet on preoperative exercises and advice
Aytekin et al., 2018	Patients allocated to the intervention group received general education about OA and TKA, with specific home-based exercise program (ankle pumping, knee range of motion, quadriceps isometric, stretching and strengthening).	Regular activities until surgery

BRPES: Borg Rating of Perceived Exertion Scale.

3.5.2. Clinical Outcome Data

Preoperative strengthening showed a positive effect on perioperative outcomes in several of the included studies. In the study by Evgeniadis et al., SF-36 score was better for the study group, in the immediate preoperative setting, though this difference was not significant [19]. Similarly, no significant difference occurred in SF-36 in the paper by Gill et al., as well as the functional outcomes, assessed through WOMAC score [18]. A progressive resistance training program, administered in the study by Skoffer et al. [16], showed improved functional recovery in the patients of the study group assessed through TUG test, 30 s chair stand test (30sCST) and determination of knee flexion strength; however, there was no difference in KOOS, VAS and on a 100-point quality of life rating scale. Similarly, no difference was observed in WOMAC score after a preoperative proprioceptive training in another recent study [17]. Contrary to these results, the progressive strength training program advocated in the study by VanLeeuwen et al. yielded comparable functional results between groups in terms of 6MWT and chair stand [12]. Similarly, in the paper by Aytekin et al. [20], KOOS and VAS were comparable between intervention group (home-based strengthening and stretching exercises) and controls. In the case series by Twiggs et al. [7], a significant correlation was found between preoperative step count and KOOS (activity of daily living subscore) immediately before surgery (rho = 0.282, $p < 0.05$). A trial reported that the ROM and the Iowa Level of Assistance Scale (ILAS) were significantly better in the study group after the completion of the supervised program, 8 weeks after surgery [19]. Conversely, the paper by Matassi et al. [14] reported a better recovery of knee ROM after a preoperative home-based general strengthening program. Nevertheless, a study reported no difference among groups in ROM and VAS in the early postoperative days after a pre-surgery home-based strengthening program [15]. Similarly, no difference in ROM was observed in the trial by Beaoupre et al. [11]. Hospital length of stay was assessed in five papers. The article by Huang et al. [15] reported a significantly lower medical expenditure for the patients that participated in the home-based preoperative program (7 ± 2 vs. 8 ± 1 days; $p = 0.001$). A shorter hospital stay was also reported by Matassi et al. (9.1 ± 2.1 vs. 9.9 ± 2.3 days) [14] and in the study by Williamson et al. for those patients that underwent home-based [14] or supervised (6.5 vs. 7.7 days) [13] strengthening programs. The major difference registered, though not statistically significant, occurred in the study by Aytekin et al., where the average length of stay was longer in the intervention group (5.5 ± 2 vs. 7.9 ± 2.3 days; $p > 0.05$) [20]. A prospective case series by Twiggs et al. [7] showed a poor positive correlation (rho $= -0.114$, $p > 0.05$) between preoperative step count and hospital length of stay.

3.5.3. Methodological Evaluation

Nine of the included studies concerning TKA were level I RCT, and one was a level IV CS. The methodological assessment was carried out through Cochrane Risk of Bias Assessment Tool for the nine trials and the MINOR score for the non-comparative series. According to the evaluation, the studies all had some major flaws in methodology, except for one [16], where only blinding bias was considered high. Among trials, the evaluation showed that major limitations were observed concerning the blinding bias because blinding of physical activity is actually impossible to achieve. Furthermore, several studies did not describe any statistical method for addressing incomplete data, thus a high risk of bias in this field was also reported. Selective reporting was also a bias of several studies, which focused only on one or a few aspects of postoperative recovery.

3.6. Total Hip Arthroplasty

3.6.1. Main intervention

Considering the studies reporting outcomes of THA, three papers [8–10] showed outcomes of patients that underwent a program of muscular strengthening. Specifically, a personalized activity divided into progressive phases [8] was administered, either home-based or supervised [9,10]. The timing of the activity program ranged between 6 and 3 weeks before surgery, with a schedule of two sessions per week. In Table 3 specific programs were summarized in comparison to control group activity.

3.6.2. Clinical Outcome Data

Although in one trial no difference occurred between study and control groups [8], the other two papers [9,10] reported better functional outcomes in the intervention group. Specifically, the time up and go (TUG) test and 6-minute walking test (6MWT) were better performed at 6 weeks after surgery by those patients managed with preoperative program of strengthening [9]. Similarly, 6MWT was improved in the study group at 12 and 24 weeks, and a greater stride length and increased gait speed were observed at 3, 12 and 24 weeks after surgery in those patients treated with a personalized activity program [9]. In the study by Hoogeboom et al., no difference was observed in length of stay, with an average time of 6 days in the study group (range 5–22 days) and of 6 days in the control group (range 4–7 days), with a $p = 0.228$ [8].

3.6.3. Methodological Evaluation

All the included studies concerning THA were level I RCT. The methodological assessment was carried out through Cochrane Risk of Bias Assessment Tool (Table 4). According to the evaluation, the three studies had one or more major flaws in methodology; therefore, the risk of bias within a single trial was high for the three studies. Among trials, evaluation also showed some major limitations, especially concerning allocation concealment, which was at high risk of bias. Furthermore, selective reporting was at high risk of bias for two studies [9,10] where only functional outcomes were reported, and no data concerning length of stay and perioperative outcomes were shown.

Table 4. Cochrane Risk of Bias Assessment Tool.

Study	Sequence Generation	Allocation Concealment	Blinding	Incomplete Data Addressed	Selective Reporting	Other Bias
Evgeniadis, 2008	L	L	U	H	H	H
Gills, 2009	H	H	H	U	L	H
Gstoettner, 2011	L	L	H	U	L	L
Hoogeboom, 2010	L	H	H	U	H	H
Huang, 2012	L	L	H	U	H	H
Matassi, 2012	L	L	H	H	H	H
Oosting, 2012	H	H	H	H	H	H
Skoffer, 2015	L	L	H	U	L	L
VanLeeuwen, 2014	L	L	H	H	H	L
Wang, 2002	H	H	H	U	L	H
Williamson, 2007	L	L	H	U	H	L
Aytekin, 2018	H	H	H	U	L	L

L: Low, H: High, U: Uncertain.

4. Discussion

The primary endpoint of the present investigation was to assess whether a preoperative activity program impacts on the functional recovery. Concerning TKA, discordant results were reported concerning functional assessment with 6MWT and TUG, either considering studies reporting similar protocols of preoperative exercise [12,16]. However, most of the studies demonstrated a comparable trend of postoperative improvement of VAS, ROM and functional scores (KOOS and WOMAC) and those of quality of life (SF-36). Conversely, clear evidence can be observed concerning the postoperative length of stay, as all the studies analyzing length of stay demonstrated a shorter length of stay in those patients undergoing the preoperative activity program. Regarding the studies on THA, stronger evidence is available on the positive influence of preoperative activity on functional recovery [9,10]. Conversely, length of stay was comparable between groups, although only one study reported these data. As in previous review works, these results do not achieve clinical relevance, although most are statistically significant [23,24].

The preoperative exercise programs were significantly variable and differed especially for the type of exercise, while the duration was similar, as almost all the studies reported a protocol of activity within the 6 weeks preceding the index surgery. The most relevant point concerning the activity program was supervision of the exercises by a trainer or a physical therapist. Some of the studies advocated a home-based program [9,14,15], while several other administered supervised training sessions [8,13,16–20]. A slight modification of the exercise program did not yield significant differences in results, in fact in the trial by VanLeeuwen et al. [12] no difference occurred between groups where progressive strength training was added to standard muscle strengthening. Conversely, progressive resistance training compared to daily life activities led to significantly better functional results [16]. These differences in study protocols made it difficult to compare results among the trials and prevented the authors to carry out a meta-analysis of the reported data. Although the conclusion of the single trials is often clear and the evidence seems to be defined, the summary of the results cannot be considered conclusive given the inhomogeneity of the study protocols.

Strength of the quadriceps muscle is one of the most important contributors to functioning of the knee, specifically in people with knee OA [22,25]. However, currently investigated studies failed to show the effectiveness of preoperative strengthening programs in enhancing postoperative recovery after TKA. The American College of Sports Medicine guidelines reported that to improve strength, muscle mass and endurance, exercises with a resistance of ~ 60% to 80% of the individual's 1 repetition maximum and titratable progression are required [26]. Moreover, a previous study showed that an 8-week period of exercise is necessary to produce significant improvements in pain and function and in objective measurements of muscle functioning in OA patients [27]. All the studies analyzed in the present review reported an intervention length ranging between 2 and 6 weeks, which is shorter than the minimum length, and most of them used home-based exercise programs, so it is difficult to have trustable data on whether the patients followed the indications for resistance thresholds or not. Those two factors may be responsible for not obtaining significantly better outcomes in patients who underwent prehabilitation compared to those who did not.

Concerning methodology, almost all the papers included had several biases assessed through the Cochrane Risk of Bias Assessment Tool. This evaluation highlighted that most of the trials included had several methodological flaws, especially concerning allocation concealment and blinding of the participants. However, it is relevant to understand that for active exercise programs blinding is actually impossible. Apart from this incongruity, the trials were designed in an appropriate manner and always included a control group for which normal daily activities were advised in the time before surgery. In addition, other relevant biases that affect the quality of the included trials are the selective report and the small cohorts of included patients. Especially the paucity of the cohort affects significantly the final result of a study, and the power analysis was not reported in most of the included papers. This may lead to an unpredictable overestimation or underestimation of the results. Furthermore, lack of appropriate power prevents the reader to truly understand and weigh the importance of the presented data in view of a clinical application of the evidence. Selective reporting was also a source of frequent bias, with many studies reporting data on functional outcomes (including WOMAC, KOOS) without reporting information about quality of daily life (SF-12 or SF-36) or vice-versa. This does not allow a thorough evaluation of the patients. All of these biases should be taken into account to carry out novel studies on this topic.

Potential limitations of the present systematic review include the narrow electronic research frame, as only two online databases have been searched. Furthermore, given the language capabilities of the author, only studies published in English have been retrieved and analyzed. This is a bias which may have reduced the pool of retrieved papers. However, the main strength of this study is the systematic methodology, strictly adhering to PRISMA guidelines and PICO process for formulation of the research question. Furthermore, as an added value in comparison to previous similar works, our study strictly focuses on elderly patients, for which outcomes seem to be more homogeneous and consistent than those in other age groups. This is especially true for studies concerning total knee arthroplasty.

5. Conclusions

Although there are insufficient data to draw definitive conclusions, prehabilitation for patients undergoing total knee arthroplasty leads to a shorter length of stay, but not to an enhanced postoperative recovery. Similarly, concerning total hip arthroplasty, although currently available data showed significantly better outcomes in patients who underwent prehabilitation programs, there is a lack of robust evidence in its favor. Although the presented results do not achieve appropriate clinical relevance, it is useful to know that in small cohorts preoperative physical training shortens the length of stay in the hospital, which is a remarkable result in an era of increased attention to healthcare expenses. Thus, considering prehabilitation measures are non-invasive and low-cost activities, it would be worthwhile to suggest them to patients undergoing total joint arthroplasty.

Author Contributions: Conceptualization, R.P. and V.D.; methodology, G.T.; writing—original draft preparation, G.T. and S.V.; writing—review and editing, F.V., G.P., B.Z., and M.B.; supervision, S.C. and C.F.; funding acquisition, R.P. All authors have read and agreed to the published version of the manuscript.

References

1. Chen, H.; Li, S.; Ruan, T.; Liu, L.; Fang, L. Is it necessary to perform prehabilitation exercise for patients undergoing total knee arthroplasty: Meta-analysis of randomized controlled trials. *Phys. Sportsmed.* **2018**, *46*, 36–43. [CrossRef] [PubMed]
2. Singh, J.A.; Cleveland, J.D. Socioeconomic status and healthcare access are associated with healthcare utilization after knee arthroplasty: A U.S. national cohort study. *Jt. Bone Spine Rev. Rhum.* **2019**, *87*, 157–162. [CrossRef]
3. Henderson, K.G.; Wallis, J.A.; Snowdon, D.A. Active physiotherapy interventions following total knee arthroplasty in the hospital and inpatient rehabilitation settings: A systematic review and meta-analysis. *Physiotherapy* **2018**, *104*, 25–35. [CrossRef] [PubMed]
4. Farrokhi, S.; Jayabalan, P.; Gustafson, J.A.; Klatt, B.A.; Sowa, G.A.; Piva, S.R. The influence of continuous versus interval walking exercise on knee joint loading and pain in patients with knee osteoarthritis. *Gait Posture* **2017**, *56*, 129–133. [CrossRef]
5. Withers, T.M.; Lister, S.; Sackley, C.; Clark, A.; Smith, T.O. Is there a difference in physical activity levels in patients before and up to one year after unilateral total hip replacement? A systematic review and meta-analysis. *Clin. Rehabil* **2017**, *31*, 639–650. [CrossRef] [PubMed]
6. Shamseer, L.; Moher, D.; Clarke, M.; Ghersi, D.; Liberati, A.; Petticrew, M.; Shekelle, P.; Stewart, L.A. Preferred reporting items for systematic review and meta-analysis protocols (PRISMA-P) 2015: Elaboration and explanation. *BMJ.* **2015**, *349*, g7647. [CrossRef]
7. Twiggs, J.; Salmon, L.; Kolos, E.; Bogue, E.; Miles, B.; Roe, J. Measurement of physical activity in the pre- and early post-operative period after total knee arthroplasty for Osteoarthritis using a Fitbit Flex device. *Med. Eng. Phys.* **2018**, *51*, 31–40. [CrossRef]
8. Hoogeboom, T.J.; Dronkers, J.J.; van den Ende, C.H.; Oosting, E.; van Meeteren, N.L. Preoperative therapeutic exercise in frail elderly scheduled for total hip replacement: A randomized pilot trial. *Clin. Rehabil.* **2010**, *24*, 901–910. [CrossRef]
9. Oosting, E.; Jans, M.P.; Dronkers, J.J.; Naber, R.H.; Dronkers-Landman, C.M.; Appelman-de Vries, S.M.; van Meeteren, N.L. Preoperative Home-Based Physical Therapy Versus Usual Care to Improve Functional Health of Frail Older Adults Scheduled for Elective Total Hip Arthroplasty: A Pilot Randomized Controlled Trial. *Arch. Phys. Med. Rehabil.* **2012**, *93*, 610–616. [CrossRef]

10. Wang, A.W.; Gilbey, H.J.; Ackland, T.R. Perioperative Exercise Programs Improve Early Return of Ambulatory Function After Total Hip Arthroplasty: A Randomized, Controlled Trial. *Am. J. Phys. Med. Rehabil.* **2002**, *81*, 801–806. [CrossRef]

11. Beaupre, L.A.; Lier, D.; Davies, D.; Johnston, D. The effect of a preoperative exercise and education program on functional recovery, health related quality of life, and health service utilization following primary total knee arthroplasty. *J. Rehumatology* **2004**, *31*, 1166–1173.

12. van Leeuwen, D.M.; de Ruiter, C.J.; Nolte, P.A.; de Haan, A. Preoperative Strength Training for Elderly Patients Awaiting Total Knee Arthroplasty. *Rehabil. Res. Pract.* **2014**, *2014*, 1–9. [CrossRef] [PubMed]

13. Williamson, L.; Wyatt, M.R.; Yein, K.; Melton, J.T.K. Severe knee osteoarthritis: A randomized controlled trial of acupuncture, physiotherapy (supervised exercise) and standard management for patients awaiting knee replacement. *Rheumatology* **2007**, *46*, 1445–1449. [CrossRef] [PubMed]

14. Matassi, F.; Duerinckx, J.; Vandenneucker, H.; Bellemans, J. Range of motion after total knee arthroplasty: The effect of a preoperative home exercise program. *Knee Surg. Sports Traumatol. Arthrosc.* **2014**, *22*, 703–709. [CrossRef]

15. Huang, S.-W.; Chen, P.-H.; Chou, Y.-H. Effects of a preoperative simplified home rehabilitation education program on length of stay of total knee arthroplasty patients. *Orthop. Traumatol. Surg. Res.* **2012**, *98*, 259–264. [CrossRef] [PubMed]

16. Skoffer, B.; Dalgas, U.; Mechlenburg, I. Progressive resistance training before and after total hip and knee arthroplasty: A systematic review. *Clin. Rehabil.* **2015**, *29*, 14–29. [CrossRef]

17. Gstoettner, M.; Raschner, C.; Dirnberger, E.; Leimser, H.; Krismer, M. Preoperative proprioceptive training in patients with total knee arthroplasty. *The Knee* **2011**, *18*, 265–270. [CrossRef]

18. Gill, S.D.; McBurney, H.; Schulz, D.L. Land-Based Versus Pool-Based Exercise for People Awaiting Joint Replacement Surgery of the Hip or Knee: Results of a Randomized Controlled Trial. *Arch. Phys. Med. Rehabil.* **2009**, *90*, 388–394. [CrossRef]

19. Evgeniadis, G.; Beneka, A.; Malliou, P.; Mavromoustakos, S.; Godolias, G. Effects of pre- or postoperative therapeutic exercise on the quality of life, before and after total knee arthroplasty for osteoarthritis. *J. Back Musculoskelet. Rehabil.* **2008**, *21*, 161–169. [CrossRef]

20. Aytekin, E.; Sukur, E.; Oz, N.; Telatar, A.; Eroglu Demir, S.; Sayner Caglar, N.; Ozturkmen, Y.; Ozgonenel, L. The effect of a 12 week prehabilitation program in pain and function for patients undergoing total knee arthroplasty: A prospective controlled study. *J. Clin Orthop Trauma.* **2018**. e-pub ahead of print. [CrossRef]

21. Ferrara, P.; Rabini, A.; Maggi, L.; Piazzini, D.; Logroscino, G.; Magliocchetti, G.; Amabile, E.; Tancredi, G.; Aulisa, A.; Padua, L.; et al. Effect of pre-operative physiotherapy in patients with end-stage osteoarthritis undergoing hip arthroplasty. *Clin. Rehabil.* **2008**, *22*, 977–986. [CrossRef] [PubMed]

22. McKay, C.; Prapavessis, H.; Doherty, T. The Effect of a Prehabilitation Exercise Program on Quadriceps Strength for Patients Undergoing Total Knee Arthroplasty: A Randomized Controlled Pilot Study. *PM&R* **2012**, *4*, 647–656.

23. Peer, M.; Rush, R.; Gallacher, P.; Gleeson, N. Pre-surgery exercise and post-operative physical function of people undergoing knee replacement surgery: A systematic review and meta-analysis of randomized controlled trials. *J. Rehabil. Med.* **2017**, *49*, 304–315. [CrossRef] [PubMed]

24. Wang, L.; Lee, M.; Zhang, Z.; Moodie, J.; Cheng, D.; Martin, J. Does preoperative rehabilitation for patients planning to undergo joint replacement surgery improve outcomes? A systematic review and meta-analysis of randomised controlled trials. *BMJ Open* **2016**, *6*, e009857. [PubMed]

25. Mizner, R.L.; Petterson, S.C.; Stevens, J.E.; Axe, M.J.; Snyder-Mackler, L. Preoperative quadriceps strength predicts functional ability one year after total knee arthroplasty. *J. Rheumatol.* **2005**, *32*, 1533–1539.

26. Thompson, P.D.; Arena, R.; Riebe, D.; Pescatello, L.S. American College of Sports Medicine ACSM's new preparticipation health screening recommendations from ACSM's guidelines for exercise testing and prescription, ninth edition. *Curr. Sports Med. Rep.* **2013**, *12*, 215–217. [CrossRef]

27. Jan, M.-H.; Lin, J.-J.; Liau, J.-J.; Lin, Y.-F.; Lin, D.-H. Investigation of Clinical Effects of High- and Low-Resistance Training for Patients With Knee Osteoarthritis: A Randomized Controlled Trial. *Phys. Ther.* **2008**, *88*, 427–436. [CrossRef]

5

The Effects of Physical Exercise on Balance and Prevention of Falls in Older People

Giuseppe Francesco Papalia [1,*], Rocco Papalia [1], Lorenzo Alirio Diaz Balzani [1], Guglielmo Torre [1], Biagio Zampogna [1], Sebastiano Vasta [1], Chiara Fossati [2], Anna Maria Alifano [1] and Vincenzo Denaro [1]

[1]   Department of Orthopaedic and Trauma Surgery, Campus Bio-Medico University of Rome, 00128 Rome, Italy; r.papalia@unicampus.it (R.P.); l.diaz@unicampus.it (L.A.D.B.); g.torre@unicampus.it (G.T.); b.zampogna@unicampus.it (B.Z.); s.vasta@unicampus.it (S.V.); a.alifano@unicampus.it (A.M.A.); denaro@unicampus.it (V.D.)

[2]   Department of Movement, Human and Health Sciences, University of Rome "Foro Italico", 00100 Rome, Italy; chiara.fossati@uniroma4.it

*   Correspondence: g.papalia@unicampus.it

Abstract: The aims of this systematic review and meta-analysis were to evaluate the effects of physical exercise on static and dynamic balance in the elderly population, and to analyze the number of falls and fallers. A systematic literature search was conducted using PubMed–Medline, Cochrane Central, and Google Scholar to select randomized clinical trials that analyzed the role of exercise on balance and fall rate in patients aged 65 or older. Sixteen articles were included in this review. Applying the Cochrane risk-of-bias tool, three studies were determined to be at low risk of bias, nine at unclear risk of bias, and four at high risk of bias. The meta-analysis showed improvements in dynamic balance ($p = 0.008$), static balance ($p = 0.01$), participants' fear of falling ($p = 0.10$), balance confidence ($p = 0.04$), quality of life ($p = 0.08$), and physical performance ($p = 0.30$) in patients who underwent physical exercise compared to controls. The analysis of the total numbers of falls showed a decreased likelihood of falls in patients who participated in exercise programs ($p = 0.0008$). Finally, the number of patients who fell at least once was significantly reduced in the intervention group ($p = 0.02$). Physical exercise is an effective treatment to improve balance and reduce fall rates in the elderly.

Keywords: physical exercise; balance; falls; older people; systematic review; meta-analysis

1. Introduction

Increasingly, attention is being paid by the scientific community to aging, and especially to successful aging. Several interventions aimed to improve the physical and psychosocial status of the elderly have been developed [1]. The decline in physical performance and cognitive capabilities with age causes progressive impairment of muscle strength, coordination, and balance [2], exposing people to a higher risk of falls [3,4]. Human balance is a complex multidimensional concept related to postural control, and it refers essentially to the ability to maintain a posture (e.g., sitting or standing), move between postures, and not fall when reacting to an external disturbance [5]. Apart from the risk of fractures [6] associated with falls, balance represents one of the main features of a plethora of daily activities, both professional and recreational; thus, an impairment of this ability could have a detrimental effect on quality of life [7]. A clear definition has been proposed for a "fall", namely "inadvertently coming to rest on the ground, floor or other lower level, excluding intentional change in position to rest in furniture, wall or other objects" [8]. Almost one out of three elderly people experience a fall every year [9,10], while a person who experiences at least two falls within 6 months is defined as a "recurrent faller" [11,12]. Falls in older people are concerning events that could result in fractures, residual disability, chronic pain, and loss of independence, leading to important social and public health consequences requiring expensive long-term treatments [13] and accounting for 40% of all injury-related deaths in this group. The severity of the injuries derived from falls vary considerably from minor cutaneous injuries to major fractures, and, in some cases, to fatal traumas [14]. For those patients affected by osteoporosis, the risk of femoral fractures or vertebral body fractures is high, especially for ground-level falls or falls on stairs. The risk for head trauma is consistent across the whole elderly population, and such injuries may result in intracranial pathology with functional sequelae [15]. Progressive physical impairment can happen because of inactivity, which is recognized to be a factor in decreased body function in the elderly [16,17]. Indeed, physical exercise (PE) plays a fundamental role in the prevention of several age-related pathologies, such as metabolic and cardiovascular disease, cancer, and loss of bone quality, to such an extent that the proclamation "exercise is medicine" has been made [18,19]. There is overwhelming evidence that physical exercise can lower the risk of falling in elderly people, averting muscle mass reduction, and improving balance control. In particular, leg strength training seems to be crucial in preventing falls, as lower-limb weakness has been identified as a significant risk factor for falling [20]. In particular, the risk of falling can be assessed using postural control markers. For instance, it has been demonstrated that the risk of a fall is more than doubled when the timed up-and-go (TUG) test requires ≥ 13.5 s to be completed, the gait speed is <1 m/s, and the modified Romberg test shows a standing time of ≤ 19 s [21,22]. Furthermore, balance training (BT) has been investigated in recent years [23,24] as an important intervention to slow the physiological decline of balance control in the elderly, and has been revealed to be an effective option for improving balance and postural control [25,26]. Aging involves some changes that affect balance; these include rigidity and reduced range of articular motion, sarcopenia and impaired muscle strength [27,28] cognitive decline, and changes in sensory systems, such as poor vision and hearing [29]. Thus, many systematic reviews and meta-analyses have reported that BT plays a crucial role and it is recommended among other interventions to reduce the risk and rate of falls in older adults [24,30]. We present an updated systematic review and meta-analysis with the aim to analyze the effect of physical exercise on static and dynamic balance in patients aged 65 years or over. The primary endpoint was the improvement of balance performance after various types of physical exercise. The secondary endpoint was the number of falls and/or fallers before and after a course of physical exercise.

2. Materials and Methods

This systematic review was conducted in accordance with the Preferred Reporting Items for Systematic Reviews and Meta-Analysis (PRISMA) guidelines [31] and was performed using the PRISMA checklist (Table S1). In this manuscript, we included randomized clinical trials (RCTs) that evaluated the effect of physical exercise on static and dynamic balance and on the number of falls and fallers in the elderly.

2.1. Inclusion Criteria

The inclusion criteria were RCTs in the English language published in the past decade, which analyzed the effects of land-based or aquatic exercise on balance and falls rate on patients aged 65 or older, according to the World Health Organization (WHO) definition of the elderly. Exclusion criteria were studies that involved patients with Parkinson's or Alzheimer's disease, dementia, hemiplegia, cancer, fibromyalgia, or following a stroke, spinal cord injuries, or fractures. We excluded studies that evaluated activities such as tai chi, yoga, pilates, or dance.

2.2. Search Methods

A systematic literature search was conducted using the following online databases: PubMed–Medline, Cochrane Central, and Google Scholar. We used the following search strings:

("Balance" (Journal) OR "balance"(All Fields)) AND ("exercise"(MeSH Terms) OR "exercise"(All Fields) OR ("physical"(All Fields) AND "activity"(All Fields)) OR "physical activity"(All Fields)) AND ("aged"(MeSH Terms) OR "aged"(All Fields) OR "elderly"(All Fields)). Moreover, the following filters were used: randomized controlled trial (article types); 2010/01/01 to 2020/05/01 (publication dates); aged: 65+ years (ages); English (languages); humans (species). The reference lists of the included RCTs were checked in order to select further studies for inclusion. After duplicates were removed, two reviewers (G.P. and S.V.) independently read the abstracts of studies appropriate for inclusion. Differences of opinion were resolved by discussion with the third review author (R.P.). Finally, the full articles were checked by two investigators (G.P. and S.V.) in order to choose the studies to be included in the review and meta-analysis.

2.3. Data Collection, Analysis, and Outcomes

Two review authors (G.P. and S.V.) independently performed data extraction. The following data were extracted from the included studies: authors, year of publication, type of study, level of evidence, numbers of participants and their age and sex in both study and control groups, previous falls, follow-up, and intervention(s) in the experimental and in the control group. Many outcomes were analyzed for the assessment of static and dynamic balance, participants' fear of falling, physical performance, quality of life, and risk of falls. Finally, total number of falls, number of fallers, and fall rate (falls per person-year) were compared between exercise and control groups.

2.4. Risk of Bias Assessment

The risk of bias of the included RCTs was independently assessed by two investigators (G.P. and S.V.) by the Cochrane risk-of-bias tool [32]. This tool consists of seven items: random sequence generation, allocation concealment, blinding of participants and personnel, blinding for outcome assessment, incomplete outcome data, selective reporting, and other sources of bias. Each item was graded as having a low, unclear, or high risk of bias. Thus, the trials presented low risk of bias if six or seven domains were reported to have low risk of bias, unclear risk of bias if four of five domains were at low risk of bias, or high risk of bias if fewer than four domains were at low risk of bias.

2.5. Statistical Analysis

A meta-analysis was conducted using the Review Manager (RevMan) software Version 5.3. Continuous outcomes were used to assess effects on static and dynamic balance, fear of falling, physical performance, quality of life, and risk of falls between the experimental and the control groups. Dichotomous outcomes were used to assess the total number of falls and the number of fallers between the two groups. Due to the use of different scores for the various outcomes, the continuous data are shown as standard mean difference (SMD) with 95% confidence intervals. Negative values of SMD indicate a benefit for the intervention group. Dichotomous data are presented as odds ratio (OR) with 95% confidence intervals. For the calculation of the weight of the samples of the trials, falls or fallers per month of follow-up were used instead of the total events. The I^2 test was used to evaluate heterogeneity. In the presence of low heterogeneity ($I^2 < 55\%$), we used a fixed-effect model; otherwise, a random-effect model was applied. The statistical significance of the results was set at $p < 0.05$.

2.6. Quality Assessment

The GRADE (Grading of Recommendations Assessment, Development, and Evaluation) assessment was used to evaluate the quality of the evidence of the outcomes and strength of recommendation [33]. This tool evaluates five items for each outcome: risk of bias, inconsistency, indirectness, imprecision, and publication bias. Each component was classified as not serious, serious, or very serious. The GRADE allocates the quality of evidence for the outcomes as high, moderate, low, or very low. RCTs were assigned an initial ranking of high, which could be downgraded for the items mentioned above.

3. Results

3.1. Results of the Search

The literature search yielded 1397 articles. After the removal of duplicates, the titles and abstracts of 1267 of these were examined, leading to the selection of 69 eligible papers that were read in full. Subsequently, 53 studies were excluded for the following reasons: not reporting selected outcomes ($n = 17$), not evaluating land-based or aquatic exercise ($n = 11$), patients aged below 65 years ($n = 9$), protocols of RCT ($n = 7$), and case reports ($n = 2$). Finally, 16 articles were included in this review and meta-analysis (Figure 1).

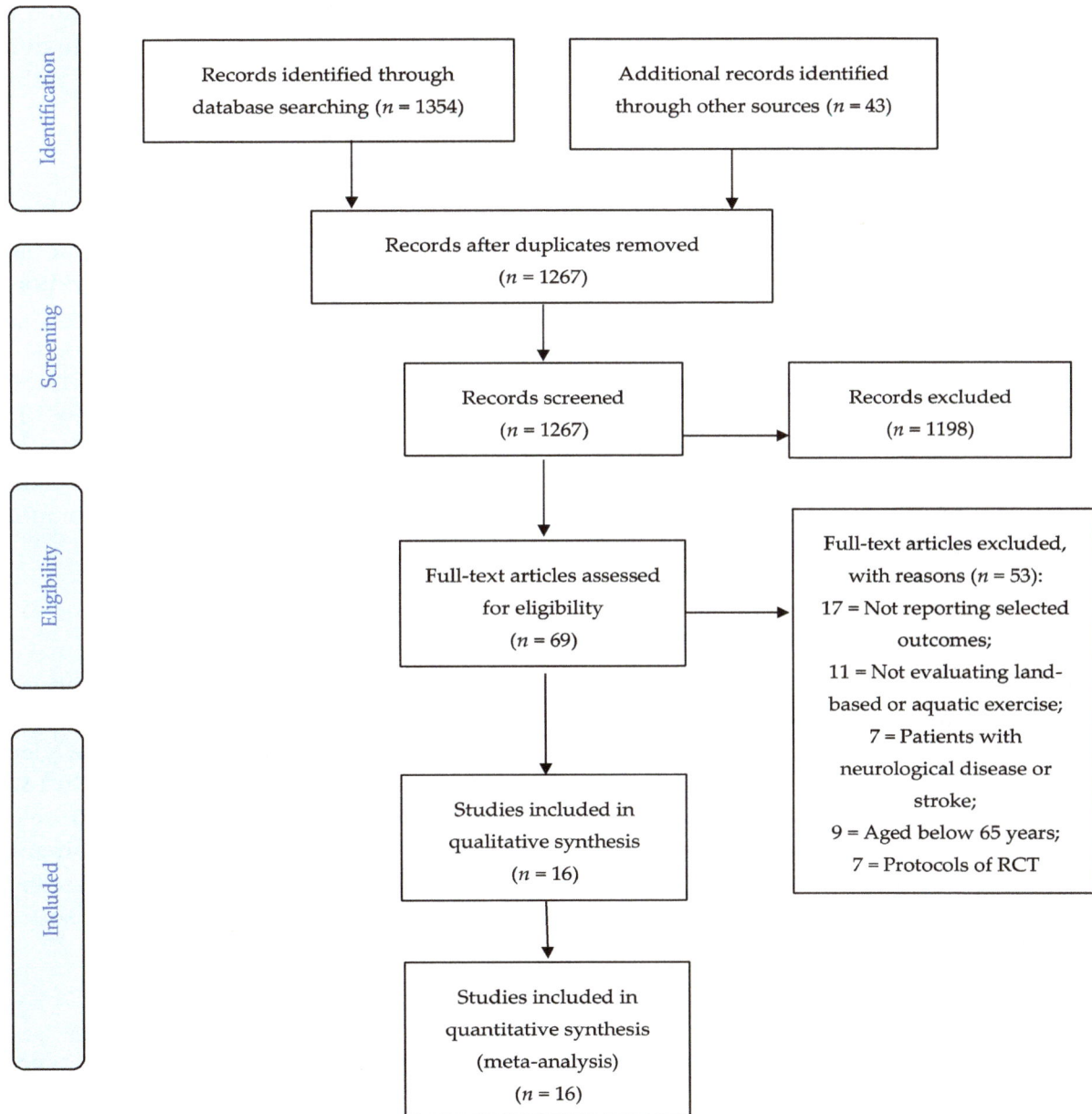

Figure 1. Preferred Reporting Items for Systematic Review and Meta-Analysis (PRISMA) flow diagram.

3.2. Demographic Data

The total number of participants in all the included studies was 2960, of which 1521 were in the combined exercise group and 1439 in the combined control group. The ages of the patients ranged from 67.3 to 86 years in the intervention groups, and from 67.2 to 86 in the control groups. The percentages of women in the trials ranged from 50% to 100% in the experimental groups and from 44% to 100% in the control groups. These data indicate a higher inclusion of females for the evaluation of the reported outcomes, and there were four studies that included only elderly women. The percentage of patients that had fallen at least once in the previous year was heterogeneous between the studies, ranging from 13.6% to 62% in the exercise groups and from 12.4% to 69% in the control groups. The demographic characteristics of the patients at baseline are reported in Table 1.

3.3. Physical Activity Program

Fourteen studies evaluated land-based exercise, while the remaining two studies [34,35] examined aquatic exercise (Table 2). Regarding exercise protocols, the patients in three trials participated in the Otago Exercise Program (OEP) [36–38], while in the other studies, the patients participated in different types of strength and balance training exercise programs. The mean follow-up was 9.2 months and ranged from 4 weeks to 2 years.

3.4. Clinical Outcome Data

The mean outcome measures before and after treatment are reported in Table 3. Dynamic balance was assessed in nine studies, using timed up-and-go (TUG) test [35,37–41], TUG-motor [42], TUGcog [34], or 8 foot up-and-go test [43]. Static balance was evaluated via Berg balance score (BBS) in six studies [34,37,40,41,43,44]. Participants' fear of falling was assessed in five studies, using the Falls Efficacy Scale—International (FES-I) [39,45], Modified Falls Efficacy Scale (MFES) [46], Falls Efficacy Scale, Swedish version (FES(S)) [36], and Thai Falls Efficacy Scale (Thai FES-I) [37]. Balance confidence was reported in four studies, using the Activities-Specific Balance Confidence (ABC) Scale [34,35,46] and short-ABC [47]. Quality of life was assessed in three studies using the Short-Form-36 (SF-36) [39,45] or Short-Form-12 (SF-12) [40] Health Survey. Physical performance was evaluated in three studies, using the Short Physical Performance Battery (SPPB) [36,38,45].

3.5. Methodological Evaluation

Upon applying the Cochrane risk-of-bias tool, three studies (18.75%) were determined to be at low risk of bias (A), nine studies (56.25%) were at unclear risk of bias (B), and four studies (25%) were at a high risk of bias (C) (Table 4). More specifically, random sequence generation was adequate in all the studies except one (93.75%). Allocation concealment was considered adequate in 14 trials (87.5%). Blinding for participants and personnel appeared to be impossible due to the nature of the intervention; thus, it was inadequate in 15 studies (93.75%). Blinding for outcome assessment was graded as adequate in 13 studies (81.25%). Incomplete outcome data were judged as adequate in eight studies (50%). Selective reporting was considered adequate in 11 studies (68.75%). Other sources of bias were adequate in eight trials (50%).

Table 1. Demographic characteristics of the patients at baseline.

Author (Year)	Type of Study	LOE	Study Group			Control Group			Fell at least Once in Past Year	
			n	Age	Sex	n	Age	Sex	Study	Control
Ansai et al., (2015) [42]	RCT	I	23	81.9 y	73.9% F, 26.1% M	23	82.6 y	65.2% F, 34.8%	10 (43.5%) *	8 (34.8%) *
			23	82.8 y	65.2% F, 34.8% M				7 (30.4%) *	
Arkkukangas et al., (2019) [36]	RCT	I	61	83 y	67% F, 33% M	56	82 y	73% F, 27% M	24 (39%)	21 (37%)
Arnold et al., (2010) [34]	RCT	I	28	73.2 y	71.4% F, 28.6% M	25	75.8 y	64% F, 36% M	14 (50%)	9 (36%)
			26	74.4 y	77% F, 23% M				16 (62%)	
Boongird et al., (2017) [37]	RCT	I	219	74.08 y	83.6% F, 16.4% M	220	73.94 y	81.4% F, 18.6% M		
Clemson et al., (2010) [46]	RCT	I	18	81 y	50% F, 50% M	16	82 y	44% F, 56% M	7 (39%) †	4 (25%) †
El-Khoury et al., (2015) [39]	RCT	I	352	79.8 y	100% F	354	79.6 y	100% F	137 (39%)	159 (45%)
Gianoudis et al., (2014) [48]	RCT	I	81	67.7 y	64% F, 36% M	81	67.2 y	73% F, 27% M	11 (13.6%)	10 (12.4%)
Hale et al., (2012) [35]	RCT	I	23	73.6 y	74% F, 26% M	16	75.7 y	75% F, 25% M	13 (61%)	11 (69%)
Hewitt et al., (2018) [45]	RCT	I	113	86 y	62.8% F, 37.2% M	108	86 y	68.2% F, 31.8% M	69 (61%)	54 (50.5%)
Jacobson et al., (2011) [43]	RCT	I	14	83.05 y	57.1% F, 42.9% M	11	81.37 y	72.7% F, 27.3% M		
Leiros-Rodriguez et al., (2014) [40]	RCT	I	14	69 y	100% F	14	68 y	100% F		
Liu-Ambrose et al., (2019) [38]	RCT	I	172	81.2 y	64% F, 36% M	172	81.9 y	69% F, 31% M	43 (25%)	60 (35%)
Miko et al., (2018) [41]	RCT	I	50	69.33 y	100% F	50	69.10 y	100% F		
Patil et al., (2015) [49]	RCT	I	205	74.4 y	100% F	204	74 y	100% F		
Patti et al., (2017) [44]	RCT	I	49	67.32 y	53% F, 47% M	43	68.93 y	55.8% F, 44.2% M		
Smulders et al., (2010) [47]	RCT	I	50	70.5 y	90% F, 10% M	46	71.6 y	97.8% F, 2.2% M		

RCT: randomized clinical trial; LOE: levels of evidence; N.: number of participants; y: years; F: female; M: male. * = fall in the past 3 months; † = frequent falls (≥ 3) in the past 12 months.

Table 2. Clinical results of the included studies.

Author	Intervention(s)	Control	Follow-up	Results
Ansai	Multicomponent training: protocol consisting of warm-up, aerobic, strength, balance, and cool-down exercises for 16 weeks	No intervention	22 w	There were no significant differences between groups and assessments in any variable.
	Resistance training: leg press, chest press, calf, back extension, abdominal, and rowing for 16 weeks			
Arkkukangas	OEP: home-based exercise program designed to improve strength, balance, and endurance over 12 weeks	No intervention	12 w	In the short-term perspective, there were no benefits of an exercise program regarding physical performance, fall self-efficacy, activity level, hand-grip strength, and fall frequency in comparison to a CG.
Arnold	AE protocol consisted of lower- and upper-extremity strengthening, trunk-control, and balance exercises twice a week for 11 weeks (preceded by educational session in the aquatics and education group)	No intervention	11 w	Significant improvement in fall risk factors ($p = 0.038$) with the combination of aquatic exercise and education.
Boongird	Modified OEP: five combined leg-muscle strengthening, balance retraining, and stretching exercises, which progressed in difficulty, and a walking plan	Fall prevention education	12 m	The incidence of falls was 0.30 falls per person year in the EG, compared with 0.40 in the CG. The fear of falling was significantly lower in the EG than CG ($p = 0.003$).
Clemson	Lifestyle Approach to Reducing Falls through Exercise (LiFE) program: home-based balance and strengthening exercise program for fall prevention	No intervention	6 m	The relative risk analysis demonstrated a significant reduction in falls in EG (RR = 0.23). Dynamic balance improved for the LiFE program participants ($p = 0.04$).
El-Khoury	Ossébo program: weekly supervised group sessions of progressive balance training for two years, supplemented by individually prescribed home exercises	No intervention	24 m	The injurious fall rate was 19% lower in the EG than in the CG ($p = 0.04$). The EG fared significantly better than the CG in all balance and gait performance tests.
Gianoudis	Multimodal program incorporating high-velocity progressive resistance training, weight-bearing impact and/or balance training, and fall-prevention exercises, performed three days per week for 12 months	Standard care self-management	12 m	There were no significant differences in fall incidence between the groups, or in the number of participants sustaining one or more falls or multiple falls.
Hale	Water-based exercise classes twice weekly for 12 weeks	Time-matched computer training program for 12 weeks	12 w	Water-based exercise did not reduce falls risk compared with attending a computer-skills training class.
Hewitt	Resistance training plus balance exercises performed in a group setting for 50 h over a 25-week period (Sunbeam program), followed by a maintenance period for 6 months	Regular activity schedule	12 m	Overall incidence of falls in the EG of 1.31 per person-year, compared with 2.91 in the CG. A significantly greater improvement was found in physical performance in the EG than in the CG ($p = 0.02$).

Table 2. *Cont.*

Author	Intervention(s)	Control	Follow-up	Results
Jacobson	Standing, static balancing, and mild leg exercise, 12 min per session, three times per week for 12 weeks.	Regular group exercise	12 w	Significant (p < 0.01) improvement for the EG over the CG in the 30 s chair test repetitions, 8-foot up and go test, balance assessment, and leg-function assessments.
Leiros-Rodríguez	12 sessions of balance exercises for 50 min	No intervention	4 w	Berg Balance Scale, timed up-and-go test, and SF-12 showed statistically significant differences in the EG (p < 0.05).
Liu-Ambrose	Usual care plus OEP (a home-based strength and balance retraining exercise program) for 12 months	Fall-prevention care	11 m	Fall rates were lower in the EG compared with CG (IRR, 0.64; p = 0.009). The estimated fall rate incidence was 1.4 per person-year in the EG and 2.1 in the CG (p = 0.006).
Miko	12-month of balance-training exercise program (three times a week for 30 min)	No intervention	12 m	TUG and BBS test scores showed a statistically significant difference between EG and CG (p < 0.005). The event rate for the number of patients who fell was 0.122 in the EG and 0.229 in the CG, thus the relative risk of falls was 0.534 (p = 0.17).
Patil	Group exercise classes twice a week for 12 months and once a week for the subsequent 12 months and home exercises	Current physical activity	24 m	Timed up-and-go and grip strength did not differ between groups. There was no difference in the total falls incidence rate ratio (IRR = 1.0).
Patti	Joint mobility, cardiovascular exercise, strengthening of core stability, proprioceptive training, and eye-hand/eye-foot coordinative exercises for 13 weeks	No intervention	14 w	Only the EG group demonstrated significant improvements in balance skills (p < 0.0001).
Smulders	11 sessions over 5.5 weeks of education, obstacle course, walking exercises, weight-bearing exercises, correction of gait abnormalities, and training in fall technique	No intervention	12 m	The fall rate in the exercise group was 39% lower than for the control group (0.72 vs 1.18 falls/person-year; risk ratio of 0.61).

OEP: Otago Exercise Program; AE: aquatic exercise; w: weeks; m: months; CG: control group; EG: experimental group.

Table 3. Outcome measures before and after treatment.

Study		TUG (s)	BBS (pts)	FES (pts)	ABC (pts)	SF-36/SF-12 (pts)	SPPB [9] (pts)
Ansai	I	30.4 ± 12.2 29.8 ± 13.1					
		29.0 ± 15.5 26.7 ± 22.2					
	C	25.3 ± 8.4 25.3 ± 9.3					
Arkukangas	I			103.3 ± 21.3 [1] 106.5 ± 20.9		7.9 ± 2.4 8.1 ± 2.8	
	C			100.2 ± 26.5 106.2 ± 20.6		7.6 ± 2.5 8.2 ± 2.6	
Arnold	I	14.9 ± 5.6 12.6 ± 3.9	30.4 ± 3.8 31.4 ± 3.2		69.2 + 19.9 [5] 75.0 ± 15.2		
		15.8 ± 9.1 15.1 ± 9.5	29.3 ± 5.2 30.5 + 5.1		70.4 ± 21.9 69.6 ± 24.4		
	C	14.3 ± 6.7 14.5 ± 7.1	31.1 ± 2.7 30.9 + 3.8		65.3 ± 18.1 62.9 ± 20.8		

Table 3. *Cont.*

Study		TUG (s) Pre	TUG (s) Post	BBS (pts) Pre	BBS (pts) Post	FES (pts) Pre	FES (pts) Post	ABC (pts) Pre	ABC (pts) Post	SF-36/SF-12 (pts) Pre	SF-36/SF-12 (pts) Post	SPPB [9] (pts) Post	SPPB [9] (pts) Pre
Boongird	I	16.75	16.7	21.68	21.6	27.11 [2]	24.7						
	C	16.6	16.8	21.48	21.7	26.84	27						
Clemson	I					45.3 ± 8.2 [3]	50.3 ± 5.18	925 ± 341 [6]	1125 ± 233				
	C					45.1 ± 8.7	46.6 ± 4.81	825 ± 372	830 ± 149				
El-Khoury	I	12.38 ± 2.76	11.93 ± 3.23			25.52 ± 7.06 [4]	26.58 ± 6.37			57.05 ± 15.80 [7]	55.65 ± 14.87		
	C	12.39 ± 3.09	12.69 ± 3.22			26.02 ± 6.97	27.46 ± 6.33			54.72 ± 16.05	53.56 ± 14.71		
Hale	I	11.0 ± 3.13	10.1 ± 2.9					64.2 ± 19.3 [5]	67.0 ± 19.95				
	C	10.7 ± 5.78	10.7 ± 6.84					66.4 ± 19.8	66.7 ± 13.23				
Hewitt	I					27.75 ± 10.08 [4]	30.01 ± 9.67			65.72 ± 18.30 [7]	74.66 ± 18.51	5.16 ± 2.57	5.81 ± 3.02
	C					31.28 ± 13.03	30.57 ± 9.69			64.96 ± 16.98	72.43 ± 16.60	4.30 ± 2.90	4.13 ± 2.92
Jacobson	I	16.97 ± 5.63	12.71 ± 3.07	26.91 ± 3.65	40.67 ± 6.10								
	C	16.20 ± 3.67	18.26 ± 5	27.24 ± 4.64	24.42 ± 7.78								
Leiros-Rodríguez	I	11 ± 1.3	6.71 ± 0.73	45.86 ± 2.91	54.07 ± 1.98					49.36 ± 3.2 [8]	54.93 ± 1.8		
	C	11.14 ± 1.68	10.93 ± 1.49	47.79 ± 3.38	47.71 ± 2.89								
Liu-Ambrose	I	16.3 ± 7	16.1 ± 6							50.29 ± 2.5	50.79 ± 2.3	7.9 ± 2.2	7.9 ± 2.2
	C	16.9 ± 6.4	16.6 ± 8.5									7.8 ± 2.3	7.8 ± 2.4
Miko	I	8.89 ± 7.38	6.74 ± 3.13										
	C	9.95 ± 12.02	10.64 ± 13.84										
Patti	I			51.83 ± 4.17	54.36 ± 2.15								
	C			51.09 ± 3.89	51.67 ± 4.49								
Smulders	I							54.3 ± 19.7 [5]	61.9 ± 16.9				
	C							55.5 ± 22.1	55.5 ± 22.8				

I: intervention group; C: control group; TUG: timed up-and-go; BBS: Berg Balance Score; FES: Falls Efficacy Scale; ABC: Activities-Specific Balance Confidence; SF-36/SF-12: Short Form-36/Short Form-12 Health Survey; SPPB: Short Physical Performance Battery; s: seconds; pts: points. FES: [1] = FES Swedish version (0–130); [2] = Thai Falls Efficacy Scale (16–64); [3] = Modified Falls Efficacy Scale (0–140); [4] = FES-I (16–64); ABC: [5] = ABC (0–100); [6] = ABC (0–1600); SF-36: [7] = SF-36 (0–100); SF-12: [8] = SF-12 (0–100); SPPB: [9] = SPPB (0–12).

Table 4. Cochrane risk-of-bias tool for randomized controlled trials.

Study	Random Sequence Generation	Allocation Concealment	Blinding (Participants and Personnel)	Blinding (Outcome Assessment)	Incomplete Outcome Data	Selective Reporting	Other Sources of Bias	Risk of Bias
Ansai	L	L	H	L	L	H	U	B
Arkkukangas	L	L	H	L	L	L	U	B
Arnold	L	L	H	L	L	U	L	B
Boongird	L	L	H	L	U	L	L	B
Clemson	L	L	H	L	H	L	U	B
El-Khoury	L	L	H	L	L	L	L	A
Gianoudis	L	U	H	U	U	L	L	C
Hale	L	L	H	L	U	L	L	B
Hewitt	L	L	H	L	L	L	L	A
Jacobson	L	L	H	H	L	H	L	B
Leiros-Rodriíguez	L	U	H	U	L	L	U	C
Liu-Ambrose	U	L	H	L	L	L	L	A
Miko	L	L	H	L	H	L	U	B
Patil	L	L	U	L	H	U	U	C
Patti	L	L	H	L	H	U	U	C

L: low; U: unclear; H: high.

3.6. Effect of Intervention

The meta-analysis showed the effect of exercise on dynamic balance, static balance, participants' fear of falling, balance confidence, quality of life, and physical performance compared to controls (Figure 2). TUG times decreased significantly in the intervention group, demonstrating significant improvements in dynamic balance in comparison with the control group (SMD -0.51, 95% CI -0.88 to -0.13, $p = 0.008$). BBS showed significant improvements in static balance for the exercise group (SMD -1.29, 95% CI -2.29 to -0.29, $p = 0.01$). FES showed better fear-of-falling outcomes in patients who did physical exercise compared to controls (SMD -0.13, 95% CI -0.28 to 0.03), but no significant differences ($p = 0.10$). Balance confidence, assessed by ABC, showed significant differences in favor of the experimental group (SMD -0.52, 95% CI -1.01 to -0.03, $p = 0.04$). Short-Form Health Survey results showed greater improvements in quality of life in the experimental groups (SMD -0.48, 95% CI -1.01 to -0.05), without significant differences ($p = 0.08$). SPPB showed no significant differences in physical performance between the two groups ($p = 0.30$), but better outcomes in the exercise group (SMD -0.19, 95% CI -0.56 to 0.17). Summarily, analyzing all the reported scores, a significant difference was shown in favor of the physical exercise group compared to the controls ($p > 0.00001$).

Study or Subgroup	Exercise Mean	SD	Total	Control Mean	SD	Total	Weight	Std. Mean Difference IV, Random, 95% CI
1.1.1 TUG								
Arnold 2010	13.8	7.27	54	14.5	7.1	25	4.1%	-0.10 [-0.57, 0.38]
El-Khoury 2015	11.93	3.23	271	12.69	3.22	277	5.8%	-0.24 [-0.40, -0.07]
Hale 2012	10.1	2.9	20	10.7	6.84	15	3.1%	-0.12 [-0.79, 0.55]
Jacobson 2011	12.71	3.07	14	18.26	5	11	2.2%	-1.33 [-2.22, -0.45]
Leiros-Rodriguez 2014	6.71	0.73	14	10.93	1.49	14	1.4%	-3.49 [-4.73, -2.26]
Liu-Ambrose 2019	16.1	6	129	16.6	8.5	133	5.5%	-0.07 [-0.31, 0.17]
Miko 2018	6.74	3.13	49	10.64	13.84	48	4.5%	-0.39 [-0.79, 0.01]
Subtotal (95% CI)			551			523	26.6%	-0.51 [-0.88, -0.13]
Heterogeneity: Tau² = 0.18; Chi² = 35.47, df = 6 (P < 0.00001); I² = 83%								
Test for overall effect: Z = 2.64 (P = 0.008)								
1.1.2 BBS								
Arnold 2010	-31	4.25	54	-30.9	3.8	25	4.1%	-0.02 [-0.50, 0.45]
Jacobson 2011	-40.67	6.1	14	-24.42	7.78	11	1.8%	-2.28 [-3.33, -1.24]
Leiros-Rodriguez 2014	-54.07	1.98	14	-47.71	2.89	14	1.8%	-2.49 [-3.51, -1.47]
Patti 2017	-54.36	2.15	49	-51.67	4.49	43	4.4%	-0.77 [-1.20, -0.35]
Subtotal (95% CI)			131			93	12.1%	-1.29 [-2.29, -0.29]
Heterogeneity: Tau² = 0.89; Chi² = 28.40, df = 3 (P < 0.00001); I² = 89%								
Test for overall effect: Z = 2.52 (P = 0.01)								
1.1.3 FES								
Arkkukangas 2019	-106.5	20.9	61	-106.2	20.6	56	4.8%	-0.01 [-0.38, 0.35]
Clemson 2010	-50.3	5.18	16	-46.6	4.81	18	2.9%	-0.72 [-1.42, -0.03]
El-Khoury 2015	26.58	6.37	267	27.46	6.33	270	5.8%	-0.14 [-0.31, 0.03]
Hewitt 2018	30.01	9.67	91	30.57	9.69	79	5.1%	-0.06 [-0.36, 0.24]
Subtotal (95% CI)			435			423	18.7%	-0.13 [-0.28, 0.03]
Heterogeneity: Tau² = 0.00; Chi² = 3.41, df = 3 (P = 0.33); I² = 12%								
Test for overall effect: Z = 1.62 (P = 0.10)								
1.1.4 ABC								
Arnold 2010	-72.4	20.3	54	-62.9	20.8	25	4.1%	-0.46 [-0.94, 0.02]
Clemson 2010	-1,125	233	16	-830	149	18	2.6%	-1.49 [-2.26, -0.72]
Hale 2012	-67	19.95	20	-66.7	13.23	15	3.1%	-0.02 [-0.69, 0.65]
Smulders 2010	-61.9	16.9	44	-55.5	22.8	40	4.4%	-0.32 [-0.75, 0.11]
Subtotal (95% CI)			134			98	14.1%	-0.52 [-1.01, -0.03]
Heterogeneity: Tau² = 0.16; Chi² = 8.97, df = 3 (P = 0.03); I² = 67%								
Test for overall effect: Z = 2.09 (P = 0.04)								
1.1.5 SF-36 / SF-12								
El-Khoury 2015	-55.65	14.87	349	-53.56	14.71	353	5.9%	-0.14 [-0.29, 0.01]
Hewitt 2018	-74.66	18.51	88	-72.43	16.6	80	5.1%	-0.13 [-0.43, 0.18]
Leiros-Rodriguez 2014	-54.93	1.8	14	-50.79	2.3	14	2.1%	-1.95 [-2.87, -1.02]
Subtotal (95% CI)			451			447	13.2%	-0.48 [-1.01, 0.05]
Heterogeneity: Tau² = 0.17; Chi² = 14.46, df = 2 (P = 0.0007); I² = 86%								
Test for overall effect: Z = 1.76 (P = 0.08)								
1.1.6 SPPB								
Arkkukangas 2019	-8.1	2.8	61	-8.2	2.6	56	4.8%	0.04 [-0.33, 0.40]
Hewitt 2018	-5.81	3.02	93	-4.13	2.92	86	5.2%	-0.56 [-0.86, -0.26]
Liu-Ambrose 2019	-7.9	2.2	128	-7.8	2.4	132	5.5%	-0.04 [-0.29, 0.20]
Subtotal (95% CI)			282			274	15.4%	-0.19 [-0.56, 0.17]
Heterogeneity: Tau² = 0.08; Chi² = 8.87, df = 2 (P = 0.01); I² = 77%								
Test for overall effect: Z = 1.04 (P = 0.30)								
Total (95% CI)			1984			1858	100.0%	-0.43 [-0.59, -0.27]
Heterogeneity: Tau² = 0.11; Chi² = 117.72, df = 24 (P < 0.00001); I² = 80%								
Test for overall effect: Z = 5.15 (P < 0.00001)								
Test for subgroup differences: Chi² = 10.31, df = 5 (P = 0.07), I² = 51.5%								

Favours [exercise]   Favours [control]

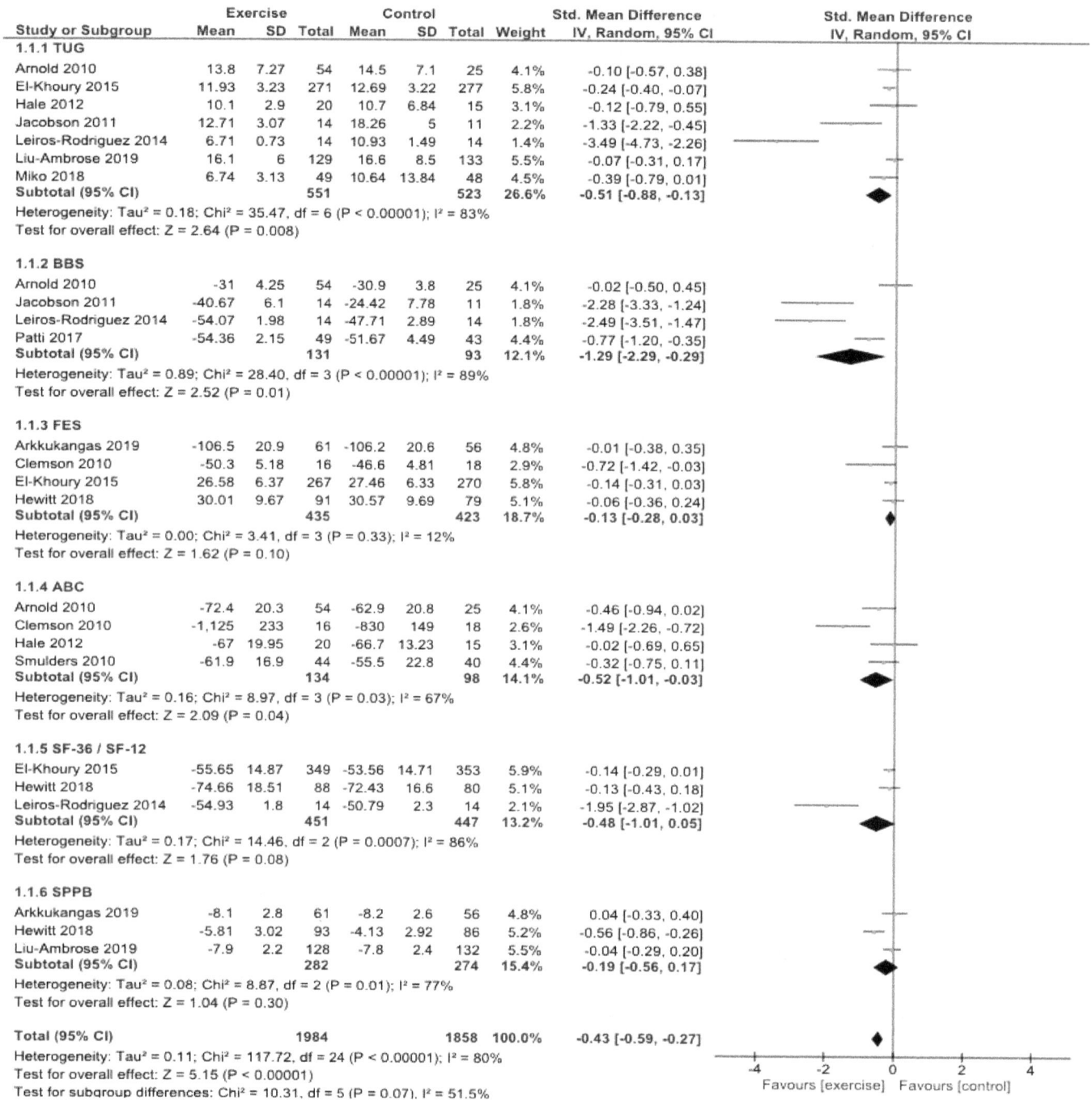

Figure 2. Outcome measurements.

The analysis of the total numbers of falls showed a statistically significant decreased likelihood of falls in patients who participated in exercise programs (OR 0.64, 95% CI 0.49 to 0.83, $p = 0.0008$) (Figure 3).

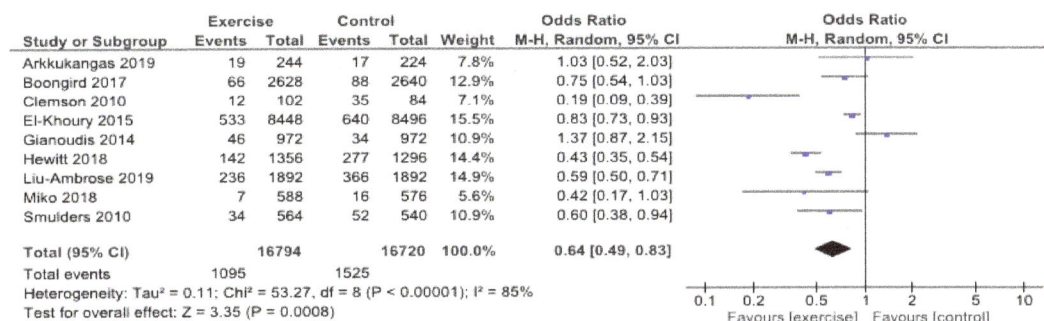

Figure 3. Total number of falls.

Finally, the number of patients who fell at least once was significantly reduced in the intervention group compared to the control group (OR 0.88, 95% CI 0.79 to 0.98, p = 0.02) (Figure 4).

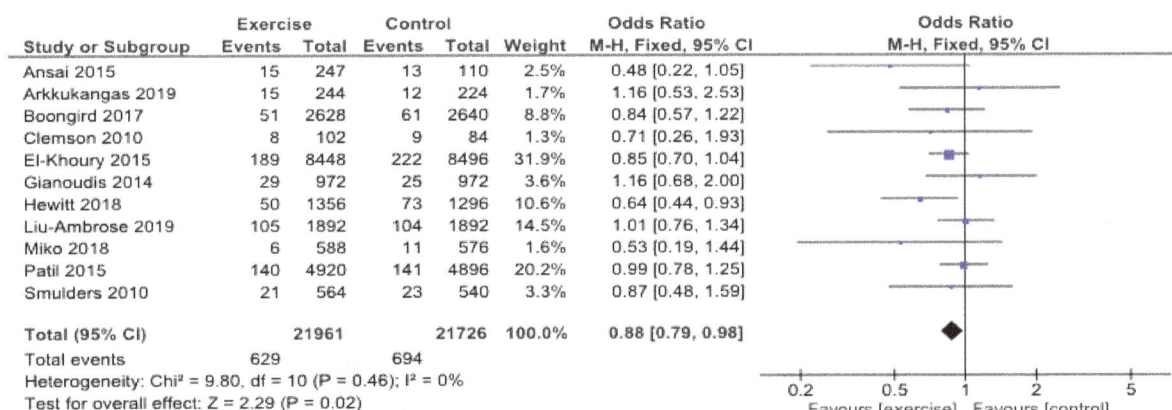

Figure 4. Number of fallers (≥1 falls).

3.7. Quality Assessment

The GRADE was used to assess the quality of the evidence provided in the included trials (Table 5). There were six comparisons for continuous data and two for dichotomous data. Regarding scores, TUG and BBS were downgraded by one level due to inconsistency of the results; thus, they reported a moderate quality. FES, ABC, and SPPB showed moderate quality because they were downgraded by one level for serious risk of bias. Finally, SF-36/SF-12 was downgraded by two levels due to serious risk of bias and inconsistency; thus, it presented low quality. In contrast, the outcomes of both total number of falls and fallers maintained a high quality of evidence.

Table 5. GRADE

Outcomes	Number of Participants (Studies)	Risk of Bias	Inconsistency	Indirectness	Imprecision	Other Considerations	Quality
TUG	1074 (7 RCTs)	not serious	serious	not serious	not serious	not serious	⊕⊕⊕◯ moderate
BBS	224 (4 RCTs)	not serious	serious	not serious	not serious	not serious	⊕⊕⊕◯ moderate
FES	858 (4 RCTs)	serious	not serious	not serious	not serious	not serious	⊕⊕⊕◯ moderate
ABC	232 (4 RCTs)	serious	not serious	not serious	not serious	not serious	⊕⊕⊕◯ moderate
SF-36/SF-12	898 (3 RCTs)	serious	serious	not serious	not serious	not serious	⊕⊕◯◯ low
SPPB	556 (3 RCTs)	serious	not serious	not serious	not serious	not serious	⊕⊕⊕◯ moderate
Total number of falls	2158 (9 RCTs)	not serious	not serious	not serious	not serious	not serious	⊕⊕⊕⊕ high
Number of fallers (≥1 falls)	2632 (11 RCTs)	not serious	not serious	not serious	not serious	not serious	⊕⊕⊕⊕ high

TUG: timed up-and-go; BBS: Berg Balance Score; FES: Falls Efficacy Scale; ABC: Activities-Specific Balance Confidence; SF-36/SF-12: Short Form-36/Short Form-12 Health Survey; SPPB: Short Physical Performance Battery; RCT: randomized clinical trial.

4. Discussion

The primary aim of this systematic review and meta-analysis was to evaluate the improvement of balance performance in the elderly population after various types of physical exercise. A secondary endpoint analyzed was the number of falls and/or fallers before and after an exercise program. Physical exercise was shown to be very beneficial for older people in terms of dynamic and static balance, fear of falling, balance confidence, quality of life, and physical performance, with a significant improvement reported for all the considered scores in patients who participated in a physical treatment compared to controls. The meta-analysis proved that the parameters for dynamic and static balance, such as TUG and BBS, demonstrated the best improvements after PE, with the most statistical significance compared to controls. In fact, balance training led to higher confidence in the participants' ability to perform various daily activities without falling, better patient mobility and safety at speed, greater ability to perform balance-related tasks, and lessened difficulties with activities of daily living. PE seemed to be particularly useful in reducing falls via the increase of postural control, more than improving quality of life and physical performance in older people. Moreover, with the exception of SF-36/SF-12 which was low, all the other outcomes presented a moderate quality of evidence as assessed by GRADE, thus supporting a recommendation of physical exercise in the geriatric population with risk of falls. The number of falls was recorded using daily fall calendars, which were returned to the blinded investigators. Regarding the evaluation of the number of falls and fallers, almost all the studies showed great improvements in the patients who underwent PE. Furthermore, the data showed both high quality and strength of recommendation according to GRADE for the benefit of balance and postural control exercises to reduce the rate of falls in the elderly. Only one study [48] reported no benefit in terms of falls and fallers after the exercise program, although it represented an effective approach for the improvement of multiple musculoskeletal and functional performance in older adults with risk factors for falls. Moreover, the meta-analysis showed that in patients who performed physical exercise, there was a statistically significant decrease in both the number of falls and fallers (respectively $p = 0.0008$ and $p = 0,02$). Furthermore, PE was more effective in reducing the total number of falls than the number of fallers, showing that improving muscle tropism and postural balance through specific protocol of exercises reduced the risk of falls, but it did not completely eradicate the risk of falling at least once. These data seem to strengthen the concept that PE represents a crucial aspect of prevention for reducing the risk of falls, which can lead to fractures and consequently to hospitalization, surgical procedures, and prolonged immobilization, with an increase in national healthcare costs. In contrast, a study by Lee et al. analyzed the effectiveness of exercise interventions on the rate of falls and number of fallers in care facilities, and they showed significant differences between all exercise interventions and control groups in the rate of falls, but they did not find differences in the number of fallers between all exercise interventions and control groups [50]. Similarly, Zhao et al. [51] showed that exercise had a positive effect on the reduction of fall-related fractures, with improvements in the rate of falls and leg strength in older people; however, they reported only a marginally beneficial effect of exercise on balance. Although the study population was represented by elderly people, the mean ages of the patients were different in the various studies. However, there was not a marked correlation found between age and greater improvements in the outcomes after balance training. Moreover, four studies enrolled only women, while the others included both sexes at various percentages. It seemed that in studies with only women, there were better improvements in the selected outcomes; therefore, the role of physical exercise and balance training could be greater in elderly women, and in the prevention of osteoporosis, reducing the risk of fracture following falls. In this systematic review, we included only RCTs in order to evaluate the role of physical activity compared to usual care. However, it was not possible to compare different kinds of physical activity in order to determine which is better for older people. In particular, only two studies analyzed aquatic therapy [34,35], which seems to be an interesting alternative to land-based exercise for the geriatric population, permitting low-impact and low-weight-bearing exercise. In fact, Guillamon et al. [52] presented some evidence that aquatic exercise can improve modifiable risk factors of falls, although the quality of this evidence was low, and there was a lack of consistency between studies. A limitation of this systematic review was the high variability of the training protocols of the included studies. Only few studies reported a fall-prevention program with a standardized protocol. The Otago Exercise Program was applied in three studies [36–38]; this is an individualized home-based program of balance and strength retraining exercises designed specifically to prevent falls [53]. Hewitt et al. [45] tested the Sunbeam program, which consists of individually prescribed progressive resistance training plus balance exercise. The Ossébo intervention, used by El-Khoury et al. [39], is composed of exercises designed to improve postural stability, muscle extensibility, balance, reaction time, coordination, and internal sense of spatial orientation [54]. The Lifestyle Approach to Reducing Falls through Exercise (LiFE) program, reported on by Clemson et al. [46], is a home-based, lifestyle-integrated balance and muscle-strengthening exercise training program specifically developed for fall prevention. Otherwise, the other studies did not refer to standardized exercise protocols, but they reported various generic exercises for postural balance, stationary strengthening [43], weight bearing [49], aerobic elements [41], and proprioceptive training and eye–hand/eye–foot coordinative [44]. Finally, Leiros-Rodríguez et al. [40] evaluated balance exercises as a recreational activity in public parks. Therefore, quite all the studies differed in terms of the applied exercise program; thus, it was difficult to compare the different results for the balance scores. Moreover, there was high heterogeneity among the studies in terms of the volume of training, due to different numbers of training weeks, sessions per week, exercises per session, repetitions per set, and sets per exercise, which resulted in varying loads of balance and strength training and fall-prevention exercises. Another limitation was the relatively short follow-up of some studies: it was one year or less in 87.5% of the studies, and may not allow the long-term effects of PA on dynamic and static balance to be determined. However, the overall quality of the included studies was good, with only four studies at a high risk of bias. The only critical item regarded the blinding for participants and personnel, which was at a high risk of bias in all the studies except one [49], but this was comprehensible for RCTs that compared clinical outcomes and the details of falls in patients who participated in specific exercise programs or no intervention. Instead, almost all studies used a clearly randomized allocation sequence and concealment, and the outcomes and falls were classified by qualified examiners (e.g., geriatricians or physical therapists) blinded to group assignment. Furthermore, the adherence to treatment in the studies was high and the patients lost to follow-up were few, demonstrating that PE protocols were well accepted by patients, despite their elderly age. In the literature search, we excluded many studies because they evaluated the role of PE only in patients with neurological or cardiovascular disease, whereas we were interested in analyzing the importance of exercise in the entire geriatric population, especially in healthy people, in order to limit the reduction of postural control and loss of muscle strength that predispose this population to an increased risk for falls [1]. We also focused on the differences between studies regarding the percentage of patients that had fallen at least once in the previous year. These data varied between 12.4% and 69% in the pretreatment measurements. Moreover, in many studies, this percentage was higher in the study group than in the control group; therefore, the result of fewer falls and fallers at follow-up in the study group acquires even more significance in light of these considerations. Valdés-Badilla et al. [55] reported the beneficial effects on quality of life, fall risk, activities of daily living, physical activity levels, and blood parameters of governmental physical activity programs for independent older adults. Finally, Tricco et al. [56] demonstrated that exercise was associated with a lower risk of injurious falls compared with usual care, but the type of physical activity used to reduce falls should be selected on the basis of patient and caregiver values. Sherrington et al. [24], in their systematic review and meta-analysis, demonstrated that a high dose of exercise, particularly involving balance training, can prevent falls in older people. In a more recent meta-analysis [57], the same group showed that exercise reduced the rate of falls in community-dwelling older people by 21%, and had a fall-prevention effect in community-dwelling people with Parkinson's disease or cognitive impairment. In contrast to these studies, we evaluated as outcomes not only the rate of falls or number of fallers, but also the clinical scores for dynamic and static balance, participants' fear of falling, physical performance, and quality of life in order to analyze the improvements in performing daily activities with less risk and fear of falling. Moreover, we focused on elderly people without neurological or cardiovascular disease, to recommend PE as an effective treatment for all the elderly population which could prevent impairment of muscle strength and a higher likelihood of falling. Furthermore, we analyzed various kinds of specific BT programs, including aquatic exercise, which could represent valid alternative or complementary activity to land-based exercise.

5. Conclusions

This systematic review proved that physical exercise is an effective treatment to improve static and dynamic balance and reduce the number of falls and fallers for patients aged 65 or over. The meta-analysis reports strong evidence that exercise programs can reduce fall rates in the geriatric population. Balance and postural exercises should be included in training protocols for the elderly in order to prevent the risk of falls, and they should be performed in the entire healthy population, not only as rehabilitation after stroke, fractures, or for patients affected by neurodegenerative disease. However, further large-scale trials with longer follow-up are needed to estimate the long-term effects of balance programs on decreasing the rate of falls. Moreover, more studies involving aquatic exercise or comparing aquatic versus land-based programs are necessary to promote innovative strategies to prevent falls in older people, which can be delivered by exercise trainers.

Author Contributions: Conceptualization, R.P. and V.D.; methodology, G.F.P. and S.V.; writing—original draft preparation, G.F.P. and L.A.D.B.; writing—review and editing, G.T., L.A.D.B. and A.M.A.; supervision, B.Z., and C.F.; funding acquisition, R.P. All authors have read and agreed to the published version of the manuscript.

References

1. Turner, A.; Chander, H.; Knight, A. Falls in Geriatric Populations and Hydrotherapy as an Intervention: A Brief Review. *Geriatrics* **2018**, *3*, 71. [CrossRef]
2. Thomas, E.; Battaglia, G.; Patti, A.; Brusa, J.; Leonardi, V.; Palma, A.; Bellafiore, M. Physical activity programs for balance and fall prevention in elderly: A systematic review. *Medicine* **2019**, *98*, e16218. [CrossRef]
3. Zecevic, A.A.; Salmoni, A.W.; Speechley, M.; Vandervoort, A.A. Defining a Fall and Reasons for Falling: Comparisons Among the Views of Seniors, Health Care Providers, and the Research Literature. *Gerontologist* **2006**, *46*, 367–376. [CrossRef]
4. Kendrick, D.; Kumar, A.; Carpenter, H.; Zijlstra, G.A.R.; Skelton, D.A.; Cook, J.R.; Stevens, Z.; Belcher, C.M.; Haworth, D.; Gawler, S.J.; et al. Exercise for reducing fear of falling in older people living in the community. *Cochrane Database Syst. Rev.* **2014**. [CrossRef]
5. Pollock, A.S.; Durward, B.R.; Rowe, P.J.; Paul, J.P. What is balance? *Clin. Rehabil.* **2000**, *14*, 402–406. [CrossRef]
6. Sherrington, C.; Tiedemann, A.; Fairhall, N.; Close, J.C.T.; Lord, S.R. Exercise to prevent falls in older adults: An updated meta-analysis and best practice recommendations. *NSW Public Health Bull.* **2011**, *22*, 78. [CrossRef]
7. Karinkanta, S.; Heinonen, A.; Sievänen, H.; Uusi-Rasi, K.; Kannus, P. Factors Predicting Dynamic Balance and Quality of Life in Home-Dwelling Elderly Women. *Gerontology* **2005**, *51*, 116–121. [CrossRef]
8. Organisation Mondiale de la Santé. *WHO Global Report on Falls Prevention in Older Age*; World Health Organization: Geneva, Switzerland, 2008; ISBN 978-92-4-156353-6.
9. Desforges, J.F.; Tinetti, M.E.; Speechley, M. Prevention of Falls among the Elderly. *N. Engl. J. Med.* **1989**, *320*, 1055–1059. [CrossRef]
10. Guideline for the prevention of falls in older persons. American Geriatrics Society, British Geriatrics Society, and American Academy of Orthopaedic Surgeons Panel on Falls Prevention. *J. Am. Geriatr. Soc.* **2001**, *49*, 664–672.

11. Graafmans, W.C.; Ooms, M.E.; Hofstee, H.M.A.; Bezemer, P.D.; Bouter, L.M.; Lips, P. Falls in the Elderly: A Prospective Study of Risk Factors and Risk Profiles. *Am. J. Epidemiol.* **1996**, *143*, 1129–1136. [CrossRef]

12. Tromp, A.M.; Pluijm, S.M.F.; Smit, J.H.; Deeg, D.J.H.; Bouter, L.M.; Lips, P. Fall-risk screening test. *J. Clin. Epidemiol.* **2001**, *54*, 837–844. [CrossRef]

13. Scuffham, P. Incidence and costs of unintentional falls in older people in the United Kingdom. *J. Epidemiol. Community Health* **2003**, *57*, 740–744. [CrossRef]

14. Schick, S.; Heinrich, D.; Graw, M.; Aranda, R.; Ferrari, U.; Peldschus, S. Fatal falls in the elderly and the presence of proximal femur fractures. *Int. J. Leg. Med.* **2018**, *132*, 1699–1712. [CrossRef]

15. Timler, D.; Dworzyński, M.; Szarpak, Ł.; Gaszyńska, E.; Dudek, K.; Gałązkowski, R. Head Trauma in Elderly Patients: Mechanisms of Injuries and CT Findings. *Adv. Clin. Exp. Med.* **2015**, *24*, 1045–1050. [CrossRef]

16. Inouye, S.K.; Studenski, S.; Tinetti, M.E.; Kuchel, G.A. Geriatric Syndromes: Clinical, Research, and Policy Implications of a Core Geriatric Concept: (See Editorial Comments by Dr. William Hazzard on pp 794–796). *J. Am. Geriatr. Soc.* **2007**, *55*, 780–791. [CrossRef]

17. Thomas, E.; Martines, F.; Bianco, A.; Messina, G.; Giustino, V.; Zangla, D.; Iovane, A.; Palma, A. Decreased postural control in people with moderate hearing loss. *Medicine* **2018**, *97*, e0244. [CrossRef]

18. Haskell, W.L.; Lee, I.-M.; Pate, R.R.; Powell, K.E.; Blair, S.N.; Franklin, B.A.; Macera, C.A.; Heath, G.W.; Thompson, P.D.; Bauman, A. Physical Activity and Public Health: Updated Recommendation for Adults from the American College of Sports Medicine and the American Heart Association. *Med. Sci. Sports Exerc.* **2007**, *39*, 1423–1434. [CrossRef]

19. Garber, C.E.; Blissmer, B.; Deschenes, M.R.; Franklin, B.A.; Lamonte, M.J.; Lee, I.-M.; Nieman, D.C.; Swain, D.P. Quantity and Quality of Exercise for Developing and Maintaining Cardiorespiratory, Musculoskeletal, and Neuromotor Fitness in Apparently Healthy Adults: Guidance for Prescribing Exercise. *Med. Sci. Sports Exerc.* **2011**, *43*, 1334–1359. [CrossRef]

20. Moreland, J.D.; Richardson, J.A.; Goldsmith, C.H.; Clase, C.M. Muscle Weakness and Falls in Older Adults: A Systematic Review and Meta-Analysis: Muscle weakness and falls in older adults. *J. Am. Geriatr. Soc.* **2004**, *52*, 1121–1129. [CrossRef]

21. Agmon, M.; Belza, B.; Nguyen, H.Q.; Logsdon, R.; Kelly, V.E. A systematic review of interventions conducted in clinical or community settings to improve dual-task postural control in older adults. *Clin. Interven. Aging* **2014**, *9*, 477–492. [CrossRef]

22. Lesinski, M.; Hortobágyi, T.; Muehlbauer, T.; Gollhofer, A.; Granacher, U. Dose-Response Relationships of Balance Training in Healthy Young Adults: A Systematic Review and Meta-Analysis. *Sports Med.* **2015**, *45*, 557–576. [CrossRef]

23. Howe, T.E.; Rochester, L.; Neil, F.; Skelton, D.A.; Ballinger, C. Exercise for improving balance in older people. *Cochrane Database Syst. Rev.* **2011**. [CrossRef]

24. Sherrington, C.; Whitney, J.C.; Lord, S.R.; Herbert, R.D.; Cumming, R.G.; Close, J.C.T. Effective Exercise for the Prevention of Falls: A Systematic Review and Meta-Analysis: Effective exercise for the prevention of falls. *J. Am. Geriatr. Soc.* **2008**, *56*, 2234–2243. [CrossRef]

25. Granacher, U.; Muehlbauer, T.; Gruber, M. A Qualitative Review of Balance and Strength Performance in Healthy Older Adults: Impact for Testing and Training. *J. Aging Res.* **2012**, *2012*, 1–16. [CrossRef]

26. Lesinski, M.; Hortobágyi, T.; Muehlbauer, T.; Gollhofer, A.; Granacher, U. Effects of Balance Training on Balance Performance in Healthy Older Adults: A Systematic Review and Meta-analysis. *Sports Med.* **2015**, *45*, 1721–1738. [CrossRef]

27. Daubney, M.E.; Culham, E.G. Lower-extremity muscle force and balance performance in adults aged 65 years and older. *Phys. Ther.* **1999**, *79*, 1177–1185. [CrossRef]

28. Doherty, T.J.; Vandervoort, A.A.; Brown, W.F. Effects of Ageing on the Motor Unit: A Brief Review. *Can. J. Appl. Physiol.* **1993**, *18*, 331–358. [CrossRef]

29. Howe, T.; Waters, M.; Dawson, P.; Rochester, L. Exercise for improving balance in older people. In *Cochrane Database of Systematic Reviews*; The Cochrane Collaboration, Ed.; John Wiley & Sons, Ltd.: Chichester, UK, 2004. [CrossRef]

30. Gillespie, L.D.; Robertson, M.C.; Gillespie, W.J.; Sherrington, C.; Gates, S.; Clemson, L.M.; Lamb, S.E. Interventions for preventing falls in older people living in the community. *Cochrane Database Syst. Rev.* **2012**. [CrossRef]

31. Page, M.J.; Moher, D. Evaluations of the uptake and impact of the Preferred Reporting Items for Systematic reviews and Meta-Analyses (PRISMA) Statement and extensions: A scoping review. *Syst. Rev.* **2017**, *6*, 263. [CrossRef]

32. Higgins, J.P.T.; Altman, D.G.; Gotzsche, P.C.; Juni, P.; Moher, D.; Oxman, A.D.; Savovic, J.; Schulz, K.F.; Weeks, L.; Sterne, J.A.C.; et al. The Cochrane Collaboration's tool for assessing risk of bias in randomised trials. *BMJ* **2011**, *343*, d5928. [CrossRef]

33. Gopalakrishna, G.; Mustafa, R.A.; Davenport, C.; Scholten, R.J.P.M.; Hyde, C.; Brozek, J.; Schünemann, H.J.; Bossuyt, P.M.M.; Leeflang, M.M.G.; Langendam, M.W. Applying Grading of Recommendations Assessment, Development and Evaluation (GRADE) to diagnostic tests was challenging but doable. *J. Clin. Epidemiol.* **2014**, *67*, 760–768. [CrossRef] [PubMed]

34. Miko, I.; Szerb, I.; Szerb, A.; Bender, T.; Poor, G. Effect of a balance-training programme on postural balance, aerobic capacity and frequency of falls in women with osteoporosis: A randomized controlled trial. *J. Rehabil. Med.* **2018**, *50*, 542–547. [CrossRef] [PubMed]

35. Clemson, L.; Singh, M.F.; Bundy, A.; Cumming, R.G.; Weissel, E.; Munro, J.; Manollaras, K.; Black, D. LiFE Pilot Study: A randomised trial of balance and strength training embedded in daily life activity to reduce falls in older adults. *Aust. Occup. Ther. J.* **2010**, *57*, 42–50. [CrossRef]

36. Leirós-Rodríguez, R.; García-Soidan, J.L. Balance Training in Elderly Women Using Public Parks. *J. Women Aging* **2014**, *26*, 207–218. [CrossRef]

37. Patil, R.; Uusi-Rasi, K.; Tokola, K.; Karinkanta, S.; Kannus, P.; Sievänen, H. Effects of a Multimodal Exercise Program on Physical Function, Falls, and Injuries in Older Women: A 2-Year Community-Based, Randomized Controlled Trial. *J. Am. Geriatr. Soc.* **2015**, *63*, 1306–1313. [CrossRef] [PubMed]

38. Liu-Ambrose, T.; Davis, J.C.; Best, J.R.; Dian, L.; Madden, K.; Cook, W.; Hsu, C.L.; Khan, K.M. Effect of a Home-Based Exercise Program on Subsequent Falls Among Community-Dwelling High-Risk Older Adults After a Fall: A Randomized Clinical Trial. *JAMA* **2019**, *321*, 2092. [CrossRef]

39. Arkkukangas, M.; Söderlund, A.; Eriksson, S.; Johansson, A.-C. Fall Preventive Exercise with or without Behavior Change Support for Community-Dwelling Older Adults: A Randomized Controlled Trial with Short-Term Follow-up. *J. Geriatr. Phys. Ther.* **2019**, *42*, 9–17. [CrossRef]

40. Jacobson, B.H.; Thompson, B.; Wallace, T.; Brown, L.; Rial, C. Independent static balance training contributes to increased stability and functional capacity in community-dwelling elderly people: A randomized controlled trial. *Clin. Rehabil.* **2011**, *25*, 549–556. [CrossRef]

41. Patti, A.; Bianco, A.; Karsten, B.; Montalto, M.A.; Battaglia, G.; Bellafiore, M.; Cassata, D.; Scoppa, F.; Paoli, A.; Iovane, A.; et al. The effects of physical training without equipment on pain perception and balance in the elderly: A randomized controlled trial. *Work* **2017**, *57*, 23–30. [CrossRef]

42. El-Khoury, F.; Cassou, B.; Latouche, A.; Aegerter, P.; Charles, M.-A.; Dargent-Molina, P. Effectiveness of two year balance training programme on prevention of fall induced injuries in at risk women aged 75–85 living in community: Ossébo randomised controlled trial. *BMJ* **2015**, *351*. [CrossRef]

43. Hewitt, J.; Goodall, S.; Clemson, L.; Henwood, T.; Refshauge, K. Progressive Resistance and Balance Training for Falls Prevention in Long-Term Residential Aged Care: A Cluster Randomized Trial of the Sunbeam Program. *J. Am. Med. Dir. Assoc.* **2018**, *19*, 361–369. [CrossRef]

44. Arnold, C.M.; Faulkner, R.A. The Effect of Aquatic Exercise and Education on Lowering Fall Risk in Older Adults With Hip Osteoarthritis. *J. Aging Phys. Act.* **2010**, *18*, 245–260. [CrossRef] [PubMed]

45. Gianoudis, J.; Bailey, C.A.; Ebeling, P.R.; Nowson, C.A.; Sanders, K.M.; Hill, K.; Daly, R.M. Effects of a Targeted Multimodal Exercise Program Incorporating High-Speed Power Training on Falls and Fracture Risk Factors in Older Adults: A Community-Based Randomized Controlled Trial: Targeted multimodal exercise: Effects on fall and fracture risk factors. *J. Bone Miner. Res.* **2014**, *29*, 182–191. [CrossRef] [PubMed]

46. Ansai, J.H.; Aurichio, T.R.; Gonçalves, R.; Rebelatto, J.R. Effects of two physical exercise protocols on physical performance related to falls in the oldest old: A randomized controlled trial: Exercises protocols in oldest old. *Geriatr. Gerontol. Int.* **2016**, *16*, 492–499. [CrossRef] [PubMed]

47. Hale, L.A.; Waters, D.; Herbison, P. A Randomized Controlled Trial to Investigate the Effects of Water-Based Exercise to Improve Falls Risk and Physical Function in Older Adults With Lower-Extremity Osteoarthritis. *Arch. Phys. Med. Rehabil.* **2012**, *93*, 27–34. [CrossRef] [PubMed]

48. Boongird, C.; Keesukphan, P.; Phiphadthakusolkul, S.; Rattanasiri, S.; Thakkinstian, A. Effects of a simple home-based exercise program on fall prevention in older adults: A 12-month primary care setting, randomized controlled trial: Simple home-based exercise. *Geriatr. Gerontol. Int.* **2017**, *17*, 2157–2163. [CrossRef] [PubMed]

49. Smulders, E.; Weerdesteyn, V.; Groen, B.E.; Duysens, J.; Eijsbouts, A.; Laan, R.; van Lankveld, W. Efficacy of a Short Multidisciplinary Falls Prevention Program for Elderly Persons With Osteoporosis and a Fall History: A Randomized Controlled Trial. *Arch. Phys. Med. Rehabil.* **2010**, *91*, 1705–1711. [CrossRef]

50. Lee, S.H.; Kim, H.S. Exercise Interventions for Preventing Falls Among Older People in Care Facilities: A Meta-Analysis: Exercise Interventions for Preventing Falls Among Older People. *Worldviews Evid. Based Nurs.* **2017**, *14*, 74–80. [CrossRef]

51. Zhao, R.; Feng, F.; Wang, X. Exercise interventions and prevention of fall-related fractures in older people: A meta-analysis of randomized controlled trials. *Int. J. Epidemiol.* **2016**, *46*, 149–161. [CrossRef]

52. Martínez-Carbonell Guillamón, E.; Burgess, L.; Immins, T.; Martínez-Almagro Andreo, A.; Wainwright, T.W. Does aquatic exercise improve commonly reported predisposing risk factors to falls within the elderly? A systematic review. *BMC Geriatr.* **2019**, *19*, 52. [CrossRef]

53. Martins, A.C.; Santos, C.; Silva, C.; Baltazar, D.; Moreira, J.; Tavares, N. Does modified Otago Exercise Program improves balance in older people? A systematic review. *Prev. Med. Rep.* **2018**, *11*, 231–239. [CrossRef] [PubMed]

54. Dargent-Molina, P.; Khoury, F.E.; Cassou, B. The 'Ossébo' intervention for the prevention of injurious falls in elderly women: Background and design. *Glob. Health Promot.* **2013**, *20*, 88–93. [CrossRef] [PubMed]

55. Valdés-Badilla, P.A.; Gutiérrez-García, C.; Pérez-Gutiérrez, M.; Vargas-Vitoria, R.; López-Fuenzalida, A. Effects of Physical Activity Governmental Programs on Health Status in Independent Older Adults: A Systematic Review. *J. Aging Phys. Act.* **2019**, *27*, 265–275. [CrossRef] [PubMed]

56. Tricco, A.C.; Thomas, S.M.; Veroniki, A.A.; Hamid, J.S.; Cogo, E.; Strifler, L.; Khan, P.A.; Robson, R.; Sibley, K.M.; MacDonald, H.; et al. Comparisons of Interventions for Preventing Falls in Older Adults: A Systematic Review and Meta-analysis. *JAMA* **2017**, *318*, 1687. [CrossRef] [PubMed]

57. Sherrington, C.; Michaleff, Z.A.; Fairhall, N.; Paul, S.S.; Tiedemann, A.; Whitney, J.; Cumming, R.G.; Herbert, R.D.; Close, J.C.T.; Lord, S.R. Exercise to prevent falls in older adults: An updated systematic review and meta-analysis. *Br. J. Sports Med.* **2017**, *51*, 1750–1758. [CrossRef] [PubMed]

6

Central and Peripheral Neuromuscular Adaptations to Ageing

Riccardo Borzuola [1], Arrigo Giombini [1], Guglielmo Torre [2,*], Stefano Campi [2], Erika Albo [2], Marco Bravi [3], Paolo Borrione [1], Chiara Fossati [1] and Andrea Macaluso [1]

[1] Department of Movement, Human and Health Sciences, University of Rome "Foro Italico", 00135 Rome, Italy; riccardo.borzuola@uniroma4.it (R.B.); arrigo.giombini@uniroma4.it (A.G.); paolo.borrione@uniroma4.it (P.B.); chiara.fossati@uniroma4.it (C.F.); andrea.macaluso@uniroma4.it (A.M.)

[2] Department of Orthopaedic And Trauma Surgery, Campus Bio-Medico University of Rome, 00128 Rome, Italy; s.campi@unicampus.it (S.C.); e.albo@unicampus.it (E.A.)

[3] Department of Physical Medicine and Rehabilitation, Campus Bio-Medico University of Rome, 00128 Rome, Italy; m.bravi@unicampus.it

* Correspondence: g.torre@unicampus.it

Abstract: Ageing is accompanied by a severe muscle function decline presumably caused by structural and functional adaptations at the central and peripheral level. Although researchers have reported an extensive analysis of the alterations involving muscle intrinsic properties, only a limited number of studies have recognised the importance of the central nervous system, and its reorganisation, on neuromuscular decline. Neural changes, such as degeneration of the human cortex and function of spinal circuitry, as well as the remodelling of the neuromuscular junction and motor units, appear to play a fundamental role in muscle quality decay and culminate with considerable impairments in voluntary activation and motor performance. Modern diagnostic techniques have provided indisputable evidence of a structural and morphological rearrangement of the central nervous system during ageing. Nevertheless, there is no clear insight on how such structural reorganisation contributes to the age-related functional decline and whether it is a result of a neural malfunction or serves as a compensatory mechanism to preserve motor control and performance in the elderly population. Combining leading-edge techniques such as high-density surface electromyography (EMG) and improved diagnostic procedures such as functional magnetic resonance imaging (fMRI) or high-resolution electroencephalography (EEG) could be essential to address the unresolved controversies and achieve an extensive understanding of the relationship between neural adaptations and muscle decline.

Keywords: aging; cerebral cortex; dynapenia; elderly; motor unit; muscle strength; neural; neuroplasticity; sarcopenia

1. Introduction

Ageing is associated with loss in muscle mass and strength. Originally, scientists conceptualised the term "sarcopenia" to describe the age-related loss of skeletal muscle mass [1,2]. Others coined the term "dynapenia" to indicate the decline in muscle strength [3–6]. More recently, numerous investigators introduced the term "muscle quality" to describe the relationship between muscle strength and size in older adults [7–10]. However, whereas the large majority of the research has focused on the intrinsic skeletal muscle properties and mechanisms to explain muscle weakness in older adults, relatively little recognition has been given to the potential role of the central nervous system as a fundamental component of the decline in muscle function [11].

Researchers have suggested that the age-related decay in muscle quality can be attributed to many neural factors, including a decline in the function of the human cortex, spinal cord and neuromuscular junction [12]. Investigating the role of neural factors in preserving muscle properties and contraction capacities is key to developing a more comprehensive understanding of the causes leading to the decline in muscle function occurring at advancing age. In this review, we highlight the neurological and neuromuscular adaptations that primarily cause impairments in the skeletal muscle function and performance of the aged population.

2. Supraspinal Age-Related Adaptations

Premotor and primary motor cortical areas comprise a large number of excitatory and inhibitory neurons, including glutamatergic neurons, axonal projections and pyramidal neurons [13]. Besides projecting to the cortical areas of the central nervous system, these neurons form a long axonal connection with the lower motor neurons in the ventral horn of the spinal cord [13]. Several studies have shown that the premotor and the primary motor cortex (M1) incur cortical atrophy [14–17]. The total volume of the cortical area has been shown to decrease (between 4% and 16%) with age [14–16]. In the past, it was commonly assumed that this was attributed to a decrease in the number of M1 neurons during ageing. However, recent evidence suggested that, rather than a numerical decay in cortical neurons, M1 cortex decline is related to a volumetric reduction in premotor and primary motor neuron cell body size and synaptic density [16–18]. This adaptation has been referred to as neural atrophy [19]. A study on cadaveric dissections [20] demonstrated that the elderly population had an average of 43% volumetric reduction in the motor cortex cell body size compared to young adults. These findings have been more recently supported by studies performed on living humans using high-resolution magnetic resonance. Salat et al. [17] found that the cerebral cortex, including M1 cortex, incurs a substantial reduction in volume due to the morphometric changes in the neural cells. Several studies evidenced a strong correlation between cortical atrophy and fine movements, such as mirror drawing [21]. Other motor tasks appear to be substantially influenced by grey matter atrophy. Rosano et al. [22] reported a decline in gait performance during GaitMat walking proportional to the decrease in grey matter volume. Similarly, Sridharan et al. [23] illustrated a strong correlation between lower grey matter volumes and impaired reaching movements in aged rhesus monkeys.

Neural atrophy, however, is not the only morphometric adaptation that occurs during ageing. A major alteration involves the cortical white matter, which exhibits a significant decrease in subjects over 65 years old [24,25]. White matter is predominantly made up of glial cells and myelinated axons, and it is responsible for the cortico-cortical and cortico-spinal connectivity. Cross-sectional studies indicate a profound disruption in the integrity of the white matter [25], which declines with age at an average rate of 2.5% every ten years [26,27]. The experimental investigation of Marner et al. [28] indicated that myelinated nerve fibre length in the white matter significantly decreased in aged population compared to younger individuals. Age-related morphometric adaptations of the motor cortex may therefore carry a considerable effect on the connectivity within the cortical areas as well as between the cortex and the rest of the central nervous system [29]. Several studies have indicated that a decrease in white matter integrity is associated with slower motor performances on interhemispheric transfer task such as alternating finger tapping [30] and other fine finger movement tasks [31]. Zahr et al. [32] demonstrated that greater white matter integrity correlates with improved motor performance for both fine and gross motor skills. Other researchers indicated that white matter hyperintensities lead to poorer stability, expressed as greater sway path and impaired static balance [33].

Age-related decline in motor functions has also been imputed to impaired neurotransmission, which is regulated by neurochemical factors. Evidence suggests that alterations in neurotransmitters (NT) and their specific receptors are directly associated with impairments of the cognitive and motor function in the elderly population. Abnormalities in the NT-regulated systems such as serotonergic [34,35], cholinergic [36], adrenergic [35], dopaminergic, GABAergic and glutamatergic [37–40] have been highlighted in ageing individuals. Although a comprehensive understanding of how each system responds to ageing remains unclear, several investigators suggested that the interaction between glutamate, dopamine and GABA plays a critical role in the decline of cortical and motor functions in the elderly [40]. The NT-regulated systems' alterations have been associated with increased neural noise, which has been defined as a random background activity in the brain signal [11].

Failures of the glutamatergic system have been ascribed as one of the neurochemical mechanisms responsible for the increase in neural noise since glutamate is directly involved in the modulation of the excitatory inputs in the central nervous system. The study of Arnth-Jensen et al. [41] demonstrated that ageing is accompanied by a significant reduction in the glutamate uptake. They found an excessive quantity of extracellular glutamate around cortical neurons and observed a significant increase in neural noise which is expressed by abnormal and unpredictable neural background activity even during simple motor tasks.

Furthermore, evidence exists that increased neural noise can be attributed to a decline of the dopaminergic system [42]. A previous investigation evidenced a considerable loss of dopamine transporters in the central nervous system with a 6.6% decay per decade in healthy individuals [43]. MacDonald et al. [44] used position emission tomography (PET) and found that increased reaction times in the aged population is closely related to the loss of dopamine receptors. Using imaging techniques like PET, researchers have reported a strong correlation between level of striatal dopamine transmission and motor decline in balance and gait parameters [45,46]. Moreover, the dopaminergic system has proven to be associated also with fine motor control, especially in older adults [47,48]. It has been suggested that failure of the dopaminergic system in aging might underlie the reduced velocity and control of fine movements [48]. Other researchers suggested that the alterations of the dopaminergic system can be due to the reduced inhibitory modulation which is regulated by the GABA neurons [40]. Inhibition of dopamine release and glutamate uptake occurring could potentially affect the ability to produce force and to preserve motor control in the elderly [11].

The GABAergic inhibitory system also plays an important role in isolating movements and retain brain neuroplasticity. A few investigators have suggested that neuroplasticity can be preserved almost entirely in the ageing brain [49–52]. Nevertheless, many researchers have reported that brain neuroplastic and neuromodulatory capabilities substantially decrease in the elderly population [53–55]. The GABAergic inhibitory system has been generally analysed in research using transcranial magnetic stimulation (TMS) [56,57], which has been proven to be a reliable method to assess neural inhibition and cortical excitability. Many TMS studies evidenced that the elderly population is characterised by a severely impaired sensorimotor integration of afferent input [54–56,58]. Fujiyama et al. [55] showed that a reduced capacity of GABA-mediated inhibition has a clear impact on short-interval intracortical inhibition during response preparation for a motor exercise. These findings were more recently supported by those of other authors [59–64]. Nonetheless, the effect of ageing on the GABAergic system has raised many questions and many discrepancies have emerged in the literature as recently described in a comprehensive review [65].

As previously stated, several TMS studies reported that ageing is associated with a decline in intracortical inhibition. Conversely, three studies reported an increased inhibition in older adults [66–68]. Furthermore, other researchers found very little to no effect of ageing on intracortical inhibition [54,69–71]. These inconsistencies between studies may be related to methodological differences, such as different TMS protocols, as well as differences between resting-state and task-related TMS assessments. To improve the interpretation of the cortical inhibitory-excitatory circuits, the TMS technique has been recently combined with electroencephalography (EEG) as in the study of Opie et al. [68] or brain imaging techniques such as magnetic resonance spectrometry (MRS) [65] and functional magnetic resonance imaging (fMRI), although the latter is limited by the inability to distinguish between inhibition and excitation [72].

Although GABAergic system failures can represent a valid and plausible reason to the age-related loss in cortical plasticity and corticospinal excitability, other factors, such as a decline in long-term potentiation [59] or altered gene expression [73], must be considered and further analysed.

3. Spinal Age-Related Adaptation

Advanced age is accompanied by a spinal neurodegenerative process, which includes both a structural and functional reorganisation at the spinal level. The most critical morphological alteration occurring in the spinal region is represented by spinal atrophy. This is primarily related to the loss of spinal motor neurons due to the apoptosis of the neural cells. In addition, the loss of motor neurons appears to be associated with an increase in the number of astrocytes as well as an alteration of the dendritic networks [74]. Several human studies also reported a reduction in the density and diameter of myelinated and unmyelinated axons in the ventral horns of the spinal cord of aged individuals [75–80]. Jacobs and Love [81] demonstrated that old adults show a decline in myelinated and unmyelinated fibres of 38% compared to young adults. Similarly, a study performed on aged rodents revealed that ageing is characterised by a loss of around 40% in the myelinated and unmyelinated fibres compared to young individuals [82]. Consistently, these authors reported a reduced axonal density and myelin thickness along with a considerable infiltration of connective tissue and increase of infolded and outfolded myelin loops [81–83].

One of the reasons for the age-related neurodegeneration at the spinal level has been attributed to a reduction of the endocrine and paracrine production of insulin-like growth factor-1 (IGF-1). IGF-1 provides not only an effective prevention mechanism, but also a compensation mechanism for the loss of spinal motor neurons with advancing age. Investigators have shown that IGF-1 plays an important role in motor neuron apoptosis, motor axon myelination, stimulation of axonal sprouting and repair of axons [84]. Although the mechanism underpinning the reduction of IGF-1 is still poorly understood, it appears that the inflammatory response which characterised the majority of elderly individuals may affect the local production of IGF-1. Grounds [85] observed an elevated level of inflammatory cytokines TNF-a and TNF-b in older adults and reported a strong correlation between the inflammatory response and the impaired IGF-1-mediated effects on motor neuron regeneration and axonal repair. The importance of IGF-1 on facilitating axonal sprouting has been demonstrated in animal experiments. In a study on young mice, a higher concentration of IGF-1 was accompanied by a greater capacity to reinnervate denervated muscle fibres after motor neurons loss [86]. The authors claimed that reinnervation through axonal sprouting can compensate for the loss of almost 50% of the original motor neurons.

Disfunction of spinal motor neurons, as well as reduced axonal myelination and reduced internodal length, have been considered responsible, at least in part, for the age-related decrease in nerve conduction velocity. Reductions in peripheral efferent and afferent axon action potential conduction velocity have been often reported in the literature [82,87–91]. Rivner et al. [92] demonstrated that advancing age highly correlates with variations of nerve conduction velocity and both motor and sensory responses. The analysis of the Hoffman (H) reflex via electromyography (EMG) and nerve stimulation has been proven to be a valid method to assess the efficacy of spinal circuitry function [93]. H-reflex primarily indicates the efficacy of Ia sensory afferent fibres to activate spinal motor neurons. Furthermore, EMG and nerve stimulation allow the analysis of the motor (M) wave which measures the direct activation of peripheral motor axons and, therefore, the magnitude of the motor response.

Many investigators revealed a significant reduction in the amplitude of the H-reflex response in old compared to young individuals. [94–99] This suggests that ageing may determine a decline in spinal motor neurons excitability although other factors such as pre-synaptic inhibition must be taken in consideration [100]. Along with a reduced H-reflex amplitude, the authors demonstrated that ageing is associated with an increased H-reflex latency [89,98]. These findings may help interpret the decline in peripheral nerve conduction velocity occurring at an advanced age. Interestingly, the research of Scaglioni et al. [89] revealed that M-wave latency was not different between young and aged individuals, in contrast to what emerged for the H-reflex latency. The same authors suggested that ageing could, therefore, affect sensory afferent fibres to a greater extent compared to efferent motor axons [89].

Another mechanism that seems to contribute to the spinal circuitry failures in aged individuals is the impaired modulation of the pre- and post-synaptic spinal inhibition [101]. Some investigators indicated that healthy young adults increase their muscle force by down-regulating their pre-synaptic inhibition, which, in turn, leads to enhanced excitatory afferent input. The research of Earles and co-workers [96] demonstrated that during an isometric voluntary contraction of a leg muscle, older participants exhibited a reduced modulation of spinal pre-synaptic inhibition although they were able to modulate the force similarly to young participants. Similarly, the work of Baudry et al. [102] indicated that older individuals did not modulate the amount of pre-synaptic inhibition of Ia afferents during a wrist extension task but rather increased the coactivation of the antagonist muscle. This appears to be related to a deterioration of the spinal afferent input and suggests that the elderly tend to rely less on spinal mechanisms and more on supraspinal mechanism in order to increase force [103].

4. Neuromuscular Junction

The progressive neuromuscular decline during ageing, as previously stated, can be accompanied by failures of the de-innervation–re-innervation mechanism, which normally compensates for neuronal loss and the related impairment in muscle strength and control. It appears that age-related neuromuscular junction (NMJ) dysfunction can primarily explain the progressive decline of the re-innervation process. As the majority of the human structures, also NMJ occurs in morphological remodelling and functional impairment as individuals age. Structural changes generally occur in the pre-synaptic area (motor nerve terminal) and post-synaptic area (muscle fibre surface and membrane), where the number of post-junctional folds in the motor endplate is significantly reduced, resulting in slower conduction velocity and decreased magnitude of the muscle action potentials [104,105]. Alterations of the nerve terminal region primarily include a numerical reduction of mitochondria in the plaque of the motor neuron terminal bouton. Mitochondria play a fundamental role in regulating metabolism, signal transduction and cell apoptosis and produce oxygen free radicals [106]. In addition, axonal mitochondria also function as a buffer for the calcium ion loads essential for excitation–contraction coupling [107].

Investigators have reported several morphological adaptations of the axonal mitochondria. Garcia et al. [108] indicated that mitochondria in the NMJ of the ageing population may incur cristae disruption, swelling and multiple fusions [109]. Studies regarding the pre-synaptic plaque have shown high levels of oxidative damage and nitrosylation. This appears to be directly responsible for the deterioration of the pre-synaptic mitochondria [110]. Some authors suggested that in the motor nerve terminals and the post-synaptic endplate, which are highly metabolically active, mitochondrial dysfunction may induce an even greater impairment [111,112]. In addition, Ibebunjo et al. [113] have recently indicated the presence of downregulation of mitochondrial energy metabolism in rats with NMJ disruption. However, the impact of oxidative stress on age-related adaptations of the peripheral nervous system remains still unclear and requires further investigation [108,114].

An author reported that in aged mitochondria located in the NMJ, there is evidence of altered calcium buffering and reduced ATP production, which may negatively affect both neurotransmission and vesicular recycling [115]. This suggests that the impaired excitation–contraction coupling occurring in elderly individuals could be closely related to the dysfunction of axonal mitochondria. However, some investigators have argued that the neurotransmission dysfunction is mainly associated with the age-related reorganisation of neurotransmitters receptors such as nicotine acetylcholine receptors (nAChR), which are found in the post-synaptic membrane, dihydropyridine receptors (DHPRs), which are located in the sarcolemma, and ryanodine receptors (RyRs) of the sarcoplasmic reticulum [116]. In particular, excitation–contraction uncoupling appears to be related to the mismatch between DHPRs and RyRs found in aged individuals. The interaction between DHPRs and RYRs plays a crucial role in the regulation of the calcium ions during contraction stimuli. Severe dysfunctions of these two receptors lead, in turn, to a decreased calcium release after an action potential, thus an impaired contraction [117,118].

Delbono [119] indicated that IGF-1 has a role in preventing the age-related failure of neurotransmitters receptors. A recent animal study suggested that overexpression of IGF-1 in mice can significantly reverse the numerical decrease of DHP receptors, thus preventing the dysfunction of the post-synaptic NMJ [120]. As previously described at the spinal level, there is strong evidence that IGF-1 can improve nerve regeneration and prevent neuronal loss. Moreover, many authors have highlighted the importance of IGF-1 in maintaining the integrity of the NMJ [121] and promote the re-innervation of previously de-innervated motor units in aged individuals [122].

The age-related structural and functional adaptations occurring at the NMJ have been further associated with other neuromuscular alterations such as reduced number of synaptic vesicles [123], reduced amounts of released neurotransmitters [115], a decline in satellite cell proliferation [124] and fragmentation of Schwann cells [125,126]. Several recent studies on Schwann cells emphasised their critical importance in neurodegenerative prevention, particularly concerning the NMJ synapse. In light of their capacity to regulate axonal regeneration, assist neural re-myelination fibres and provide functional recovery, degeneration of these cells might strongly contribute to ineffective re-innervation and neuromuscular dysfunction in ageing [127–129].

Authors have suggested that many NMJ impairments can be related to the high level of circulating inflammatory markers, such as cytokines and interleukines, which are commonly found in aged individuals. Elderly people generally incur chronic low-grade inflammation, also referred to as "inflammaging" [130], which represent a considerable risk factor for an accelerated decline of the neuromuscular structures, including NMJ. Previous literature clearly indicated that individuals suffering from chronic inflammation show evidence of muscle wasting and weakness [131,132]. In the NMJ, two mechanisms have been mainly identified in association with ageing inflammation. In the work of Saheb-Al Zamani et al. [133], overexpression of the interleukine 6 (IL-6) was found closely correlated with degeneration of Schwann cells in elderly, underlining the negative effect of inflammation on axonal regeneration. Furthermore, as reported in the previous paragraph, high levels of cytokines (TNF-a and TNF-b) in the aged population appear to down-regulate the production of IGF-1 and impair its regeneration activity [84].

Although there is indisputable evidence that elderly people present signs of muscle denervation and NMJ dysfunction, there is still no clear agreement if this process anticipates muscle sarcopenia or is a result of the decline of muscle fibres. Unfortunately, direct studies of the NMJ in humans are extremely challenging due to the delicate accessibility of its structures. The animal studies reported in this review have always required invasive surgical interventions (such as muscle needle biopsies) which are not commonly performed for research purposes in humans.

In living humans, insight into the NMJ decline during ageing is mostly reported via EMG assessments of single motor unit action potentials [134]. Current works on ageing NMJ have revealed severe alterations in the EMG recordings of single motor units. These consisted of abnormally large intervals between action potentials of two fibres of the same motor unit (Jitter) and higher variability in the shape of a single motor unit during consecutive discharges (Jiggle) [135,136]. Developing new neurophysiological techniques could be key to fully understanding the mechanisms underpinning the age-related neurodegeneration of the human NMJ. Substantial signs of progress have been made in the understanding of the molecular basis behind NMJ dysfunction through the analysis of circulating biomarkers as addressed in this paragraph. This area of investigation has a strong translational potential although the role of biomarkers, and their correlation with ageing neurodegeneration is not fully understood.

5. Muscle Fibre

Motor unit remodelling characterises elderly individuals and results in a considerable loss of innervated muscle fibres and a decrease in active fibres size [136,137]. Rates of fibres denervation greatly overcome re-innervation, and the decline in fibre size is closely related to the increase of oxidative stress and cell apoptosis, with significant reductions in the number of satellite cell responsible for muscle fibres regeneration [138,139].

Old humans generally exhibit muscle atrophy, which consists of smaller fibres in the active motor units compared to young adults. [140–142]. Reduced fibre cross-sectional area appears to occur across all fibres, although studies have reported contrasting results with significant variability determined by muscle type and sex of participants [137,143]. Age-related atrophy has been often associated with decreased protein synthesis and fewer satellite cells particularly in type II fibres [144–146]. In addition, histochemical studies in both humans and animals showed that older individuals tend to exhibit multiple myosin heavy chain (MHC) isoforms in single fibres [147]. The expression of multiple MHC isoform in older adults could often impede the conventional categorisation of muscle fibres in type I and type II.

Some studies indicated that muscle-specific tension may be retained with ageing despite the decrease in muscle fibre size [142,148]. Nonetheless, several works on old and very old individuals reported lower specific tension across different muscles at advancing age, especially in participants of 80 years or more [149,150]. The authors suggested that lower specific tension could be related to a decreased level of intracellular calcium and calcium sensitivity which characterise older individuals [151,152]. Animal studies have shown reductions of specific tension associated with excitation coupling impairments as comprehensively reviewed by Delbono [153]. The discrepancies in the findings on specific tension of single fibres in aged muscles seem to be related to sampling bias due to neglect of lifestyle modifiers such as physical activity and nutrition. Physical activity appears to strongly influence specific tension [150], thus studies with participants matched for physical activity are required to better understand the extent of specific tension decline at advancing age.

In old individuals, contractile properties of the muscle fibres equally decline as age increases [141]. In particular, old adults show reduced contractile speed compared with young people with several studies reporting lower rates of force development [154] and decreased maximal shortening velocity in single muscle fibres [149,155]. This decline has normally been associated with an impairment of the cross-bridge kinetics [143]. Authors have suggested that any age-related shift from type II to type I fibres can induce a compelling reduction in peak power and contractile speed up to six times lower compared to young adults [148].

Similar to contractile speed, also the rate of muscle relaxation appears to be reduced with ageing [156–158]. Authors indicated that alterations of the cross-bridge mechanics as well as reduced calcium uptake and calcium-ATPase activity are primarily responsible for impaired muscle relaxation in older people [159].

6. Conclusions and Perspectives

In this review, we analysed the most updated literature regarding central and peripheral adaptation occurring during the ageing process. The increased aged population has required and requires a more comprehensive understanding of the mechanisms involved in muscular decline due to its strong correlation with disability and mortality. When possible, we have highlighted the studies in which physiological changes were associated with functional outcomes.

The emerging picture is that ageing determines a structural and functional reorganisation at the central and peripheral level which, in turn, causes impairments in voluntary activation capacity and reduction in motor performance. Although studies have reported large variability in voluntary activation within older adults, there is evidence that elderly individuals show impairments in voluntary activation which varies in magnitude depending on the task performed and the muscle groups involved [160–162].

Neural factors, such as cortical adaptations appear to play a fundamental role in the deterioration of muscle quality, although a strong theoretical rationale often has not been accompanied by equally valuable evidence. Whilst the majority of scientists widely agrees on the structural remodelling of the ageing brain and the resulting motor impairments, further research is required to fully understand whether age-related reorganisation of inhibitory and excitatory circuits derive from neural malfunction or serve as a compensatory mechanism to preserve motor control in older individuals. Unanswered questions and literature inconsistencies may be addressed by combining newly developed diagnostics techniques and optimised procedures such as TMS in combination with novel brain imaging techniques (fMRI, MRS, magnetoencephalography) and electrophysiological monitoring techniques as, for instance, high-resolution EEG [163].

Age-related impairments occurring at the spinal level and in the NMJ area have been extensively analysed in the past and more recent research, but yet, a lack of agreement has arisen between different investigators. Introducing novel neurophysiological techniques as well as improving the understanding of the relationship between neuromuscular mechanisms such as pre- and post-synaptic inhibition and muscular voluntary activation could help resolve the discrepancies emerged in the literature. As previously described, the analysis of circulating biomarkers has carried a notable insight on the molecular basis behind the neurodegenerative process involving the spinal circuitry function and the NMJ. Further research is required to fully understand this process and the related mechanisms, in consideration of the strong translational potential of this area of research.

In order to understand the neuromuscular adaptations occurring at advancing age, several researchers have suggested the need to analyse the changes in neural drive to the muscles [164]. Surface EMG can provide some information on the neural drive to the muscles although the conventional procedures have been long debated and led to controversial conclusions, mainly due to the unavailability of motor unit population data. Recently, a novel, high-density EMG technique has been introduced to improve the estimation of the neural drive to the muscles [165]. Through the use of an array of electrodes rather than the usual bipolar configuration, a more accurate decomposition of the EMG signal appears to be feasible and it has shown promising results with regards to neural drive and motor unit properties estimation. Only few studies that used high-density EMG have been performed on elderly adults [166,167]. They reported evidence of impaired motor unit discharge characteristics which indicates a reduced integrity of the motor unit firing modulation [165,166]. Developing this technique could be key to more extensively interpreting the neural and intrinsic changes occurring with ageing.

Acknowledgments: In this section you can acknowledge any support given which is not covered by the author contribution or funding sections. This may include administrative and technical support, or donations in kind (e.g., materials used for experiments).

References

1.   Evans, W.J. What is sarcopenia? *J. Gerontol. A Biol. Sci. Med. Sci.* **1995**, *50*, 5–8. [CrossRef] [PubMed]
2.   Rosenberg, I.H. Sarcopenia: Origins and clinical relevance. *J. Nutr.* **1997**, *127*, 990–991. [CrossRef] [PubMed]
3.   Clark, B.C.; Manini, T.M. Sarcopenia =/= dynapenia. *J. Gerontol. A Biol. Sci. Med. Sci.* **2008**, *63*, 829–834. [CrossRef] [PubMed]
4.   Janssen, I. Evolution of sarcopenia research. *Appl. Physiol. Nutr. Metab.* **2010**, *35*, 707–712. [CrossRef]
5.   Glover, E.I.; Phillips, S.M. Resistance exercise and appropriate nutrition to counteract muscle wasting and promote muscle hypertrophy. *Curr. Opin. Clin. Nutr. Metab. Care* **2010**, *13*, 630–634. [CrossRef]
6.   Barbat-Artigas, S.; Dupontgand, S.; Fex, A.; Karelis, A.D.; Aubertin-Leheudre, M. Relationship between dynapenia and cardio-respiratory functions in healthy postmenopausal women: A novel clinical criteria. *Menopause* **2011**, *18*, 400–405. [CrossRef]
7.   Newman, A.B.; Haggerty, C.L.; Goodpaster, B.; Harris, T.; Kritchevsky, S.; Nevitt, M.; Miles, T.P.; Visser, M. Strength and muscle quality in a well functioning cohort of older adults: The Health, Aging and Body Composition Study. *J. Am. Geriatr. Soc.* **2003**, *51*, 323–330. [CrossRef]

8.   Katsiaras, A.; Newman, A.B.; Kriska, A.; Brach, J.; Krishnaswami, S.; Feingold, E.; Kritchevsky, S.B.; Li, R.;
     Harris, T.B.; Schwartz, A.; et al. Skeletal muscle fatigue, strength, and quality in the elderly: The Health ABC
     Study. *J. Appl. Physiol.* **2005**, *99*, 210–216. [CrossRef]
9.   Brooks, N.; Layne, J.E.; Gordon, P.L.; Roubenoff, R.; Nelson, M.E.; Castaneda-Sceppa, C. Strength training
     improves muscle quality and insulin sensitivity in Hispanic older adults with type 2 diabetes. *Int. J. Med.
     Sci.* **2006**, *4*, 19–27. [CrossRef]
10. Delmonico, M.J.; Harris, T.B.; Visser, M.; Park, S.W.; Conroy, M.B.; Velasquez-Mieyer, P.; Boudreau, R.;
     Manini, T.M.; Nevitt, M.; Newman, A.B.; et al. Longitudinal study of muscle strength, quality, and adipose
     tissue infiltration. *Am. J. Clin. Nutr.* **2009**, *90*, 1579–1585.
11. Manini, T.M.; Hong, S.L.; Clark, B.C. Aging and muscle: A neuron's perspective. *Curr. Opin. Clin. Nutr.
     Metab. Care* **2013**, *16*, 21–26. [CrossRef] [PubMed]
12. Russ, D.W.; Gregg-Cornell, K.; Conaway, M.J.; Clark, B.C. Evolving concepts on the age-related changes in
     "muscle quality". *J. Cachexia Sarcopenia Muscle* **2012**, *3*, 95–109. [CrossRef] [PubMed]
13. Kandel, E.J.; Schwartz, J.H.; Jessel, T.M. *Principles of Neural Science*, 5th ed.; McGraw-Hill: New York, NY,
     USA, 2012.
14. Bartzokis, G.; Beckson, M.; Lu, P.H.; Nuechterlein, K.H.; Edwards, N.; Mintz, J. Age-related changes in frontal
     and temporal lobe volumes in men: A magnetic resonance imaging study. *Arch. Gen. Psychiatry* **2001**, *58*,
     461–465. [CrossRef] [PubMed]
15. Raz, N.; Gunning-Dixon, F.; Head, D.; Rodrigue, K.M.; Williamson, A.; Acker, J.D. Aging, sexual dimorphism,
     and hemispheric asymmetry of the cerebral cortex: Replicability of regional differences in volume. *Neurobiol.
     Aging* **2004**, *25*, 377–396. [CrossRef]
16. McGinnis, S.M.; Brickhouse, M.; Pascual, B.; Dickerson, B.C. Age-related changes in the thickness of cortical
     zones in humans. *Brain Topogr.* **2011**, *24*, 279–291. [CrossRef]
17. Salat, D.H.; Buckner, R.L.; Snyder, A.Z.; Greve, D.N.; Desikan, R.S.; Busa, E.; Morris, J.C.; Dale, A.M.; Fischl, B.
     Thinning of the cerebral cortex in aging. *Cereb. Cortex* **2001**, *14*, 721–730. [CrossRef]
18. Morrison, J.H.; Hof, P.R. Life and death of neurons in the aging brain. *Science* **1997**, *278*, 412–419. [CrossRef]
19. Ward, N.S. Compensatory mechanisms in the aging motor system. *Ageing. Res. Rev.* **2006**, *5*, 239–254.
     [CrossRef]
20. Haug, H.; Eggers, R. Morphometry of the human cortex cerebri and corpus striatum during aging. *Neurobiol.
     Aging* **1991**, *12*, 336–338. [CrossRef]
21. Kennedy, K.M.; Raz, N. Age, sex and regional brain volumes predict perceptual-motor skill acquisition.
     Cortex **2005**, *41*, 560–569. [CrossRef]
22. Rosano, C.; Aizenstein, H.; Brach, J.; Longenberger, A.; Studenski, S.; Newman, A.B. Special article: Gait
     measures indicate underlying focal gray matter atrophy in the brain of older adults. *J. Gerontol. A Biol. Sci.
     Med. Sci.* **2008**, *63*, 1380–1388. [CrossRef] [PubMed]
23. Sridharan, A.; Willette, A.A.; Bendlin, B.B.; Alexander, A.L.; Coe, C.L.; Voytko, M.L.; Colman, R.J.;
     Kemnitz, J.W.; Weindruch, R.H.; Johnson, S.C. Brain volumetric and microstructural correlates of executive
     and motor performance in aged rhesus monkeys. *Front. Aging Neurosci.* **2012**, *4*, 31. [CrossRef] [PubMed]
24. Ge, Y.; Grossman, R.I.; Babb, J.S.; Rabin, M.L.; Mannon, L.J.; Kolson, D.L. Age-related total gray matter
     and white matter changes in normal adult brain. part I: Volumetric MR imaging analysis. *AJNR Am. J.
     Neuroradiol.* **2002**, *23*, 1327–1333. [PubMed]
25. Madden, D.J.; Whiting, W.L.; Huettel, S.A.; White, L.E.; MacFall, J.R.; Provenzale, J.M. Diffusion tensor
     imaging of adult age differences in cerebral white matter: Relation to response time. *Neuroimage* **2004**, *21*,
     1174–1181. [CrossRef]
26. Ota, M.; Obata, T.; Akine, Y.; Ito, H.; Ikehira, H.; Asada, T.; Suhara, T. Age-related degeneration of corpus
     callosum measured with diffusion tensor imaging. *Neuroimage* **2006**, *31*, 1445–1452. [CrossRef]
27. Sullivan, E.V.; Pfefferbaum, A. Diffusion tensor imaging and aging. *Neurosci. Biobehav. Rev.* **2006**, *30*, 749–761.
     [CrossRef]
28. Marner, L.; Nyengaard, J.R.; Tang, Y.; Pakkenberg, B. Marked loss of myelinated nerve fibers in the human
     brain with age. *J. Comp. Neurol.* **2003**, *462*, 144–152. [CrossRef]
29. Pannese, E. Morphological changes in nerve cells during normal aging. *Brain Struct. Funct.* **2011**, *216*, 85–89.
     [CrossRef]

30.   Sullivan, E.V.; Adalsteinsson, E.; Hedehus, M.; Ju, C.; Moseley, M.; Lim, K.O.; Pfefferbaum, A. Equivalent disruption of regional white matter microstructure in aging healthy men and women. *Neuroreport* **2001**, *12*, 99–104. [CrossRef]

31.   Sullivan, E.V.; Rohlfing, T.; Pfefferbaum, A. Quantitative fiber tracking of lateral and interhemispheric white matter systems in normal aging: Relations to timed performance. *Neurobiol. Aging* **2010**, *31*, 464–481. [CrossRef]

32.   Zahr, N.M.; Rohlfing, T.; Pfefferbaum, A.; Sullivan, E.V. Problem solving, working memory, and motor correlates of association and commissural fiber bundles in normal aging: A quantitative fiber tracking study. *Neuroimage* **2009**, *44*, 1050–1062. [CrossRef] [PubMed]

33.   Sullivan, E.V.; Rose, J.; Rohlfing, T.; Pfefferbaum, A. Postural sway reduction in aging men and women: Relation to brain structure, cognitive status, and stabilizing factors. *Neurobiol. Aging* **2009**, *30*, 793–807. [CrossRef] [PubMed]

34.   Morgan, D.G.; May, P.C.; Finch, C.E. Dopamine and serotonin systems in human and rodent brain: Effects of age and neurodegenerative disease. *J. Am. Geriatr. Soc.* **1987**, *35*, 334–345. [CrossRef] [PubMed]

35.   Bigham, M.H.; Lidow, M.S. Adrenergic and serotonergic receptors in aged monkey neocortex. *Neurobiol. Aging* **1995**, *16*, 91–104. [CrossRef]

36.   Bartus, R.T.; Dean, R.L.; Beer, B.; Lippa, A.S. The cholinergic hypothesis of geriatic memory dysfunction. *Science* **1982**, *217*, 408–417. [CrossRef]

37.   Roth, G.S.; Joseph, J.A. Cellular and molecular mechanisms of impaired dopaminergic function during aging. *Ann. N. Y. Acad. Sci.* **1994**, *719*, 129–135. [CrossRef]

38.   Roth, G.S. Age changes in signal transduction and gene expression. *Mech. Ageing Dev.* **1997**, *98*, 231–238. [CrossRef]

39.   Segovia, G.; Porras, A.; Del Arco, A.; Mora, F. Glutamatergic neurotransmission in aging: A critical perspective. *Mech. Ageing Dev.* **2001**, *122*, 1–29. [CrossRef]

40.   Mora, F.; Segovia, G.; Del Arco, A. Glutamate-dopamine-GABA interactions in the aging basal ganglia. *Brain Res. Rev.* **2008**, *58*, 340–353. [CrossRef]

41.   Arnth-Jensen, N.; Jabaudon, D.; Scanziani, M. Cooperation between independent hippocampal synapses is controlled by glutamate uptake. *Nat. Neurosci.* **2002**, *5*, 325–331. [CrossRef]

42.   Darbin, O. The aging striatal dopamine function. *Parkinsonism Relat. Disord.* **2012**, *18*, 426–432. [CrossRef] [PubMed]

43.   Volkow, N.D. Dopamine transporters decrease with age. *J. Nucl. Med.* **1996**, *37*, 554–559. [PubMed]

44.   MacDonald, S.W.; Karlsson, S.; Rieckmann, A.; Nyberg, L.; Backman, L. Aging-related increases in behavioral variability: Relations to losses of dopamine D1 receptors. *J. Neurosci.* **2012**, *32*, 8186–8191. [CrossRef]

45.   Cham, R.; Perera, S.; Studenski, S.A.; Bohnen, N.I. Striatal dopamine denervation and sensory integration for balance in middle-aged and older adults. *Gait Posture* **2007**, *26*, 516–525. [CrossRef]

46.   Cham, R.; Studenski, S.A.; Perera, S.; Bohnen, N.I. Striatal dopaminergic denervation and gait in healthy adults. *Exp. Brain Res.* **2008**, *185*, 391–398. [CrossRef] [PubMed]

47.   Floel, A.; Garraux, G.; Xu, B.; Breitenstein, C.; Knecht, S.; Herscovitch, P.; Cohen, L.G. Levodopa increases memory encoding and dopamine release in the striatum in the elderly. *Neurobiol. Aging* **2008**, *29*, 267–279. [CrossRef]

48.   Van Dyck, C.H.; Avery, R.A.; MacAvoy, M.G.; Marek, K.L.; Quinlan, D.M.; Baldwin, R.M.; Seibyl, J.P.; Innis, R.B.; Arnsten, A.F. Striatal dopamine transporters correlate with simple reaction time in elderly subjects. *Neurobiol. Aging* **2008**, *29*, 1237–1246. [CrossRef]

49.   Skarabot, J.; Ansdell, P.; Temesi, J.; Howatson, G.; Goodall, S.; Durbaba, R. Neurophysiological responses and adaptation following repeated bouts of maximal lengthening contractions in young and older adults. *J. Appl. Physiol.* **2019**, *127*, 1224–1237. [CrossRef]

50.   Van Praag, H.; Kempermann, G.; Gage, F.H. Neural consequences of environmental enrichment. *Nat. Rev. Neurosci.* **2000**, *1*, 191–198. [CrossRef]

51.   Nithianantharajah, J.; Hannan, A.J. Enriched environments, experience-dependent plasticity and disorders of the nervous system. *Nat. Rev. Neurosci.* **2006**, *7*, 697–709. [CrossRef]

52.   Mora, F. Successful brain aging: Plasticity, environmental enrichment and lifestyle. *Dialogues Clin. Neurosci.* **2013**, *15*, 45–52. [PubMed]

53. Rogasch, N.C.; Dartnall, T.J.; Cirillo, J.; Nordstrom, M.A.; Semmler, J.G. Corticomotor plasticity and learning of a ballistic thumb training task are diminished in older adults. *J. Appl. Physiol.* **2009**, *107*, 1874–1883. [CrossRef] [PubMed]

54. Smith, A.E.; Ridding, M.C.; Higgins, R.D.; Wittert, G.A.; Pitcher, J.B. Cutaneous afferent input does not modulate motor intracortical inhibition in ageing men. *Eur. J. Neurosci.* **2011**, *34*, 1461–1469. [CrossRef] [PubMed]

55. Fujiyama, H.; Hinder, M.R.; Schmidt, M.W.; Tandonnet, C.; Garry, M.I.; Summers, J.J. Age-related differences in corticomotor excitability and inhibitory processes during a visuomotor RT task. *J. Cogn. Neurosci.* **2012**, *24*, 1253–1263. [CrossRef]

56. Kobayashi, M.; Pascual-Leone, A. Transcranial magnetic stimulation in neurology. *Lancet Neurol.* **2007**, *2*, 145–156. [CrossRef]

57. Reis, J.; Swayne, O.B.; Vandermeeren, Y.; Camus, M.; Dimyan, M.A.; Harris-Love, M.; Perez, M.A.; Ragert, P.; Rothwell, J.C.; Cohen, L.G. Contribution of transcranial magnetic stimulation to the understanding of cortical mechanisms involved in motor control. *J. Physiol.* **2008**, *586*, 325–351. [CrossRef]

58. Degardin, A.; Devos, D.; Cassim, F.; Bourriez, J.L.; Defebvre, L.; Derambure, P.; Devanne, H. Deficit of sensorimotor integration in normal aging. *Neurosci. Lett.* **2006**, *498*, 208–212. [CrossRef]

59. Burke, S.N.; Barnes, C.A. Neural plasticity in the ageing brain. *Nat. Rev. Neurosci.* **2006**, *7*, 30–40. [CrossRef]

60. Heise, K.-F.; Zimerman, M.; Hoppe, J.; Gerloff, C.; Wegscheider, K.; Hummel, F.C. The aging motor system as a model for plastic changes of GABA-mediated intracortical inhibition and their behavioral relevance. *J. Neurosci.* **2013**, *33*, 9039–9049. [CrossRef]

61. Levin, O.; Fujiyama, H.; Boisgontier, M.P.; Swinnen, S.P.; Summers, J.J. Aging and motor inhibition: A converging perspective provided by brain stimulation and imaging approaches. *Neurosci. Biobehav. Rev.* **2014**, *43*, 100–117. [CrossRef]

62. Peinemann, A.; Lehner, C.; Conrad, B.; Siebner, H.R. Age-related decrease in paired-pulse intracortical inhibition in the human primary motor cortex. *Neurosci. Lett.* **2001**, *313*, 33–36. [CrossRef]

63. Marneweck, M.; Loftus, A.; Hammond, G. Short-interval intracortical inhibition and manual dexterity in healthy aging. *Neurosci. Res.* **2011**, *70*, 408–414. [CrossRef] [PubMed]

64. Hermans, L.; Levin, O.; Maes, C.; Van Ruitenbeek, P.; Heise, K.F.; Edden, R.A.E.; Cuypers, K. GABA levels and measures of intracortical and interhemispheric excitability in healthy young and older adults: An MRS-TMS study. *Neurobiol. Aging* **2018**, *65*, 168–177. [CrossRef] [PubMed]

65. Bhandari, A.; Radhu, N.; Farzan, F.; Mulsant, B.H.; Rajji, T.K.; Daskalakis, Z.J.; Blumberger, D.M. A meta-analysis of the effects of aging on motor cortex neurophysiology assessed by transcranial magnetic stimulation. *Clin. Neurophysiol.* **2016**, *27*, 2834–2845. [CrossRef] [PubMed]

66. Kossev, A.R.; Schrader, C.; Däuper, J.; Dengler, R.; Rollnik, J.D. Increased intracortical inhibition in middle-aged humans; a study using paired-pulse transcranial magnetic stimulation. *Neurosci. Lett.* **2002**, *333*, 83–88. [CrossRef]

67. McGinley, M.; Hoffman, R.L.; Russ, D.W.; Thomas, J.S.; Clark, B.C. Older adults exhibit more intracortical inhibition and less intracortical facilitation than young adults. *Exp. Gerontol.* **2010**, *45*, 671–678. [CrossRef]

68. Opie, G.M.; Sidhu, S.K.; Rogasch, N.C.; Ridding, M.C.; Semmler, J.G. Cortical inhibition assessed using paired-pulse TMS-EEG is increased in older adults. *Brain Stimul.* **2018**, *11*, 545–557. [CrossRef]

69. Oliviero, A.; Profice, P.; Tonali, P.A.; Pilato, F.; Saturno, E.; Dileone, M. Effects of aging on motor cortex excitability. *Neurosci. Res.* **2006**, *55*, 74–77. [CrossRef]

70. Cirillo, J.; Rogasch, N.C.; Semmler, J.G. Hemispheric differences in use-dependent corticomotor plasticity in young and old adults. *Exp. Brain Res.* **2010**, *205*, 57–68. [CrossRef]

71. Stevens-Lapsley, J.E.; Thomas, A.C.; Hedgecock, J.B.; Kluger, B.M. Corticospinal and intracortical excitability of the quadriceps in active older and younger healthy adults. *Arch. Gerontol. Geriatr.* **2013**, *56*, 279–284. [CrossRef]

72. Arthurs, O.J.; Boniface, S. How well do we understand the neural origins of the fMRI BOLD signal? *Trends Neurosci.* **2002**, *25*, 27–31. [CrossRef]

73. Clayton, D.A.; Grosshans, D.R.; Browning, M.D. Aging and surface expression of hippocampal NMDA receptors. *J. Biol. Chem.* **2002**, *277*, 14367–14369. [CrossRef] [PubMed]

74. Cruz-Sánchez, F.F.; Moral, A.; Rossi, M.L.; Quintó, L.; Castejón, C.; Tolosa, E.; De Belleroche, J.C. Synaptophysin in spinal anterior horn in aging and ALS: An immunohistological study. *J. Neural. Transm.* **1996**, *103*, 1317–1329. [CrossRef] [PubMed]

75. Tomlinson, B.E.; Irving, D. The numbers of limb motor neurons in the human lumbosacral cord throughout life. *J. Neurol. Sci.* **1977**, *34*, 213–219. [CrossRef]

76. Kawamura, Y.; O'Brien, P.C.; Okazaki, H.; Dyck, P.J. Lumbar motorneurons of man. I. Numbers and diameter histograms of alpha and gamma axons and ventral roots. *J. Neuropathol. Exp. Neurol.* **1977**, *36*, 853–860. [CrossRef] [PubMed]

77. Kawamura, Y.; O'Brien, P.C.; Okazaki, H.; Dyck, P.J. Lumbar motoneurons of man. II. Numbers and diameter distributions of large- and intermediate-diameter cytons in motoneuron columns of spinal cord of man. *J. Neuropathol. Exp. Neurol.* **1977**, *36*, 861–870. [CrossRef]

78. Mittal, K.R.; Logmani, F.H. Age-related reduction in 8th cervical ventral nerve root myelinated fiber diameters and numbers in man. *J. Gerontol.* **1987**, *42*, 8–10. [CrossRef]

79. Terao, S.; Sobue, G.; Hashizume, Y.; Shimada, N.; Mitsuma, T. Age-related changes of the myelinated fibers in the human corticospinal tract: A quantitative analysis. *Acta Neuropathol.* **1994**, *88*, 137–142. [CrossRef]

80. Buchman, A.S.; Leurgans, S.E.; VanderHorst, V.G.J.M.; Nag, S.; Schneider, J.A.; Bennett, D.A. Spinal motor neurons and motor function in older adults. *J. Neurol.* **2019**, *266*, 174–182. [CrossRef]

81. Jacobs, J.M.; Love, S. Qualitative and quantitative morphology of human sural nerve at different ages. *Brain* **1985**, *108*, 897–924. [CrossRef]

82. Ceballos, D.; Cuadras, J.; Verdú, E.; Navarro, X. Morphometric and ultrastructural changes with ageing in mouse peripheral nerve. *J. Anat.* **1999**, *197*, 563–576. [CrossRef] [PubMed]

83. Verdú, E.; Ceballos, D.; Vilches, J.J.; Navarro, X. Influence of aging on peripheral nerve function and regeneration. *J. Peripher. Nerv. Syst.* **2000**, *5*, 191–208. [CrossRef] [PubMed]

84. Grounds, M.D. Reasons for the degeneration of ageing skeletal muscle: A central role for IGF-1 signalling. *Biogerontology* **2002**, *3*, 19–24. [CrossRef] [PubMed]

85. Grounds, M.D.; Radley, H.G.; Gebski, B.L.; Bogoyevitch, M.A.; Shavlakadze, T. Implications of cross-talk between tumor necrosis factor and insulin-like growth factor-1 signalling in skeletal muscle. *Clin. Exp. Pharmacol. Physiol.* **2008**, *35*, 846–851. [CrossRef]

86. Hantai, D.; Akaaboune, M.; Lagord, C.; Murawsky, M.; Houenou, L.J.; Festoff, B.W.; Vaught, J.L.; Rieger, F.; Blondet, B. Beneficial effects of insulin-like growth factor-I on wobbler mouse motoneuron disease. *J. Neurol. Sci.* **1995**, *129*, 122–126. [CrossRef]

87. Doherty, T.J.; Stashuk, D.W.; Brown, W.F. Determinants of mean motor unit size: Impact on estimates of motor unit number. *Muscle Nerve* **1993**, *16*, 1326–1331. [CrossRef]

88. Metter, E.J.; Conwit, R.; Metter, B.; Pacheco, T.; Tobin, J. The relationship of peripheral motor nerve conduction velocity to age-associated loss of grip strength. *Aging* **1998**, *10*, 471–478. [CrossRef]

89. Scaglioni, G.; Ferri, A.; Minetti, A.E.; Martin, A.; Van Hoecke, J.; Capodaglio, P.; Sartorio, A.; Narici, M.V. Plantar flexor activation capacity and H reflex in older adults: Adaptations to strength training. *J. Appl. Physiol.* **2002**, *92*, 2292–2302. [CrossRef]

90. Geertsen, S.S.; Willerslev-Olsen, M.; Lorentzen, J.; Nielsen, J.B. Development and aging of human spinal cord circuitries. *J. Neurophysiol.* **2017**, *118*, 1133–1140. [CrossRef]

91. Palve, S.S.; Palve, B.S. Impact of aging on nerve conduction velocities and late responses in healthy individuals. *J. Neurosci. Rural. Pract.* **2018**, *9*, 112–116. [CrossRef]

92. Rivner, M.H.; Swift, T.R.; Malik, K. Influence of age and height on nerve conduction. *Muscle Nerve* **2001**, *24*, 1134–1141. [CrossRef] [PubMed]

93. Burke, D. Clinical uses of H reflexes of upper and lower limb muscles. *Clin. Neurophysiol. Pract.* **2016**, *1*, 9–17. [CrossRef] [PubMed]

94. Skarabot, J.; Ansdell, P.; Brownstein, C.G.; Hicks, K.M.; Howatson, G.; Goodall, S.; Durbaba, R. Reduced corticospinal responses in older compared with younger adults during submaximal isometric, shortening, and lengthening contractions. *J. Appl. Physiol.* **2019**, *126*, 1015–1031. [CrossRef] [PubMed]

95. Koceja, D.M.; Markus, C.A.; Trimble, M.H. Postural modulation of the soleus H reflex in young and old subjects. *Electroencephalogr. Clin. Neurophysiol.* **1995**, *97*, 387–393. [CrossRef]

96. Earles, D.R.; Koceja, D.M.; Shively, C.W. Enviromental changes in soleus H reflex excitability in young and elderly subjects. *Int. J. Neurosci.* **2000**, *105*, 1–13. [CrossRef]

97. Koceja, D.M.; Mynark, R.G. Comparison of heteronymous monosynaptic Ia facilitation in young and elderly subjects in supine and standing positions. *Int. J. Neurosci.* **2000**, *103*, 1–17. [CrossRef]

98. Kido, A.; Tanaka, N.; Stein, R.B. Spinal excitation and inhibition decrease as humans age. *Can. J. Physiol. Pharmacol.* **2004**, *82*, 238–248. [CrossRef]

99. Raffalt, P.C.; Alkjær, T.; Simonsen, E.B. Changes in soleus H-reflex during walking in middle-aged, healthy subjects. *Muscle Nerve* **2015**, *51*, 419–425. [CrossRef]

100. Baudry, S.; Duchateau, J. Age-related influence of vision and proprioception on Ia presynaptic inhibition in soleus muscle during upright stance. *J. Physiol.* **2012**, *590*, 5541–5554. [CrossRef]

101. Aagaard, P.; Suetta, C.; Caserotti, P.; Magnusson, S.P.; Kjær, M. Role of the nervous system in sarcopenia and muscle atrophy with aging: Strength training as a countermeasure. *Scand. J. Med. Sci. Sports* **2010**, *20*, 49–64. [CrossRef]

102. Baudry, S.; Maerz, A.H.; Enoka, R.M. Presynaptic modulation of Ia afferents in young and old adults when performing force and position control. *J. Neurophysiol.* **2010**, *103*, 623–631. [CrossRef] [PubMed]

103. Papegaaij, S.; Taube, W.; Baudry, S.; Otten, E.; Hortobágyi, T. Aging causes a reorganization of cortical and spinal control of posture. *Front. Aging Neurosci.* **2014**, *6*, 126. [CrossRef] [PubMed]

104. Kurokawa, K.; Mimori, Y.; Tanaka, E.; Kohriyama, T.; Nakamura, S. Age-related change in peripheral nerve conduction: Compound muscle action potential duration and dispersion. *Gerontology* **1999**, *45*, 168–173. [CrossRef] [PubMed]

105. Punga, A.R.; Ruegg, M.A. Signaling and aging at the neuromuscular synapse: Lessons learnt from neuromuscular diseases. *Curr. Opin. Pharmacol.* **2012**, *12*, 340–346. [CrossRef]

106. Peterson, C.M.; Johannsen, D.L.; Ravussin, E. Skeletal muscle mitochondria and aging: A review. *J. Aging Res.* **2012**, *2012*, 194821. [CrossRef]

107. Barrett, E.F.; Barrett, J.N.; David, G. Mitochondria in motor nerve terminals: Function in health and in mutant superoxide dismutase 1 mouse models of familial ALS. *J. Bioenerg. Biomembr.* **2011**, *43*, 581–586. [CrossRef]

108. Garcia, M.L.; Fernandez, A.; Solas, M.T. Mitochondria, motor neurons and aging. *J. Neurol. Sci.* **2013**, *330*, 18–26. [CrossRef]

109. Gonzalez-Freire, M.; De Cabo, R.; Studenski, S.A.; Ferrucci, L. The neuromuscular junction: Aging at the crossroad between nerves and muscle. *Front. Aging Neurosci.* **2014**, *6*, 208. [CrossRef]

110. Banker, B.Q.; Kelly, S.S.; Robbins, N. Neuromuscular transmission and correlative morphology in young and old mice. *J. Physiol.* **1983**, *339*, 355–377. [CrossRef]

111. Li, H.; Kumar Sharma, L.; Li, Y.; Hu, P.; Idowu, A.; Liu, D.; Lu, J.; Bai, Y. Comparative bioenergetic study of neuronal and muscle mitochondria during aging. *Free Rad. Biol. Med.* **2013**, *63*, 30–40. [CrossRef]

112. Baines, H.L.; Turnbull, D.M.; Greaves, L.C. Human stem cell aging: Do mitochondrial DNA mutations have a causal role? *Aging Cell* **2014**, *13*, 201–205. [CrossRef] [PubMed]

113. Ibebunjo, C.; Chick, J.M.; Kendall, T.; Eash, J.K.; Li, C.; Zhang, Y.; Vickers, C.; Wu, Z.; Clarke, B.A.; Shi, J.; et al. Genomic and proteomic profiling reveals reduced mitochondrial function and disruption of the neuromuscular junction driving rat sarcopenia. *Mol. Cell. Biol.* **2013**, *33*, 194–212. [CrossRef] [PubMed]

114. Lin, L.F.; Doherty, D.H.; Lile, J.D.; Bektesh, S.; Collins, F. GDNF: A glial cell line-derived neurotrophic factor for midbrain dopaminergic neurons. *Science* **1993**, *260*, 1130–1132. [CrossRef] [PubMed]

115. Deschenes, M.R. Motor unit and neuromuscular junction remodeling with aging. *Curr. Aging Sci.* **2011**, *4*, 209–220. [CrossRef] [PubMed]

116. Delbono, O. Neural control of aging skeletal muscle. *Aging Cell* **2003**, *2*, 21–29. [CrossRef] [PubMed]

117. Wang, X.; Engisch, K.L.; Li, Y.; Pinter, M.J.; Cope, T.C.; Rich, M.M. Decreased synaptic activity shifts the calcium dependence of release at the mammalian neuromuscular junction in vivo. *J. Neurosci.* **2004**, *24*, 10687–10692. [CrossRef] [PubMed]

118. Shear, T.D.; Martyn, J.A.J. Physiology and biology of neuromuscular transmission in health and disease. *J. Crit. Care* **2009**, *24*, 5–10. [CrossRef]

119. Delbono, O. Regulation of excitation contraction coupling by insulin-like growth factor-1 in aging skeletal muscle. *J. Nutr. Health Aging* **2000**, *4*, 162–164.

120. Zheng, Z.; Wang, Z.M.; Delbono, O. Insulin-like growth factor-1 increases skeletal muscle dihydropyridine receptor alpha1s transcriptional activity by acting on the camp-response element-binding protein element of the promoter region. *J. Biol. Chem.* **2002**, *277*, 50535–50542. [CrossRef]

121. Vergani, L.; Di Giulio, A.M.; Losa, M.; Rossoni, G.; Muller, E.E.; Gorio, A. Systemic administration of insulin-like growth factor decreases motor neuron cell death and promotes muscle reinnervation. *J. Neurosci. Res.* **1998**, *54*, 840–847. [CrossRef]

122. Messi, M.L.; Delbono, O. Target-derived trophic effect on skeletal muscle innervation in senescent mice. *J. Neurosci.* **2003**, *23*, 1351–1359. [CrossRef] [PubMed]

123. Wang, Q.; Hebert, S.L.; Rich, M.M.; Kraner, S.D. Loss of synaptic vesicles from neuromuscular junctions in aged MRF4-null mice. *Neuroreport* **2011**, *22*, 185–189. [CrossRef] [PubMed]

124. Kirschner, K.; Chandra, T.; Kiselev, V.; Flores-Santa Cruz, D.; Macaulay, I.; Park, H.; Li, J.; Kent, D.G.; Kumar, R.; Pask, D.C.; et al. Proliferation drives aging-related functional decline in a subpopulation of the hematopoietic stem cell compartment. *Cell Rep.* **2017**, *19*, 1503–1511. [CrossRef] [PubMed]

125. Kawabuchi, M.; Tan, H.; Wang, S. Age affects reciprocal cellular interactions in neuromuscular synapses following peripheral nerve injury. *Ageing Res. Rev.* **2011**, *10*, 43–53. [CrossRef]

126. Kim, H.A.; Mindos, T.; Parkinson, D.B. Plastic fantastic: Schwann cells and repair of the peripheral nervous system. *Stem Cells Transl. Med.* **2013**, *2*, 553–557. [CrossRef]

127. Verge, V.M.; Gratto, K.A.; Karchewski, L.A.; Richardson, P.M. Neurotrophins and nerve injury in the adult. *Philos. Trans. R. Soc. Lond. B Biol. Sci.* **1996**, *351*, 423–430.

128. Kawabuchi, M.; Zhou, C.J.; Wang, S.; Nakamura, K.; Liu, W.T.; Hirata, K. The spatio temporal relationship among Schwann cells, axons and post-synaptic acetylcholine receptor regions during muscle reinnervation in aged rats. *Anat. Rec.* **2001**, *264*, 183–202. [CrossRef]

129. Gordon, T.; Udina, E.; Verge, V.M.K.; De Chaves, E.I.P. Brief electrical stimulation accelerates axon regeneration in the peripheral nervous system and promotes sensory axon regeneration in the central nervous system. *Motor Control* **2009**, *13*, 412–441. [CrossRef]

130. Franceschi, C.; Capri, M.; Monti, D.; Giunta, S.; Olivieri, F.; Sevini, F.; Panourgia, M.P.; Invidia, L.; Celani, L.; Scurti, M.; et al. Inflammaging and anti-inflammaging: A systemic perspective on aging and longevity emerged from studies in humans. *Mech. Ageing Dev.* **2007**, *128*, 92–105. [CrossRef]

131. Saini, A.; Faulkner, S.; Al-Shanti, N.; Stewart, C. Powerful signals for weak muscles. *Ageing Res. Rev.* **2009**, *8*, 251–267. [CrossRef]

132. Ferrucci, L.; Corsi, A.; Lauretani, F.; Bandinelli, S.; Bartali, B.; Taub, D.D.; Guralnik, J.M.; Longo, D.L. The origins of age-related proinflammatory state. *Blood* **2005**, *105*, 2294–2299. [CrossRef] [PubMed]

133. Saheb-Al-Zamani, M.; Yan, Y.; Farber, S.J.; Hunter, D.A.; Newton, P.; Wood, M.D.; Stewart, S.A.; Johnson, P.J.; Mackinnon, S.E. Limited regeneration in long acellular nerve allografts is associated with increased Schwann cells senescence. *Exp. Neurol.* **2013**, *247*, 165–177. [CrossRef] [PubMed]

134. Bromberg, M.B.; Scott, D.M. Single fiber EMG reference values: Reformatted in tabular form. Ad Hoc Committee of the AAEM Single Fiber Special Interest Group. *Muscle Nerve* **1994**, *17*, 820–821. [CrossRef] [PubMed]

135. Hourigan, M.L.; McKinnon, N.B.; Johnson, M.; Rice, C.L.; Stashuk, D.W.; Doherty, T.J. Increased motor unit potential shape variability across consecutive motor unit discharges in the tibialis anterior and vastus medialis muscles of healthy older subjects. *Clin. Neurophysiol.* **2015**, *126*, 2381–2389. [CrossRef]

136. Hepple, R.T.; Rice, C.L. Innervation and neuromuscular control in ageing skeletal muscle. *J. Physiol.* **2016**, *594*, 1965–1978. [CrossRef]

137. Lexell, J.; Taylor, C.C.; Sjöström, M. What is the cause of the ageing atrophy? Total number, size and proportion of different fiber types studied in whole vastus lateralis muscle from 15- to 83-year-old men. *J. Neurol. Sci.* **1988**, *84*, 275–294. [CrossRef]

138. Narasimhan, M.; Hong, J.; Atieno, N.; Muthusamy, V.R.; Davidson, C.J.; Abu-Rmaileh, N.; Richardson, R.S.; Gomes, A.V.; Hoidal, J.R.; Rajasekaran, N.S. Nrf2 deficiency promotes apoptosis and impairs PAX7/MyoD expression in aging skeletal muscle cells. *Free Radic. Biol. Med.* **2014**, *71*, 402–414. [CrossRef]

139. Blau, H.M.; Cosgrove, B.D.; Ho, A.T. The central role of muscle stem cells in regenerative failure with aging. *Nat. Med.* **2015**, *21*, 854–862. [CrossRef]

140. Lexell, J.; Taylor, C.C. Variability in muscle fibre areas in whole human quadriceps muscle: Effects of increasing age. *J. Anat.* **1991**, *174*, 239–249.

141. Macaluso, A.; De Vito, G. Muscle strength, power and adaptions to resistance training in older people. *Eur. J. Appl. Physiol.* **2004**, *91*, 450–472. [CrossRef]

142. Venturelli, M.; Saggin, P.; Muti, E.; Naro, F.; Cancellara, L.; Toniolo, L.; Tarperi, C.; Calabria, E.; Richardson, R.S.; Reggiani, C.; et al. In vivo and in vitro evidence that intrinsic upper and lower-limb skeletal muscle function is unaffected by ageing and disuse in oldest-old humans. *Acta Physiol.* **2015**, *215*, 58–71. [CrossRef] [PubMed]

143. Miller, M.S.; Bedrin, N.G.; Callahan, D.M.; Previs, M.J.; Jennings, M.E.; Ades, P.A.; Maughan, D.W.; Palmer, B.M.; Toth, M.J. Age-related slowing of myosin actin cross-bridge kinetics is sex specific and predicts decrements in whole skeletal muscle performance in humans. *J. Appl. Physiol.* **2013**, *115*, 1004–1014. [CrossRef] [PubMed]

144. Verdijk, L.B.; Koopman, R.; Schaart, G.; Meijer, K.; Savelberg, H.H.; Van Loon, L.J. Satellite cell content is specifically reduced in type II skeletal muscle fibers in the elderly. *Am. J. Physiol. Endocrinol. Metab.* **2007**, *292*, E151–E157. [CrossRef] [PubMed]

145. Kadi, F.; Ponsot, E. The biology of satellite cells and telomeres in human skeletal muscle: Effects of aging and physical activity. *Scand. J. Med. Sci. Sports* **2010**, *20*, 39–48. [CrossRef]

146. Wall, B.T.; Gorissen, S.H.; Pennings, B.; Koopman, R.; Groen, B.B.; Verdijk, L.B.; Van Loon, L.J. Aging is accompanied by a blunted muscle protein synthetic response to protein ingestion. *PLoS ONE* **2015**, *10*, e0140903. [CrossRef]

147. Purves-Smith, F.M.; Sgarioto, N.; Hepple, R.T. Fiber typing in aging muscle. *Exerc. Sport Sci. Rev.* **2014**, *42*, 45–52. [CrossRef]

148. Trappe, S.; Gallagher, P.; Harber, M.; Carrithers, J.; Fluckey, J.; Trappe, T. Single muscle fibre contractile properties in young and old men and women. *J. Physiol.* **2003**, *552*, 47–58. [CrossRef]

149. Larsson, L.; Li, X.; Frontera, W.R. Effects of aging on shortening velocity and myosin isoform composition in single human skeletal muscle cells. *Am. J. Physiol. Cell Physiol.* **1997**, *272*, C638–C649. [CrossRef]

150. Power, G.A.; Flaaten, N.; Dalton, B.H.; Herzog, W. Age-related maintenance of eccentric strength: A study of temperature dependence. *Age* **2016**, *38*, 43. [CrossRef]

151. Morgan, D.L.; Claflin, D.R.; Julian, F.J. The relationship between tension and slowly varying intracellular calcium concentration in intact frog skeletal muscle. *J. Physiol.* **1997**, *500*, 177–192. [CrossRef]

152. Lamboley, C.R.; Wyckelsma, V.L.; Dutka, T.L.; McKenna, M.J.; Murphy, R.M.; Lamb, G.D. Contractile properties and sarcoplasmic reticulum calcium content in type I and type II skeletal muscle fibres in active aged humans. *J. Physiol.* **2015**, *593*, 2499–2514. [CrossRef] [PubMed]

153. Delbono, O. Expression and regulation of excitation-contraction coupling proteins in aging skeletal muscle. *Curr. Aging Sci.* **2011**, *4*, 248–259. [CrossRef] [PubMed]

154. Bellumori, M.; Jaric, S.; Knight, C.A. Age-related decline in the rate of force development scaling factor. *Motor Control* **2013**, *14*, 370–381. [CrossRef] [PubMed]

155. Krivickas, L.S.; Suh, D.; Wilkins, J.; Hughes, V.A.; Roubenoff, R.; Frontera, W.R. Age- and gender-related differences in maximum shortening velocity of skeletal muscle fibers. *Am. J. Phys. Med. Rehabil.* **2001**, *80*, 447–457. [CrossRef]

156. Hunter, S.K.; Todd, G.; Butler, J.E.; Gandevia, S.C.; Taylor, J.L. Recovery from supraspinal fatigue is slowed in old adults after fatiguing maximal isometric contractions. *J. Appl. Physiol.* **2008**, *105*, 1199–1209. [CrossRef]

157. Callahan, D.M.; Kent-Braun, J.A. Effect of old age on human skeletal muscle force-velocity and fatigue properties. *J. Appl. Physiol.* **2011**, *111*, 1345–1352. [CrossRef]

158. Molenaar, J.P.; McNeil, C.J.; Bredius, M.S.; Gandevia, S.C. Effects of aging and sex on voluntary activation and peak relaxation rate of human elbow flexors studied with motor cortical stimulation. *Age* **2013**, *35*, 1327–1337. [CrossRef]

159. Hunter, S.K.; Thompson, M.W.; Ruell, P.A.; Harmer, A.R.; Thom, J.M.; Gwinn, T.H.; Adams, R.D. Human skeletal sarcoplasmic reticulum Ca^{2+} uptake and muscle function with aging and strength training. *J. Appl. Physiol.* **1999**, *86*, 1858–1865. [CrossRef]

160. Jacobi, J.M.; Rice, C.L. Voluntary muscle activation varies with age and muscle group. *J. Appl. Physiol.* **2002**, *93*, 457–462. [CrossRef]

161. Klass, M.; Baudry, S.; Duchateau, J. Voluntary activation during maximal contraction with advancing age: A brief review. *Eur. J. Appl. Physiol.* **2007**, *100*, 543–551. [CrossRef]

162. Hunter, S.K.; Pereira, H.M.; Keenan, K.G. The aging neuromuscular system and motor performance. *J. Appl. Physiol.* **2016**, *121*, 982–995. [CrossRef] [PubMed]

163. Berchicci, M.; Lucci, G.; Di Russo, F. Benefits of physiscal exercise on the aging brain: The role of the prefrontal cortex. *J. Gerontol. A Biol. Sci. Med. Sci.* **2013**, *68*, 1337–1341. [CrossRef] [PubMed]

164. Del Vecchio, A.; Negro, F.; Felici, F.; Farina, D. Association between motor unit action potential parameters and surface EMG features. *J. Appl. Physiol.* **2017**, *123*, 835–843. [CrossRef] [PubMed]

165. Del Vecchio, A.; Negro, F.; Falla, D.; Bazzucchi, I.; Farina, D.; Felici, F. Higher muscle fiber conduction velocity and early rate of torque development in chronically strength-trained individuals. *J. Appl. Physiol.* **2018**, *125*, 1218–1226. [CrossRef]

166. Watanabe, K.; Holobar, A.; Kouzaki, M.; Ogawa, M.; Akima, H.; Moritani, T. Age-related changes in motor unit firing pattern of vastus lateralis muscle during low-moderate contraction. *Age* **2016**, *36*, 48. [CrossRef]

167. Mani, D.; Almuklass, A.M.; Hamilton, L.D.; Vieira, T.M.; Botter, A.; Enoka, R.M. Motor unit activity, force steadiness, and perceived fatigability are correlated with mobility in older adults. *J. Neurophysiol.* **2018**, *120*, 1988–1997. [CrossRef]

7

The Role of Physical Activity as Conservative Treatment for Hip and Knee Osteoarthritis in Older People

Biagio Zampogna [1],*, Rocco Papalia [1], Giuseppe Francesco Papalia [1], Stefano Campi [1], Sebastiano Vasta [1], Ferruccio Vorini [1], Chiara Fossati [2], Guglielmo Torre [1] and Vincenzo Denaro [1]

[1] Department of Orthopaedic and Trauma Surgery, Campus Bio-Medico University of Rome, 00128 Rome, Italy; r.papalia@unicampus.it (R.P.); g.papalia@unicampus.it (G.F.P.); s.campi@unicampus.it (S.C.); s.vasta@unicampus.it (S.V.); f.vorini@unicampus.it (F.V.); g.torre@unicampus.it (G.T.); denaro@unicampus.it (V.D.)

[2] Department of Movement, Human and Health Sciences, University of Rome "Foro Italico", 00100 Rome, Italy; chiara.fossati@uniroma4.it

* Correspondence: b.zampogna@unicampus.it

Abstract: The aim of this systematic review and meta-analysis is to determine the role of physical activity as a conservative treatment for older people with knee or hip osteoarthritis. The effect on pain, physical function, stiffness, quality of life, and dynamic balance of Aquatic Exercise, Land-based Exercise, and Sports were compared in a specific population composed of osteoarthritic patients aged 65 or over. A systematic search using Pubmed-Medline, Google Scholar, and the Cochrane Library was carried out to select randomized clinical trials, observational studies, or case series that evaluated outcome measures after physical activity. Twenty randomized controlled trials (RCTs) and two case series were included in this review. Four trials were at low risk of bias (A), 12 at unclear risk of bias (B), and four at high risk of bias (C). Compared to controls, Aquatic Exercise, Land-based Exercise, Tai Chi, and Yoga showed a small to high effect for improving pain, physical function, quality of life, and stiffness. Active exercise and sport are effective to improve pain and physical function in elderly people with osteoarthritis. Nevertheless, further studies are required to validate the use of land-based exercise, aquatic exercise, or sport to treat the symptoms of older adults that suffer from knee and hip osteoarthritis.

Keywords: physical activity; active exercise; sport; land-based; aquatic; knee or hip osteoarthritis; older people; systematic review; meta-analysis

1. Introduction

Osteoarthritis (OA) is a chronic progressive disease that represents a considerable cause of impairment in elderly people [1]. It is characterized by pain, reduction of physical function with decreased range of motion (ROM), joint rigidity and swelling, muscle weakness, and joint instability [2,3]. All these conditions lead to impaired quality of life with worsening to achieve daily activities and disability, especially in older adults [4]. Knee and hip are commonly affected by OA [5] because they represent the joints most involved in heavy weight-bearing and increased activity [6,7]. The prevalence of OA is higher in women and elderly people [8]. OA requires remarkable healthcare resources and involves considerable social costs for treatment, due to its progressive and chronic condition, and those demands are bound to increase with an aging population [9]. Conservative treatment for OA consists of pharmacologic therapy (Non-Steroidal Anti-Inflammatory Drugs, cyclooxygenase inhibitors, oral or transdermal opioid, acetaminophen), injective therapy (corticosteroids, Hyaluronic acid, Platelet-Rich Plasma or Adipose-Derived Stem Cell), supportive therapy (glucosamine or chondroitin), physical therapy (Electrical Nerve Stimulation, Pulsed Electromagnetic Field, Laser Therapy, Therapeutic Ultrasound), braces, orthoses, active exercise (aquatic or land-based), physical and sport activity [10–12]. We focused our research on active exercise and sports that have been determined to be effective in pain relief, maintenance of joint integrity, and muscle strength, improvement in physical function, and lessening deformity and instability [13]. Active exercise has been proved to increase physical function and reduce knee and hip pain and disability, improving general health status and quality of life [14,15]. The role of exercise or sportive activities is to avoid or delay the necessity to recur to the knee or hip joint replacement, which must be reserved just for the final stage of OA [16], which is characterized by severe pain and deformity. Land-based exercise programs such as aerobic, strengthening, and resistance training are effective therapies for knee and hip OA [17,18]. Furthermore, the increase of lower limb muscular strength and the improvement of balance and coordination of movements are effective in achieve compensatory functional stability in older people with advanced OA in order to reduce the risk of falling [19,20]. Aquatic exercise profits by the weight-relieving properties of water to obtain pain relief, to allow easier joint movement improving physical function, to reduce muscle stiffness and to cause muscle relaxation in patients with OA [21,22]. In contact sports, there is a higher incidence of significant joint injuries or progression of osteoarthritis [23]; however, low-impact sports are suggested as a physical treatment for osteoarthritis because they prevent from maximum stress and enhance muscle strength and joint stability [24]. Therefore, sports are effective both in the prevention and in the treatment of OA, but they have to be modulated on the individual patient's physical abilities. The evidence on comparative effectiveness on pain and physical function of different types of active exercise or sport interventions or older adults with knee or hip OA is still poor. In fact, an adequate activity to conservatively treat those patients obtaining clinical benefits has not yet been identified. Therefore, the aim of this systematic review and meta-analysis is to determine the efficacy of physical activity as a conservative treatment for elderly people with knee or hip OA. The primary endpoint is to assess the effect on pain, physical function, stiffness, quality of life, and dynamic balance outcomes of different active exercise and sports. The secondary endpoint is to establish the specific benefits on the selected outcomes of the single intervention, to try to evaluate if there is an exercise or sport that leads to better enhancement in physical capacity and quality of life of older osteoarthritic adults.

2. Materials and Methods

A systematic review and meta-analysis were carried out using the Preferred Reporting Items for Systematic Reviews and Meta-analysis (PRISMA) guidelines [25]. The review was planned and conducted following the PRISMA checklist (Supplementary Materials Table S1). In this review, we included randomized clinical trial, observational studies, or case series, which evaluated the role of sport or exercises as a conservative treatment for patients aged 65 or over with all degrees of the knee and hip OA.

2.1. Criteria for Considering Studies for This Review

According to the WHO definition of the elderly, studies with patients with a mean age of 65 or over both in the experimental group(s) and the control group, if present, were included in the review. Studies that compared effects on pain, physical function, and physical performance of the aquatic exercise, land-based exercise, or sports with a control group were included in the review. In the randomized clinical trial, the patients in the control group had to receive usual care or no intervention. We excluded studies that investigated physical activity in the prevision of hip or knee surgery or after hip or knee replacements.

2.2. Search Methods for Identification of Studies

A systematic literature search was performed using the following databases: Pubmed-Medline, Google Scholar, and the Cochrane Library. For Pubmed we used the following search strategy: ("exercise"[MeSH Terms] or "exercise"[All Fields] or ("physical"[All Fields] and "activity"[All Fields]) or "physical activity"[All Fields]) and ("knee osteoarthritis"[MeSH Terms] or " knee osteoarthritis"[All Fields]); ("exercise"[MeSH Terms] OR "exercise"[All Fields] or ("physical"[All Fields] AND "activity"[All Fields]) or "physical activity"[All Fields]) AND ("hip osteoarthritis"[MeSH Terms] or "hip osteoarthritis"[All Fields]). The reference list of the identified articles was screened manually for further publications. After duplicates removed, the abstracts of all studies eligible were independently examined by two review authors (G.P. and B.Z.). Any uncertainties or disagreements (17 in total) were discussed with the third reviewer (R.P.) to reach a consensus. Two reviewers (G.P. and B.Z.) screened the full articles in order to determine those to include in the review and quantitative analysis.

2.3. Data Collection, Analysis, and Outcomes

Data extraction was independently produced by two reviewers (G.P. and B.Z.). We extracted the following study characteristics: authors, year of publication, type of study, level of evidence, numbers of participants in the intervention or control group integrated with age, gender and Body Mass Index (BMI), joint(s) involved, intervention in the study and in the control group, primary and secondary outcome measures, follow-up, and results. Any uncertainties or disagreements (four in total) were discussed with the third reviewer (R.P.) to reach a consensus. Outcomes included the severity of pain, which was measured on a visual analog scale (VAS), on the pain scale of the Western Ontario and McMaster Universities Arthritis Index (WOMAC) or the Knee injury and Osteoarthritis Outcome Score (KOOS) pain scale. Physical function was calculated by the WOMAC physical function scale, the KOOS ADL (function in daily living) scale, the 6-min walking test (6-MWT), the sit to stand test and range of motion (ROM) of the considered joint. Stiffness was checked with the WOMAC stiffness scale. The quality of life of the patients was measured through Short Form-36 (SF-36) or Short Form-12 (SF-12), and KOOS Quality of Life (QOL). Finally, the dynamic balance was assessed using the time up and go test (TUG).

2.4. Risk of Bias Assessment

Two review authors (G.P. and B.Z.) independently assessed the risk of bias of the randomized controlled trial (RCT) using the Cochrane Risk of Bias Tool [26]. We checked the following criteria: sequence generation, allocation concealment, blinding, incomplete data addressed, free of selective reporting, and free of other bias. Each domain was classified as presenting high risk of bias, low risk of bias, or unclear risk of bias. Then the trials were allocated to one of the following groups: low risk of bias if five or six criteria were judged adequate, unclear risk of bias if three to four criteria were judged as adequate or high risk of bias if less than three criteria were judged adequate. Two reviewers (G.P. and B.Z.) used the Methodological Index for Non-Randomized Studies (MINORS) score [27] to estimate the methodological quality of non-randomized studies. It consists of 8 items for non-comparative studies and 12 items for comparative studies. The score for each item ranges from 0 to 2, for a total maximum of 24 points.

2.5. Statistical Analysis

The quantitative data analysis was performed using the Review Manager (RevMan) software (Version 5.3, Cochrane Collaboration 2014, Copenhagen, Denmark). The data were pooled if at least two studies presented similar and comparable outcomes. A meta-analysis was performed to determine the effect of the different types of physical activity on pain, physical function, quality of life, stiffness, and dynamic balance. All continuous data were reported as mean difference (MD) with 95% confidence intervals when all the trials used the same score; otherwise, the standardized mean difference (SMD) with 95% confidence intervals was used when the analyzed scores were similar but not identical. Negative values of the mean difference or standardized mean difference proved the advantage of the experimental group. Heterogeneity was determined using the I^2 test. A fixed-effect model was conducted if the I^2 test demonstrated low heterogeneity ($I^2 < 55\%$); for I^2 greater than or equal to 55%, a random-effect model was performed.

2.6. Quality Assessment

To assess the quality of the evidence of the outcomes presented in the reported trials, the GRADE (Grading of Recommendations Assessment, Development, and Evaluation) was performed [28]. It consists of the following five items: risk of bias, inconsistency, indirectness, imprecision, and other considerations. Each domain was defined as not serious, serious, or very serious. The resulting quality assessment of the evidence was classified as high, moderate, low, or very low.

3. Results

3.1. Results of the Search

The literature search identified 2445 articles. Of these, 1817 were screened on title and abstract after the removal of duplicates. One hundred sixty-nine articles were read in full text, and 147 of those were excluded for the following reasons: not mainly evaluating physical activity intervention ($n = 45$), patients aged less than 65 years ($n = 67$), not specified joints that suffered from OA ($n = 14$), protocols of RCT ($n = 18$), and case reports ($n = 3$). Thus, 22 articles that met the inclusion criteria were included in this review. Finally, 19 articles were included in the meta-analysis (Figure 1).

3.2. Included and Excluded Studies

The studies were 20 RCTs and two case series. One case series involved Baduanjin, while the other one evaluated exercise [29]. Of the RCTs, six studies checked sports activity $n = 4$ Tai Chi [30–33], $n = 2$ yoga [34,35]. The remaining RCTs were focused on water-based and land-based exercises: there were three studies with three arms (hydrotherapy, land-based exercise and control group) [36–38], four studies that compared only hydrotherapy with controls [39–42], and seven studies that only evaluated land-based exercises [43–49].

3.3. Demographic Data

The overall number of participants in all the studies was 1504, allocated to either intervention or control groups. The mean age of the participants ranged from 65 to 78.9 years. All studies showed a higher female percentage (ranging from 50 to 100%) of included patients. Only one study [35] did not describe gender distribution in the groups. BMI ranged between 23.7 and 33.6. All demographic data are compiled in Table 1.

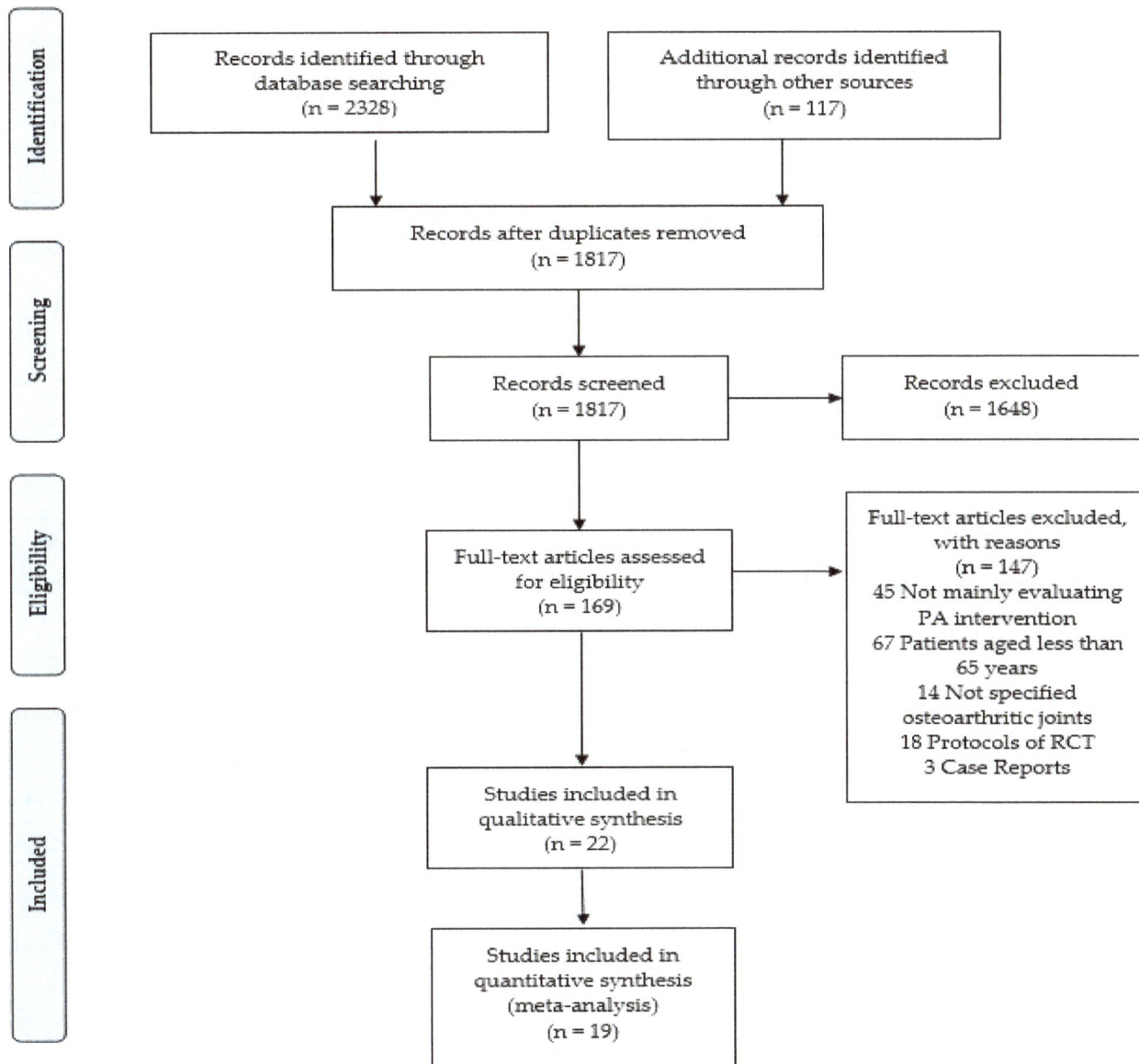

Figure 1. Flowchart of the article selection process.

Table 1. Demographic data of the included studies.

Author (Year)	Type of Study	LOE	Study Group				Control Group				Joint/s
			n	Age	Sex	BMI	*n*	Age	Sex	BMI	
Arnold et al. (2010) [42]	RCT	I	Aquatic and education: 28	73.2 y	71.4% F, 28.6% M	29.2	25	75.8 y	64% F, 36% M	30	hip OA
			Aquatic: 26	74.4 y	77% F, 23% M	30.4					
Bearne et al. (2011) [43]	RCT	I	24	65 y	62.5% F, 37.5% M	27.3	24	67 y	79% F, 21% M	26.9	hip OA
Bezalel et al. (2010) [44]	RCT	I	25	73.8 y	68% F, 32% M	/	25	73.7 y	80% F, 20% M	/	knee OA
Brismee et al. (2007) [31]	RCT	I	22	70.8 y	86.4% F, 13.6% M	28	19	68.8 y	78.9% F, 21.1% M	27.7	knee OA
Casilda-López et al. (2017) [40]	RCT	I	17	65.62 y	100% F	31.69	17	66 y	100% F	33.65	knee OA
Cheung et al. (2014) [34]	RCT	I	18	71.9 y	100% F	29.1	18	71.9 y	100% F	28.8	knee OA
Cheung et al. (2016) [35]	RCT	I	Yog: 32	68.9 y	/	29.8	23	71.8 y	/	27.8	knee OA
			Exercises: 28	74.4 y	/	29.2					
Doi et al. (2008) [46]	RCT	I	63	67.4 y	76% F, 24% M	24.8	58	71.2 y	72% F, 28% M	24.3	knee OA
Foley et al. (2003) [37]	RCT	I	Aquatic: 35	73 y	43% F, 57% M	/	35	6.8 y	57% F, 43% M	/	hip and knee OA
			Land-based: 35	69.8 y	49% F, 51% M	/					
Fransen et al. (2007) [30]	RCT	I	Aquatic: 55	70 y	73% F, 27% M	30	41	69.6 y	83% F, 17% M	30.7	hip and knee OA
			Tai chi: 56	70.8 y	68% F, 32% M	29.6					
Hale et al. (2012) [39]	RCT	I	23	73.6 y	74% F, 26% M	/	16	75.7 y	75% F, 25% M	/	hip and knee OA
Huang et al. (2017) [45]	RCT	I	128	68.07 y	79% F, 21% M	24.11	122	67.42 y	80% F, 20% M	25.01	knee OA
Hurley et al. (2007) [48]	RCT	I	Individual rehabilitation: 146	66 y	71% F, 29% M	30	140	67 y	68.5% F, 31.5% M	30.3	knee OA
			Group rehabilitation: 132	68 y	71% F, 29% M	30.18					
Lee et al. (2009) [32]	RCT	I	29	70.2 y	93.1% F, 6.9% M	26	15	66.9 y	93.3% F, 6.7% M	26	knee OA
Lund et al. (2008) [38]	RCT	I	Aquatic: 27	65 y	83% F, 17% M	27.4	27	70 y	66% F, 34% M	26.1	knee OA
			Land-based: 25	68 y	88% F, 12% M	23.7					
Marconcin et al. (2017) [47]	RCT	I	35	70.3 y	80% F, 20% M	32.3	32	67.8 y	59.4% F, 40.6% M	30.1	knee OA
Taglietti et al. (2018) [41]	RCT	I	31	67.3 y	74.2% F, 25.8% M	29.2	29	68.7 y	62.1% F, 37.9% M	30.4	knee OA
Takacs et al. (2017) [49]	RCT	I	20	66,1 y	95% F, 5% M	28.5	20	67.1 y	65% F, 35% M	28.9	knee OA
Tsai et al. (2013) [33]	RCT	I	28	78.89 y	78.6% F, 21.4% M	/	27	78.93 y	66.7% F, 33.3% M	/	knee OA
Wang et al. (2011) [36]	RCT	I	Aquatic: 26	66.7 y	84.6% F, 15.4% M	/	26	67.9 y	84.6% F, 15.4% M	/	knee OA
			Land-based: 26	68.3 y	88.5% F, 11.5% M	/					
An et al. (2013) [50]	CS	IV	22	66 y	86% F, 14% M	25	/				knee OA
Bove et al. (2017) [29]	CS	IV	7	66 y	71.5% F, 28.5% M	30.5	/				knee OA

RCT: Randomized Clinical Trial; CS: Case Series; LOE: Levels of Evidence; BMI: Body Mass Index; OA: Osteoarthritis; *n*: Number of participants; y: years; F: female; M: male.

3.4. Clinical Outcome Data

Seventeen studies included patients with knee OA alone, two studies included patients with hip OA alone, and the remaining three studies included patients with both knee and hip OA. The outcome measures evaluated in the included articles were the Western Ontario and McMaster Universities Arthritis Index (WOMAC) in 17 articles, the 6-min walk test (6-MWT) in seven articles, Knee Injury and Osteoarthritis Outcome Score (KOOS) in three articles, Visual Analog Scale (VAS) in seven articles, Short Form-36 (SF-36) in four articles, Short Form-12 (SF-12) in four articles, sit to stand test and timed up and go test in five articles (Table 2).

Table 2. Clinical outcome data of the included studies.

Author (Year)	Intervention(s)	Control	Primary Outcome Measure	Secondary Outcome Measure	Follow-Up	Results
Arnold et al. (2010) [42]	Aquatic and education: aquatic exercise twice a week with once-a-week group education for 11 weeks; Aquatic: two weeks aquatic exercise for 11 weeks	no intervention	Berg Balance Scale, 6-MWT, Timed Up and Go Test	PASE score, AIMS-2 score	11 weeks	Significant improvement in fall risk factors ($p = 0.038$) with the combination of aquatic exercise and education.
Bearne et al. (2011) [43]	Ten 75-min group exercise and self-management sessions (twice a week for five weeks)	no intervention	WOMAC physical function	WOMAC pain, WOMAC total score	Six weeks and six months	No between-group differences in any outcome measure.
Bezalel et al. (2010) [44]	Group education program once a week for four weeks, followed by a self-executed home-based exercise program	six 20-min sessions of short-wave diathermy	WOMAC total score	Sit to stand test, Timed up and go test	four and eight weeks	Significant improvement in the timed up and go test and WOMAC total ($p < 0.01$) in the exercise group.
Brismee et al. (2007) [31]	Six weeks of group Tai Chi sessions, 40 min/session, three times a week, followed by another six weeks of home-based Tai Chi training	three 40-min group sessions per week for six weeks	WOMAC pain, VAS	WOMAC stiffness and physical function	3, 6, 9, 12, 15, and 18 weeks	Less overall pain and better WOMAC physical function with Tai Chi ($p = 0.0089$ and 0.0157, respectively).
Casilda-López et al. (2017) [40]	Eight-week dance-based aquatic exercise program	global aquatic exercise program	WOMAC total score	6-MWT and VAS	Eight weeks and Three months	Postintervention differences in the WOMAC pain and aggregate ($p = 0.002$ and $p = 0.048$) in favor of the experimental group.
Cheung et al. (2014) [34]	Eight-week Hatha yoga intervention involving group and home-based exercise sessions	no intervention	WOMAC total score	SPPB, SF-12	Four weeks, eight weeks and 20 weeks	Improvement in WOMAC pain $p = 0.01$) and stiffness ($p = 0.02$) in the intervention group.
Cheung et al. (2016) [35]	Yoga: one 45-min class per week for eight weeks and additional 30 min/day, four times/week of yoga practice at home; Exercises: eight weekly group-based classes	no intervention	WOMAC total score, VAS	SPPB, SF-12	Four and eight weeks	Yoga group presented improvements in WOMAC TOTAL ($p = 0.001$) and VAS scores ($p = 0.03$) compared to exercises group.
Doi et al. (2008) [46]	Four sets of 20 repetitions of quadriceps exercise every day (knee extension movements while sitting on a chair or in a supine position)	NSAIDs	WOMAC total score and VAS	SF-36	Eight weeks	Improvements in total WOMAC, SF-36 and VAS: all $p < 0.001$ in the exercises group; WOMAC and VAS at $p < 0.001$ and SF-36 at $P < 0.03$ in the control group.
Foley et al. (2003) [37]	Three water based, or three gym-based exercise sessions a week for six weeks, including a short warm up period, lower limb stretches, and a set of resistance exercises	no intervention	WOMAC total score, 6-MWT	SF-12	Six weeks	Walking speed and distance increased in the hydrotherapy and gym groups (both $p < 0.001$). No significant changes for WOMAC function or stiffness.
Fransen et al. (2007) [30]	Aquatic or Tai Chi program (with a preliminary 10-min warm-up session): 1 h, twice a week for 12 weeks	no intervention	WOMAC pain and physical function	SF-12, DASS21	12 and 24 weeks	Improvements of 6.5 and 10.5 for pain and physical function scores with hydrotherapy and improvements of 5.2 and 9.7 with Tai Chi.
Hale et al. (2012) [44]	Water-based exercise classes twice weekly for 12 weeks	community-based computer-skills training program	PPA	Step Test, Timed Up and Go Test, WOMAC total score	12 weeks	No statistically significant between-group differences were found for any outcome measured.

Table 2. *Cont.*

Author (Year)	Intervention(s)	Control	Primary Outcome Measure	Secondary Outcome Measure	Follow-Up	Results
Huang et al. (2017) [45]	Quadriceps isometric contraction exercise (two sets of exercises in the morning and evening)	local physiotherapy and oral NSAIDs	WOMAC total score, VAS	/	One and three months	Significant improvement of WOMAC and VAS score in the experimental group ($p < 0.05$).
Hurley et al. (2007) [48]	12 supervised sessions that combined discussion on specific topics regarding self-management and coping, with an individualized, progressive exercise regimen	no intervention	WOMAC physical function	WOMAC pain, WOMAC total score	Six weeks and six months	Individual and group rehabilitated participants had better WOMAC score ($p = 0.01$) than control group.
Lee et al. (2009) [32]	Eight weeks of group Tai Chi Qigong sessions, with 60 min per session twice a week	no intervention	SF-36	WOMAC total score, 6-MWT	Eight weeks	Improvements in SF-36 ($p = 0.010$) and 6-MWT ($p = 0.005$) in the Tai Chi group.
Lund et al. (2008) [38]	Aquatic and land-based exercise programs for eight weeks with 2 sessions per week	no intervention	KOOS function and pain, VAS	Muscle Strength	Eight weeks and three months	Only in the land-based exercise group a decrease of pain was detected ($p = 0.039$). There were no significant differences between groups for KOOS.
Marconcin et al. (2017) [47]	PLE2NO program: 90-min intervention twice a week for 12 weeks	no intervention	KOOS pain	KOOS function and total score, 6-MWT	12 weeks	Significant clinical improvement was found for all KOOS (larger than 10 points) and in the 6 MWT ($p = 0.035$) in the exercise group.
Taglietti et al. (2018) [41]	Aquatic program twice a week for eight weeks	educational program: once a week for eight weeks	WOMAC total score, VAS	SF-36, Timed up and go test, Yesavage Geriatric Depression Scale	Three months	WOMAC pain reduced in favour of the aquatic exercise group ($p = 0.021$). No differences for the outcome's functional mobility or depression.
Takacs et al. (2017) [49]	Ten weeks of exercises targeting dynamic balance and strength performed four times per week	no intervention	CB&M, WOMAC physical function	Muscle Strength	10 weeks	Improvements in self-reported pain ($p = 0.005$), physical function ($p = 0.002$), and fear of movement ($p = 0.01$) in the training group.
Tsai et al. (2013) [33]	Three sessions a week of Tai Chi exercise (12-form Sun Tai Chi) for 20 weeks	no intervention	WOMAC pain	WOMAC physical function and stiffness, timed up and go test and Sit to stand test	21 weeks	WOMAC pain ($p < 0.001$), physical function ($p = 0.001$) and stiffness scores ($p = 0.001$) improved in the Tai Chi group.
Wang et al. (2011) [36]	Aquatic/land-based exercise protocol with a 60-min flexibility and aerobic training class, three times a week for 12 weeks	no intervention	KOOS total score, 6-MWT	knee ROMs	Six and 12 weeks	Aquatic and land group presented less pain than control group (respectively $p < 0.001$ and $p = 0.002$).
An et al. (2013) [50]	Short-term Baduanjin exercise: 30-min sessions five times a week for one year	/	WOMAC total score, SF-36	6-MWT	one year	WOMAC pain, stiffness and physical function subscales, SF-36 body pain and 6-MWT were significantly improved.
Bove et al. (2017) [29]	16 sessions of task-specific training at a frequency of two visits per week	/	KOOS total score	30-Second Chair Rise, Timed Stair Climb Test, Floor Transfer Test	Four, six, and eight weeks	Improvements in patient-rated and performance-based outcomes.

PASE: Physical Activity Scale for the Elderly; AIMS-2: Arthritis Impact Measurement Scales 2; WOMAC: Western Ontario and McMaster Universities Arthritis Index; VAS: Visual Analog Scale; 6-MWT: 6 min walk test; SPPB: Short Physical Performance Battery SF-12: Short Form-12; NSAIDs: Nonsteroidal anti-inflammatory drugs; DASS21: Depression, Anxiety and Stress Scale; PPA: Physiological Profile Assessment; KOOS: Knee injury and Osteoarthritis Outcome Score; CB&M: Community Balance and Mobility Scale; ROM: Range of Motion.

3.5. Methodological Evaluation

Using the Cochrane risk of bias tool for RCTs, sequence generation was considered adequate in 16 articles (80%), allocation concealment was graded as adequate in 15 studies (75%), blinding was inadequate in 15 trials (75%), outcome data addressed were regarded adequate in 16 articles (80%), reporting of selective outcome was judged as adequate in 14 (70%) trials, and the likelihood of other sources of bias was adequate in 10 (50%) of the studies. In conclusion, four trials were at low risk of bias (A), 12 included studies were at unclear risk of bias (B), and four studies were at high risk of bias (C) (Table 3). The MINORS score was calculated for two case series [29.50] included in the review. Only eight items were evaluated because the two studies were non-comparative (Table 4).

Table 3. Cochrane risk of bias tool for randomized controlled trials.

Study	Sequence Generation	Allocation Concealment	Blinding	Incomplete Data Addressed	Free of Selective Reporting	Free of Other Bias	Risk of Bias
Arnold et al. (2010)	L	L	H	L	U	L	B
Bearne et al. (2011)	L	U	H	L	U	U	C
Bezalel et al. (2010)	L	L	H	U	U	U	C
Brismee et al. (2007)	L	U	H	L	L	U	B
Casilda-López et al. (2017)	L	L	U	L	U	U	B
Cheung et al. (2014)	L	L	H	L	L	U	B
Cheung et al. (2016)	L	L	H	L	L	L	A
Doi e al. (2008)	L	L	H	H	L	U	B
Foley et al. (2003)	L	L	U	L	L	U	B
Fransen et al. (2007)	L	L	U	L	L	U	B
Hale et al. (2012)	L	L	U	U	L	L	B
Huang et al. (2017)	U	U	H	L	H	H	C
Hurley et al. (2007)	U	L	H	U	L	L	B
Lee et al. (2009)	L	L	H	L	L	L	A
Lund et al. (2008)	U	L	U	L	L	L	B
Marconcin et al. (2017)	H	U	H	L	L	U	C
Taglietti et al. (2018)	L	L	H	L	L	L	A
Takacs et al. (2017)	L	L	H	L	U	L	B
Tsai et al. (2013)	L	L	H	L	L	L	A
Wang et al. (2011)	L	U	H	L	L	L	B

Table 4. MINORS (Methodological Index for Non-Randomized Studies) score.

Study	Stated Aim	Inclusion of Patients	Collection of Data	Endpoints Appropriate to the Aim	Unbiased Assessment of the Study Endpoint	Follow-Up	Loss to Follow Up Less Than 5%	Prospective Calculation of the Study Size	Total
Am et al. (2013)	2	1	2	2	1	2	2	0	12
Bove et al. (2017)	2	1	2	2	1	1	2	0	11

3.6. Studies Included

3.6.1. Double Study Group

Five studies with two study groups were identified. Wang et al. [36] recruited 78 patients that were divided into the aquatic group, the land group, and the control group. The study demonstrated that patients in both exercise groups showed pain reduction over time. More specifically, the aquatic and the land groups presented significantly less pain than the control group at week 12 (both $p < 0.001$) and at week 6 ($p < 0.001$ for aquatic and $p = 0.002$ for land). Comparing the aquatic group with the land group, they did not show any significant difference in pain reduction at weeks 12 and 6. Foley et al. [37] evaluated 105 participants with hip or knee OA, that received water-based exercise sessions, gym-based exercise sessions, or were allocated to the control group. At follow up, walking speed and distance increased in the hydrotherapy and gym groups (both $p < 0.001$), but not in the control group. However, they did not find a significant difference between the two intervention groups for increases in physical function. Furthermore, the WOMAC pain significantly declined in the hydrotherapy group, but they did not demonstrate significant changes from baseline or between groups for WOMAC function or stiffness. Lund et al. [38] compared the efficiency of aquatic exercise and a land-based exercise program with control in 79 patients with knee OA. Only in the land-based exercise group, a decrease of pain was detected ($p = 0.039$). There were no significant differences between groups for KOOS. Fransen et al. [30] assigned 152 older patients with chronic hip or knee OA to hydrotherapy group, Tai Chi group, or a waiting list (control group). It has been shown improvements of 6.5 and 10.5 for pain and physical function scores with hydrotherapy and improvements of 5.2 and 9.7 with Tai Chi, compared with controls. Only the hydrotherapy group showed significant improvements in pain scores, SF-12, and the measures of physical performance. Cheung et al. [51] evaluated the effects of yoga and aerobic/strengthening exercises on knee OA, compared with the education control group. Patients in the yoga group presented improvements in WOMAC TOTAL ($p = 0.001$) and VAS scores ($p = 0.03$) compared to patients in exercises group.

3.6.2. Land-Based Exercise

In a study by Bearne et al. [43], 48 people with hip OA were divided into the rehabilitation group or the control group. At the term of the program, the WOMAC total score improved with a moderate effect size. But there were no differences between the two groups in any outcome measure. Bezalel et al. [44] randomly assigned 50 patients with knee OA to an exercise group or a short-wave diathermy control group. At follow-up, participants in the study group showed significant improvement in the get-up-and-go test and the WOMAC total, pain, and disability scores compared to the controls ($p < 0.01$). Huang et al. [45] enrolled 250 patients with knee OA. The test group underwent quadriceps isometric contraction exercise, while in the control group local physiotherapy and oral NSAIDs were used. At three months, WOMAC and VAS scores showed significant progress in the exercise group compared to the controls (both $p < 0.05$). In a study by Doi et al. [46], 121 patients with knee OA were allocated to an exercise group and an NSAID group. The participants in both groups presented improvements in the totality of the scores (WOMAC, SF-36, and VAS at $p < 0.001$ in the exercises group; WOMAC and VAS at $p < 0.001$ and SF-36 at $p < 0.03$ in the control group), although these increases were not statistically significant between the two groups. Therefore, they showed the "noninferiority" of exercises compared with NSAIDs as a therapy for knee OA. Marconcin et al. [47] allocated 67 patients aged 60 years or older with knee OA to a self-management and exercise intervention or an educational intervention. In the self-management and exercise group, significant improvements in all KOOS dimensions (larger than 10 points) and in the 6 MWT ($p = 0.035$) were found. In a study by Hurley et al. [48], 418 practices were randomly assigned to three groups to receive usual primary care, usual primary care plus individual rehabilitation or usual primary care plus rehabilitation in groups. Six months after the end of the schedule, the WOMAC-function scores for the individual rehabilitation and group rehabilitation classes were significantly better compared with usual care ($p = 0.01$). Although the improvements were similar for participants that made individual or group rehabilitation. Takacs et al. [49] checked 40 participants that underwent exercises targeting dynamic balance and strength or no intervention. They showed significant improvement in WOMAC physical function in the exercise group (within-group $p = 0.002$; between-group $p = 0.016$). Moreover, self-reported knee pain and fear of movement results were better in the exercise group ($p = 0.005$ and $p = 0.01$, respectively) compared to the control group. In a study by Bove et al. [29], seven patients underwent a novel task-specific training approach to exercise therapy for chronic knee pain, composed of sit to stand, floor transfer, and ascending and descending stairs training. After the treatment, the participants demonstrated important improvements in both patient-rated outcomes (for example, KOOS) and performance-based outcomes.

3.6.3. Aquatic Exercise

In a study by Hale et al. [39], 39 persons with hip or knee OA and at risk for falling underwent a water-based program (intervention group) or a time-matched computer training program (control group). After the 12-week intervention, they proved that water-based exercise did not decrease falls risk compared with a computer skills training class, with no significant disparities between the two groups for the primary outcome (PPA score) or any of the secondary outcomes measured. Casilda-Lopez et al. [40] divided 34 obese women with knee OA into a dance-based aquatic exercise program (experimental group) and a global aquatic exercise program (control group). Postintervention, they found significant differences between groups in the WOMAC pain and aggregate ($p = 0.002$ and $p = 0.048$, respectively) in favor of the aquatic dance group. Taglietti et al. [41] allocated 60 patients with knee OA to an aquatic exercise group, and an educational program group. After the treatment, they presented a significant decrease of WOMAC pain for the aquatic exercise group compared to the educational program group ($p = 0.021$). Furthermore, the WOMAC function decreased significantly in the aquatic exercise group compared to baseline ($p = 0.020$). Moreover, improvements in quality of life were detected in the aquatic exercise group ($p < 0.001$) at the follow-up. In a study by Arnold et al. [42], 79 adults, 65 years of age or older with hip OA were randomly divided into three groups: aquatic exercise and education, aquatic exercise only, and control. It has been described, a significant increase in fall risk factors ($p = 0.038$) for the patients the aquatics and education group, which increased in falls efficacy compared with controls. Moreover, they demonstrated a significant improvement of physical performance, Timed Up and Go Test, and 6-min walk in the aquatics and education group compared with both aquatics and control groups.

3.6.4. Sport

In a study by Brismée et al. [31], 41 adults with knee OA attended a Tai Chi exercise program or an attention activities program. At follow-up, the Tai Chi group presented less overall pain and better WOMAC physical function than the control group ($p = 0.0089$ and 0.0157, respectively). Moreover, the Tai Chi group had improvements in WOMAC overall, pain subscale and physical function subscale. In a study by Lee et al. [32], 44 patients with knee OA were randomized to a Tai Chi training program or a waiting list control group. The training group reported significant increments in the total SF-36 ($p = 0.010$) and 6-m walking test ($p = 0.005$). Finally, the WOMAC scores in the training group were markedly improved, although the differences were not statistically significant. Tsai et al. [33] studied the role of Tai Chi to decrease pain and stiffness in elders with knee OA and cognitive impairment, compared with controls. They demonstrated that both groups increased their WOMAC pain score ($p < 0.001$ for Tai Chi group vs. $p = 0.042$ for control group); on the other hand, the WOMAC Physical Function and Stiffness scores improved only in the Tai Chi group ($p = 0.001$ vs. $p = 0.515$ and $p < 0.001$ vs. $p = 0.324$, respectively). For all these scores, the discrepancies between the two groups improved significantly over time. Cheung et al. [34] randomly assigned 36 older women with knee OA to a yoga program or wait-list control. In their study, the differences between treatment and control groups were significant for WOMAC pain ($p = 0.01$) and stiffness scores ($p = 0.02$). An et al. [50] evaluated 22 patients (29 knees) with knee OA after one-year Baduanjin exercise. Compared with their baseline levels before exercise, patients showed significant improvements in WOMAC pain ($p = 0.000$), stiffness ($p = 0.000$) and physical function subscales ($p = 0.003$), SF-36 ($p = 0.005$), and 6-MWT ($p = 0.036$).

3.7. Effect of Intervention

3.7.1. Pain

Almost all the included studies assessed pain through WOMAC pain and KOOS pain scale. The meta-analysis showed no significant pain decrease (SMD 0.33, 95% CI 0.03 to 0.63) and no heterogeneity ($I^2 = 0\%$) when comparing aquatic exercise and land-based exercise (Figure 2). Compared to controls for pain reduction, aquatic exercise presented significant differences (SMD -0.53, 95% CI -1.25 to 0.19) and high heterogeneity ($I^2 = 91\%$) (Figure 3), land-based exercise demonstrated no significant differences (SMD -0.26, 95% CI -0.42 to -0.11) and no heterogeneity ($I^2 = 0\%$) (Figure 4), Tai Chi reported significant differences (MD -2.14, 95% CI -3.11 to -1.18) and moderate heterogeneity ($I^2 = 38\%$) (Figure 5), Yoga had significant differences (MD -1.82, 95% CI -2.96 to -0.67) without heterogeneity ($I^2 = 0\%$) (Figure 6).

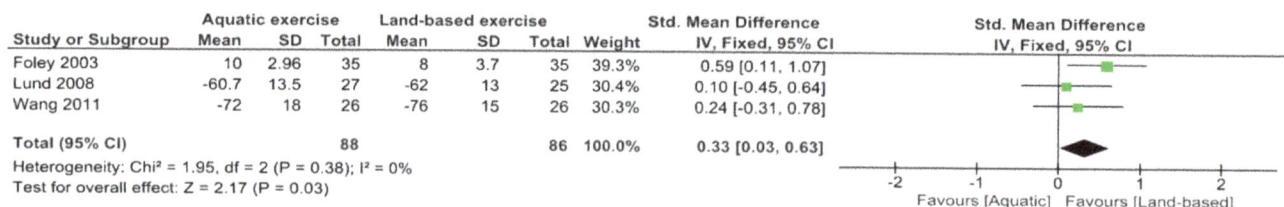

Study or Subgroup	Aquatic exercise Mean	SD	Total	Land-based exercise Mean	SD	Total	Weight	Std. Mean Difference IV, Fixed, 95% CI
Foley 2003	10	2.96	35	8	3.7	35	39.3%	0.59 [0.11, 1.07]
Lund 2008	-60.7	13.5	27	-62	13	25	30.4%	0.10 [-0.45, 0.64]
Wang 2011	-72	18	26	-76	15	26	30.3%	0.24 [-0.31, 0.78]
Total (95% CI)			88			86	100.0%	0.33 [0.03, 0.63]

Heterogeneity: Chi² = 1.95, df = 2 (P = 0.38); I² = 0%
Test for overall effect: Z = 2.17 (P = 0.03)

Figure 2. Pain: Aquatic exercise versus Land-based exercise.

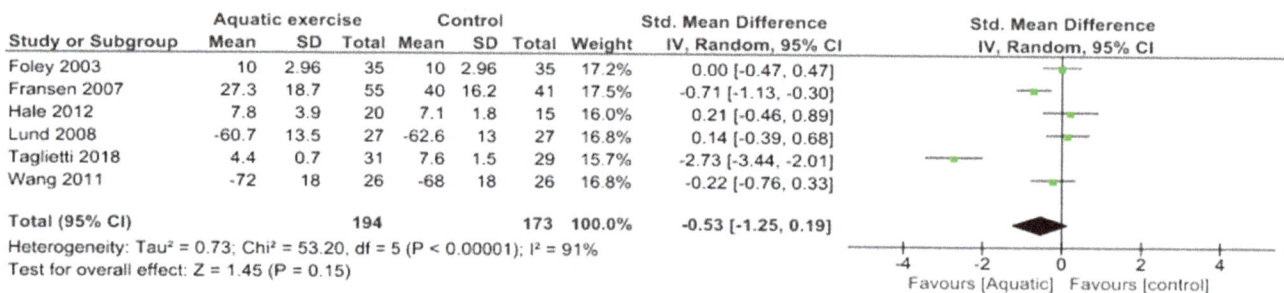

Study or Subgroup	Aquatic exercise Mean	SD	Total	Control Mean	SD	Total	Weight	Std. Mean Difference IV, Random, 95% CI
Foley 2003	10	2.96	35	10	2.96	35	17.2%	0.00 [-0.47, 0.47]
Fransen 2007	27.3	18.7	55	40	16.2	41	17.5%	-0.71 [-1.13, -0.30]
Hale 2012	7.8	3.9	20	7.1	1.8	15	16.0%	0.21 [-0.46, 0.89]
Lund 2008	-60.7	13.5	27	-62.6	13	27	16.8%	0.14 [-0.39, 0.68]
Taglietti 2018	4.4	0.7	31	7.6	1.5	29	15.7%	-2.73 [-3.44, -2.01]
Wang 2011	-72	18	26	-68	18	26	16.8%	-0.22 [-0.76, 0.33]
Total (95% CI)			194			173	100.0%	-0.53 [-1.25, 0.19]

Heterogeneity: Tau² = 0.73; Chi² = 53.20, df = 5 (P < 0.00001); I² = 91%
Test for overall effect: Z = 1.45 (P = 0.15)

Figure 3. Pain: Aquatic exercise versus Control.

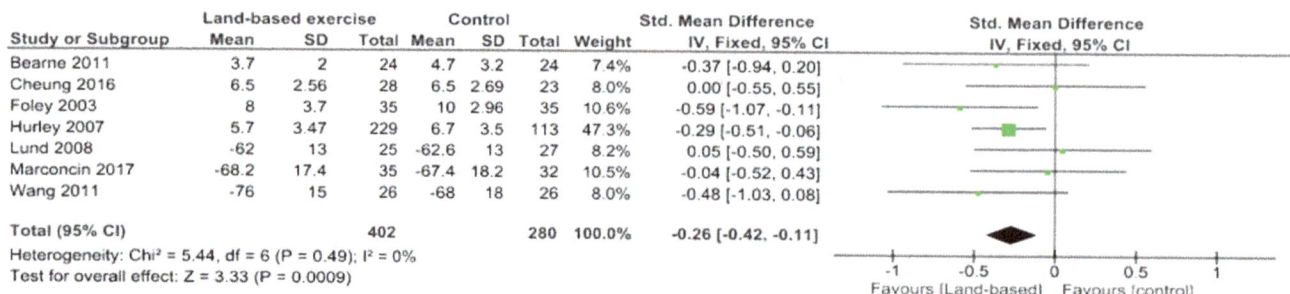

Study or Subgroup	Land-based exercise Mean	SD	Total	Control Mean	SD	Total	Weight	Std. Mean Difference IV, Fixed, 95% CI
Bearne 2011	3.7	2	24	4.7	3.2	24	7.4%	-0.37 [-0.94, 0.20]
Cheung 2016	6.5	2.56	28	6.5	2.69	23	8.0%	0.00 [-0.55, 0.55]
Foley 2003	8	3.7	35	10	2.96	35	10.6%	-0.59 [-1.07, -0.11]
Hurley 2007	5.7	3.47	229	6.7	3.5	113	47.3%	-0.29 [-0.51, -0.06]
Lund 2008	-62	13	25	-62.6	13	27	8.2%	0.05 [-0.50, 0.59]
Marconcin 2017	-68.2	17.4	35	-67.4	18.2	32	10.5%	-0.04 [-0.52, 0.43]
Wang 2011	-76	15	26	-68	18	26	8.0%	-0.48 [-1.03, 0.08]
Total (95% CI)			402			280	100.0%	-0.26 [-0.42, -0.11]

Heterogeneity: Chi² = 5.44, df = 6 (P = 0.49); I² = 0%
Test for overall effect: Z = 3.33 (P = 0.0009)

Figure 4. Pain: Land-based exercise versus Control.

	Tai Chi			Control				Mean Difference	Mean Difference
Study or Subgroup	Mean	SD	Total	Mean	SD	Total	Weight	IV, Fixed, 95% CI	IV, Fixed, 95% CI
Brismee 2007	13.95	5.81	22	15.25	3.92	19	10.3%	-1.30 [-4.30, 1.70]	
Fransen 2007	30.7	18.9	56	40	16.2	41	1.9%	-9.30 [-16.31, -2.29]	
Lee 2009	4.6	4	29	5.9	3.7	15	16.5%	-1.30 [-3.67, 1.07]	
Tsai 2013	4.36	2.55	28	6.63	1.69	27	71.4%	-2.27 [-3.41, -1.13]	
Total (95% CI)			135			102	100.0%	-2.14 [-3.11, -1.18]	

Heterogeneity: Chi² = 4.84, df = 3 (P = 0.18); I² = 38%
Test for overall effect: Z = 4.36 (P < 0.0001)

-20 -10 0 10 20
Favours [Tai Chi] Favours [control]

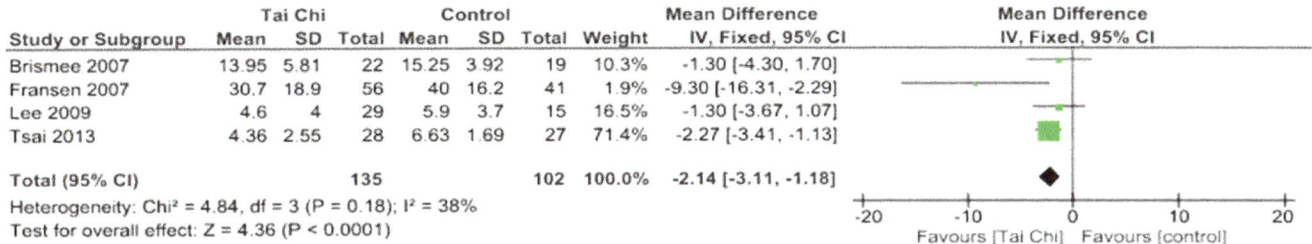

Figure 5. Pain: Tai Chi versus Control.

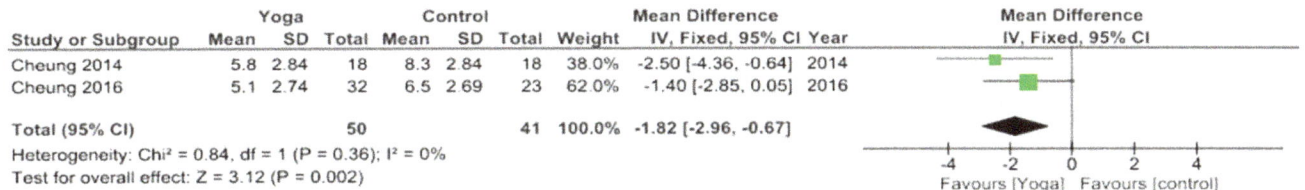

	Yoga			Control				Mean Difference		Mean Difference
Study or Subgroup	Mean	SD	Total	Mean	SD	Total	Weight	IV, Fixed, 95% CI	Year	IV, Fixed, 95% CI
Cheung 2014	5.8	2.84	18	8.3	2.84	18	38.0%	-2.50 [-4.36, -0.64]	2014	
Cheung 2016	5.1	2.74	32	6.5	2.69	23	62.0%	-1.40 [-2.85, 0.05]	2016	
Total (95% CI)			50			41	100.0%	-1.82 [-2.96, -0.67]		

Heterogeneity: Chi² = 0.84, df = 1 (P = 0.36); I² = 0%
Test for overall effect: Z = 3.12 (P = 0.002)

-4 -2 0 2 4
Favours [Yoga] Favours [control]

Figure 6. Pain: Yoga versus Control.

3.7.2. Physical Function

Physical function was assessed using the WOMAC physical function scale and KOOS ADL. It has been demonstrated no significant physical function improvements (SMD 0.35, 95% CI 0.05 to 0.65) and no heterogeneity (I^2 = 0%) between aquatic exercise and land-based exercise (Figure 7). Compared to controls for increase of physical function, aquatic exercise showed significant differences (SMD −0.39, 95% CI −0.62 to −0.16) and no heterogeneity (I^2 = 0%) (Figure 8), land-based exercise presented significant differences (SMD −0.45, 95% CI −0.74 to −0.17) and high heterogeneity (I^2 = 57%) (Figure 9), Tai Chi had significant differences (MD −6.80, 95% CI −9.88 to −3.73) and low heterogeneity (I^2 = 2%) (Figure 10), Yoga reported significant differences (MD −6.07, 95% CI −9.75 to −2.39) without heterogeneity (I^2 = 0%) (Figure 11).

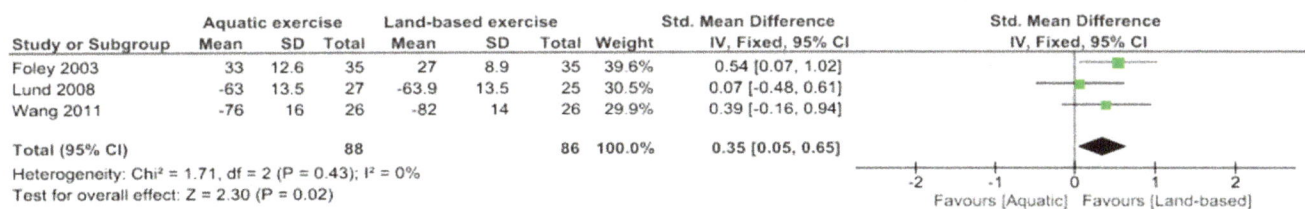

	Aquatic exercise			Land-based exercise				Std. Mean Difference	Std. Mean Difference
Study or Subgroup	Mean	SD	Total	Mean	SD	Total	Weight	IV, Fixed, 95% CI	IV, Fixed, 95% CI
Foley 2003	33	12.6	35	27	8.9	35	39.6%	0.54 [0.07, 1.02]	
Lund 2008	-63	13.5	27	-63.9	13.5	25	30.5%	0.07 [-0.48, 0.61]	
Wang 2011	-76	16	26	-82	14	26	29.9%	0.39 [-0.16, 0.94]	
Total (95% CI)			88			86	100.0%	0.35 [0.05, 0.65]	

Heterogeneity: Chi² = 1.71, df = 2 (P = 0.43); I² = 0%
Test for overall effect: Z = 2.30 (P = 0.02)

-2 -1 0 1 2
Favours [Aquatic] Favours [Land-based]

Figure 7. Function: Aquatic exercise versus Land-based exercise.

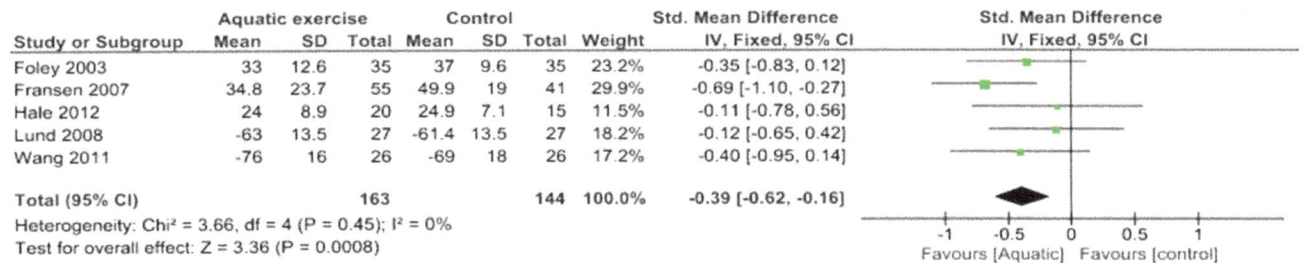

	Aquatic exercise			Control				Std. Mean Difference	Std. Mean Difference
Study or Subgroup	Mean	SD	Total	Mean	SD	Total	Weight	IV, Fixed, 95% CI	IV, Fixed, 95% CI
Foley 2003	33	12.6	35	37	9.6	35	23.2%	-0.35 [-0.83, 0.12]	
Fransen 2007	34.8	23.7	55	49.9	19	41	29.9%	-0.69 [-1.10, -0.27]	
Hale 2012	24	8.9	20	24.9	7.1	15	11.5%	-0.11 [-0.78, 0.56]	
Lund 2008	-63	13.5	27	-61.4	13.5	27	18.2%	-0.12 [-0.65, 0.42]	
Wang 2011	-76	16	26	-69	18	26	17.2%	-0.40 [-0.95, 0.14]	
Total (95% CI)			163			144	100.0%	-0.39 [-0.62, -0.16]	

Heterogeneity: Chi² = 3.66, df = 4 (P = 0.45); I² = 0%
Test for overall effect: Z = 3.36 (P = 0.0008)

-1 -0.5 0 0.5 1
Favours [Aquatic] Favours [control]

Figure 8. Function: Aquatic exercise versus Control.

Study or Subgroup	Land-based exercise Mean	SD	Total	Control Mean	SD	Total	Weight	Std. Mean Difference IV, Random, 95% CI
Bearne 2011	11.1	7.9	24	13.8	10.6	24	12.8%	-0.28 [-0.85, 0.28]
Cheung 2016	25.8	8.37	28	25.2	8.44	23	13.2%	0.07 [-0.48, 0.62]
Foley 2003	27	8.9	35	37	9.6	35	14.5%	-1.07 [-1.57, -0.57]
Hurley 2007	21.6	11.2	229	25	11.4	113	22.9%	-0.30 [-0.53, -0.07]
Lund 2008	-63.9	13.5	25	-61.4	13.5	27	13.4%	-0.18 [-0.73, 0.36]
Takacs 2017	20	11	17	28	10	19	10.5%	-0.75 [-1.43, -0.07]
Wang 2011	-82	14	26	-69	18	26	12.9%	-0.79 [-1.36, -0.23]
Total (95% CI)			384			267	100.0%	-0.45 [-0.74, -0.17]

Heterogeneity: Tau² = 0.08; Chi² = 13.94, df = 6 (P = 0.03); I² = 57%
Test for overall effect: Z = 3.17 (P = 0.002)

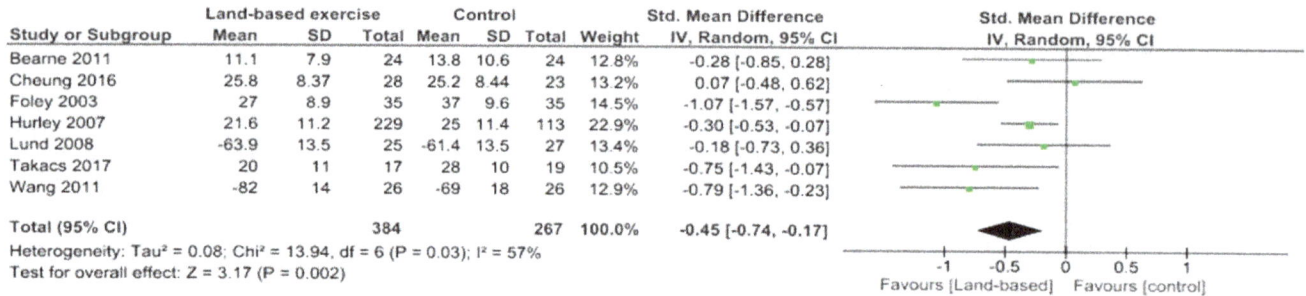

Figure 9. Function: Land-based exercise versus Control.

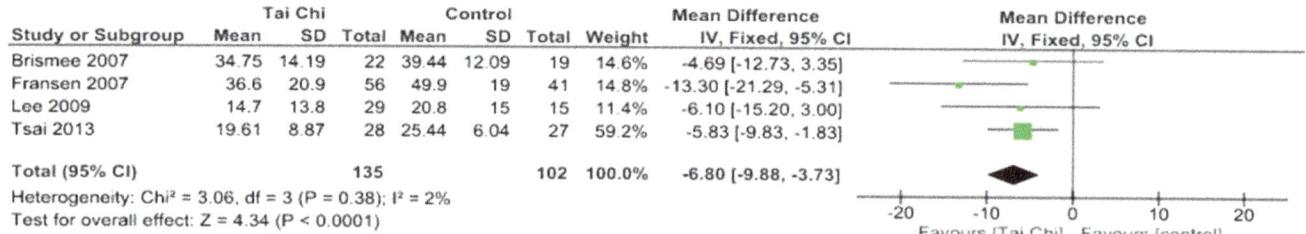

Study or Subgroup	Tai Chi Mean	SD	Total	Control Mean	SD	Total	Weight	Mean Difference IV, Fixed, 95% CI
Brismee 2007	34.75	14.19	22	39.44	12.09	19	14.6%	-4.69 [-12.73, 3.35]
Fransen 2007	36.6	20.9	56	49.9	19	41	14.8%	-13.30 [-21.29, -5.31]
Lee 2009	14.7	13.8	29	20.8	15	15	11.4%	-6.10 [-15.20, 3.00]
Tsai 2013	19.61	8.87	28	25.44	6.04	27	59.2%	-5.83 [-9.83, -1.83]
Total (95% CI)			135			102	100.0%	-6.80 [-9.88, -3.73]

Heterogeneity: Chi² = 3.06, df = 3 (P = 0.38); I² = 2%
Test for overall effect: Z = 4.34 (P < 0.0001)

Figure 10. Function: Tai Chi versus Control.

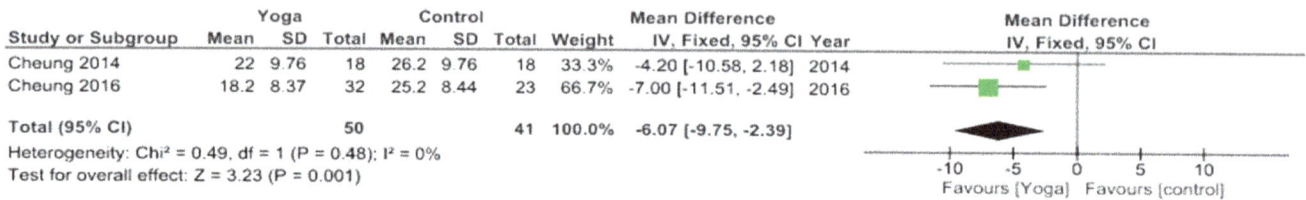

Study or Subgroup	Yoga Mean	SD	Total	Control Mean	SD	Total	Weight	Mean Difference IV, Fixed, 95% CI	Year
Cheung 2014	22	9.76	18	26.2	9.76	18	33.3%	-4.20 [-10.58, 2.18]	2014
Cheung 2016	18.2	8.37	32	25.2	8.44	23	66.7%	-7.00 [-11.51, -2.49]	2016
Total (95% CI)			50			41	100.0%	-6.07 [-9.75, -2.39]	

Heterogeneity: Chi² = 0.49, df = 1 (P = 0.48); I² = 0%
Test for overall effect: Z = 3.23 (P = 0.001)

Figure 11. Function: Yoga versus Control.

3.7.3. Quality of Life

Quality of life was evaluated by KOOS QOL and SF-12. The meta-analysis showed no significant improvement in quality of life (SMD −0.20, 95% CI −0.50 to 0.10) and moderate heterogeneity (I^2 = 54%) in the aquatic exercise compared to land-based exercise (Figure 12). Compared to controls for effect on the quality of life, aquatic exercise produced significant differences (SMD −0.43, 95% CI −0.67 to −0.19) and moderate heterogeneity (I^2 = 51%) (Figure 13), while land-based exercise reported no significant differences (SMD −0.27, 95% CI −0.54 to −0.01) and no heterogeneity (I^2 = 0%) (Figure 14).

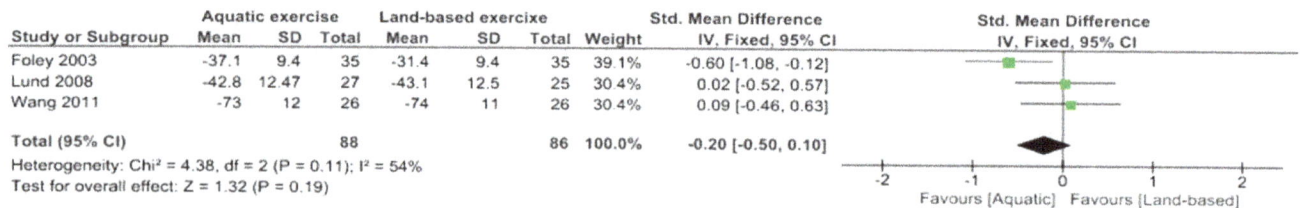

Study or Subgroup	Aquatic exercise Mean	SD	Total	Land-based exercixe Mean	SD	Total	Weight	Std. Mean Difference IV, Fixed, 95% CI
Foley 2003	-37.1	9.4	35	-31.4	9.4	35	39.1%	-0.60 [-1.08, -0.12]
Lund 2008	-42.8	12.47	27	-43.1	12.5	25	30.4%	0.02 [-0.52, 0.57]
Wang 2011	-73	12	26	-74	11	26	30.4%	0.09 [-0.46, 0.63]
Total (95% CI)			88			86	100.0%	-0.20 [-0.50, 0.10]

Heterogeneity: Chi² = 4.38, df = 2 (P = 0.11); I² = 54%
Test for overall effect: Z = 1.32 (P = 0.19)

Figure 12. Quality of Life: Aquatic exercise versus Land-based exercise.

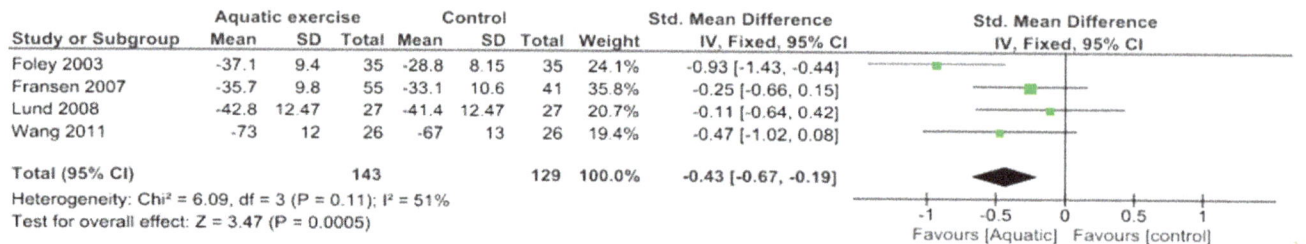

Study or Subgroup	Aquatic exercise Mean	SD	Total	Control Mean	SD	Total	Weight	Std. Mean Difference IV, Fixed, 95% CI
Foley 2003	-37.1	9.4	35	-28.8	8.15	35	24.1%	-0.93 [-1.43, -0.44]
Fransen 2007	-35.7	9.8	55	-33.1	10.6	41	35.8%	-0.25 [-0.66, 0.15]
Lund 2008	-42.8	12.47	27	-41.4	12.47	27	20.7%	-0.11 [-0.64, 0.42]
Wang 2011	-73	12	26	-67	13	26	19.4%	-0.47 [-1.02, 0.08]
Total (95% CI)			143			129	100.0%	-0.43 [-0.67, -0.19]

Heterogeneity: Chi² = 6.09, df = 3 (P = 0.11); I² = 51%
Test for overall effect: Z = 3.47 (P = 0.0005)

Figure 13. Quality of Life: Aquatic exercise versus Control.

Study or Subgroup	Land-based exercise			Control			Weight	Std. Mean Difference IV, Fixed, 95% CI
	Mean	SD	Total	Mean	SD	Total		
Cheung 2016	-53.8	9.18	28	-52.8	12.48	23	22.8%	-0.09 [-0.64, 0.46]
Foley 2003	-31.4	9.4	35	-28.8	8.15	35	31.3%	-0.29 [-0.76, 0.18]
Lund 2008	-43.1	12.5	25	-41.4	12.47	27	23.4%	-0.13 [-0.68, 0.41]
Wang 2011	-74	11	26	-67	13	26	22.5%	-0.57 [-1.13, -0.02]
Total (95% CI)			114			111	100.0%	-0.27 [-0.54, -0.01]

Heterogeneity: Chi² = 1.79, df = 3 (P = 0.62); I² = 0%
Test for overall effect: Z = 2.03 (P = 0.04)

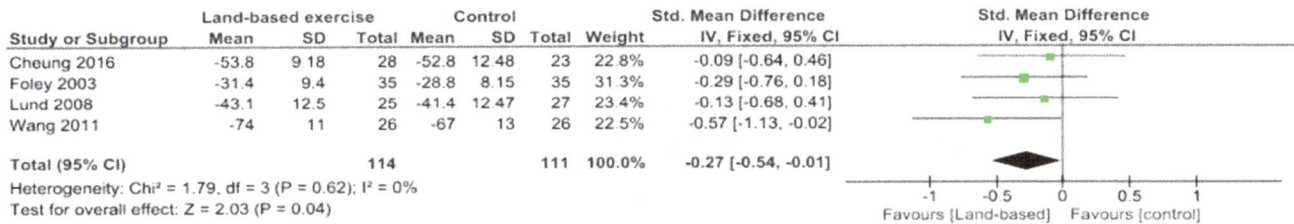

Figure 14. Quality of Life: Land-based exercise versus Control.

3.7.4. Stiffness

Stiffness was checked with the WOMAC stiffness scale. The meta-analysis presented no significant reduction of stiffness (MD 0.16, 95% CI −0.55 to 0.87) and no heterogeneity (I² = 0%) in the aquatic exercise compared to the control group (Figure 15). Similarly, in the land-based exercise, there was no significant decrease of stiffness (MD −0.05, 95% CI −0.66 to 0.56) and no heterogeneity (I² = 0%) compared to the controls (Figure 16). Compared to controls improvement of stiffness, Tai Chi showed significant differences (MD −0.74, 95% CI −1.22 to −0.26) and moderate heterogeneity (I² = 42%) (Figure 17), and Yoga reported significant differences (MD −1.06, 95% CI −1.63 to −0.50) without heterogeneity (I² = 0%) (Figure 18).

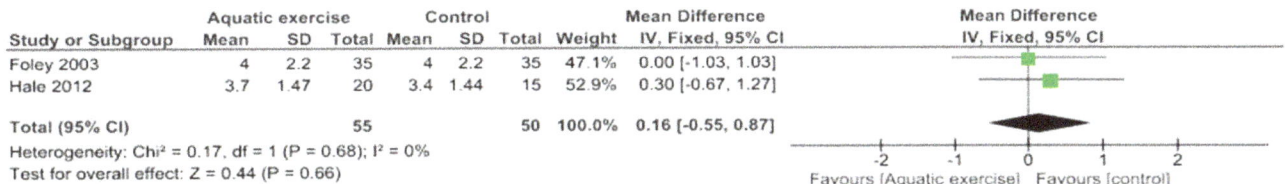

Study or Subgroup	Aquatic exercise			Control			Weight	Mean Difference IV, Fixed, 95% CI
	Mean	SD	Total	Mean	SD	Total		
Foley 2003	4	2.2	35	4	2.2	35	47.1%	0.00 [-1.03, 1.03]
Hale 2012	3.7	1.47	20	3.4	1.44	15	52.9%	0.30 [-0.67, 1.27]
Total (95% CI)			55			50	100.0%	0.16 [-0.55, 0.87]

Heterogeneity: Chi² = 0.17, df = 1 (P = 0.68); I² = 0%
Test for overall effect: Z = 0.44 (P = 0.66)

Figure 15. Stiffness: Aquatic exercise versus Control.

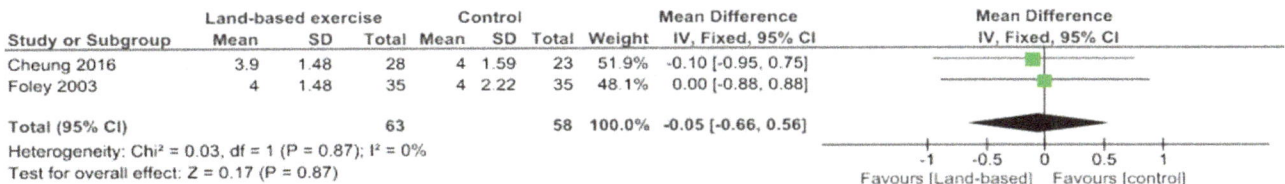

Study or Subgroup	Land-based exercise			Control			Weight	Mean Difference IV, Fixed, 95% CI
	Mean	SD	Total	Mean	SD	Total		
Cheung 2016	3.9	1.48	28	4	1.59	23	51.9%	-0.10 [-0.95, 0.75]
Foley 2003	4	1.48	35	4	2.22	35	48.1%	0.00 [-0.88, 0.88]
Total (95% CI)			63			58	100.0%	-0.05 [-0.66, 0.56]

Heterogeneity: Chi² = 0.03, df = 1 (P = 0.87); I² = 0%
Test for overall effect: Z = 0.17 (P = 0.87)

Figure 16. Stiffness: Land-based exercise versus Control.

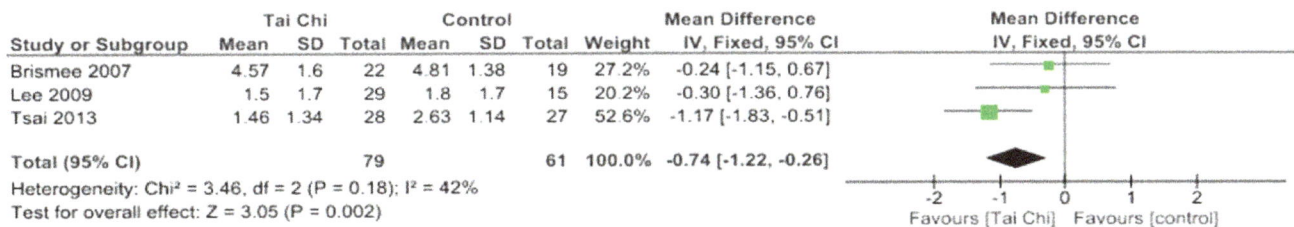

Study or Subgroup	Tai Chi			Control			Weight	Mean Difference IV, Fixed, 95% CI
	Mean	SD	Total	Mean	SD	Total		
Brismee 2007	4.57	1.6	22	4.81	1.38	19	27.2%	-0.24 [-1.15, 0.67]
Lee 2009	1.5	1.7	29	1.8	1.7	15	20.2%	-0.30 [-1.36, 0.76]
Tsai 2013	1.46	1.34	28	2.63	1.14	27	52.6%	-1.17 [-1.83, -0.51]
Total (95% CI)			79			61	100.0%	-0.74 [-1.22, -0.26]

Heterogeneity: Chi² = 3.46, df = 2 (P = 0.18); I² = 42%
Test for overall effect: Z = 3.05 (P = 0.002)

Figure 17. Stiffness: Tai Chi versus Control.

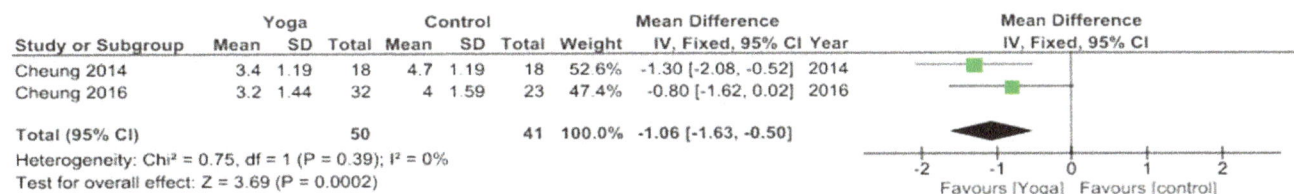

Study or Subgroup	Yoga			Control			Weight	Mean Difference IV, Fixed, 95% CI	Year
	Mean	SD	Total	Mean	SD	Total			
Cheung 2014	3.4	1.19	18	4.7	1.19	18	52.6%	-1.30 [-2.08, -0.52]	2014
Cheung 2016	3.2	1.44	32	4	1.59	23	47.4%	-0.80 [-1.62, 0.02]	2016
Total (95% CI)			50			41	100.0%	-1.06 [-1.63, -0.50]	

Heterogeneity: Chi² = 0.75, df = 1 (P = 0.39); I² = 0%
Test for overall effect: Z = 3.69 (P = 0.0002)

Figure 18. Stiffness: Yoga versus Control.

3.7.5. Dynamic Balance

Only aquatic exercise studies evaluated the dynamic balance by the Time Up and Go test. It has been reported significant improvement of dynamic balance (MD −1.62, 95% CI −1.99 to −1.25) and low heterogeneity ($I^2 = 8\%$) in the aquatic exercise in comparison with controls (Figure 19).

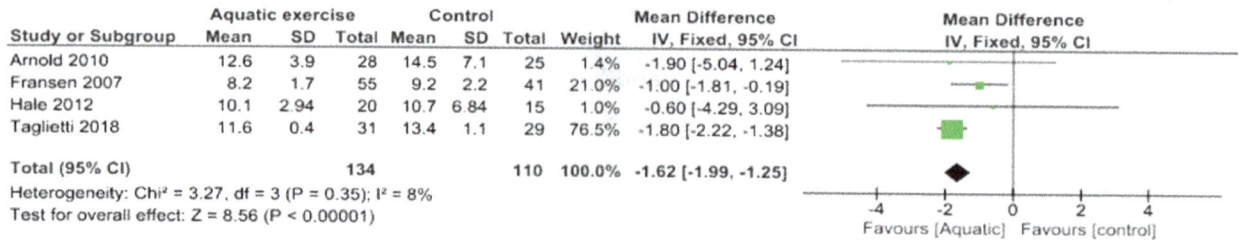

Study or Subgroup	Aquatic exercise Mean	SD	Total	Control Mean	SD	Total	Weight	Mean Difference IV, Fixed, 95% CI
Arnold 2010	12.6	3.9	28	14.5	7.1	25	1.4%	-1.90 [-5.04, 1.24]
Fransen 2007	8.2	1.7	55	9.2	2.2	41	21.0%	-1.00 [-1.81, -0.19]
Hale 2012	10.1	2.94	20	10.7	6.84	15	1.0%	-0.60 [-4.29, 3.09]
Taglietti 2018	11.6	0.4	31	13.4	1.1	29	76.5%	-1.80 [-2.22, -1.38]
Total (95% CI)			134			110	100.0%	-1.62 [-1.99, -1.25]

Heterogeneity: Chi² = 3.27, df = 3 (P = 0.35); I² = 8%
Test for overall effect: Z = 8.56 (P < 0.00001)

Figure 19. Dynamic Balance: Aquatic exercise versus Control.

3.8. Quality Assessment

The quality of the evidence of the included studies was assessed for 18 comparisons using the GRADE system (Table 5). Of these, 15 comparisons were downgraded by one level due to serious risk of bias, especially as regarded the lack of blinding; therefore, they presented a moderate quality. The remaining three comparisons were downgraded by two levels due to serious risk of bias and inconsistency because there was significant and unexplained variability in results from different trials.

Table 5. GRADE.

Outcomes	Comparisons	n of Participants (Studies)	Risk of Bias	Inconsistency	Indirectness	Imprecision	Other Considerations	Quality
Pain	Aquatic vs. Land-based	174 (3 RCT)	serious	not serious	not serious	not serious	not serious	⊕⊕⊕○ moderate
Function	Aquatic vs. Land-based	174 (3 RCT)	serious	not serious	not serious	not serious	not serious	⊕⊕⊕○ moderate
Quality of Life	Aquatic vs. Land-based	174 (3 RCT)	serious	serious	not serious	not serious	not serious	⊕⊕○○ low
Pain	Aquatic vs. Control	367 (6 RCT)	serious	serious	not serious	not serious	not serious	⊕⊕○○ low
Function	Aquatic vs. Control	307 (5 RCT)	serious	not serious	not serious	not serious	not serious	⊕⊕⊕○ moderate
Quality of Life	Aquatic vs. Control	272 (4 RCT)	serious	not serious	not serious	not serious	not serious	⊕⊕⊕○ moderate
Stiffness	Aquatic vs. Control	105 (2 RCT)	serious	serious	not serious	not serious	not serious	⊕⊕○○ low
Dynamic Balance	Aquatic vs. Control	244 (4 RCT)	serious	not serious	not serious	not serious	not serious	⊕⊕⊕○ moderate
Pain	Land-based vs. Control	682 (7 RCT)	serious	not serious	not serious	not serious	not serious	⊕⊕⊕○ moderate
Function	Land-based vs. Control	651 (7 RCT)	serious	not serious	not serious	not serious	not serious	⊕⊕⊕○ moderate
Quality of Life	Land-based vs. Control	225 (4 RCT)	serious	not serious	not serious	not serious	not serious	⊕⊕⊕○ moderate
Stiffness	Land-based vs. Control	121 (2 RCT)	serious	not serious	not serious	not serious	not serious	⊕⊕⊕○ moderate
Pain	Tai Chi vs. Control	237 (4 RCT)	serious	not serious	not serious	not serious	not serious	⊕⊕⊕○ moderate
Function	Tai Chi vs. Control	237 (4 RCT)	serious	not serious	not serious	not serious	not serious	⊕⊕⊕○ moderate
Stiffness	Tai Chi vs. Control	140 (3 RCT)	serious	not serious	not serious	not serious	not serious	⊕⊕⊕○ moderate
Pain	Yoga vs. Control	91 (2 RCT)	serious	not serious	not serious	not serious	not serious	⊕⊕⊕○ moderate
Function	Yoga vs. Control	91 (2 RCT)	serious	not serious	not serious	not serious	not serious	⊕⊕⊕○ moderate
Stiffness	Yoga vs. Control	91 (2 RCT)	serious	not serious	not serious	not serious	not serious	⊕⊕⊕○ moderate

RCT: Randomized Clinical Trial.

4. Discussion

The primary aim of this systematic review and meta-analysis was to summarize the evidence of the efficiency of various types of physical activity on pain, physical function, stiffness, quality of life, and dynamic balance in patients aged 65 or over with knee and hip OA. Another endpoint was to examine either land-based active exercise, aquatic active exercise, and sports, in order to establish greater improvements. Physical activity has shown to be very beneficial for older people with knee and hip OA in terms of pain reduction, better function, performance, and quality of life, with statistically significant improvements compared to the control group. Nevertheless, it was not possible to determine with certainty greater long-term benefits of one type of physical activity compared to the others, also considering the different rates of adherence, and adverse events. The literature review produced almost exclusively RCTs, and this could be justified by the fact that the follow-up was short, and after the follow-up, the control group could have received the same training program as the treatment group. A limitation of this study was represented by the fact that only five studies were composed of three arms, of which two intervention groups and one control group. Three studies (32–34) with two intervention groups presented in the quantitative analysis quite contrasting results about variations in pain and physical function after treatments when comparing land-based with aquatic active exercise; however, showing improvements of both interventions compared to the control group. Also, when comparing Tai Chi or Yoga with aquatic and aerobic exercise [30,35], there were uncertain results on symptom improvement, pain relief, and perceived function. In five studies [44,45,47–49], active exercise represented the only intervention group, and in all of those participants in the study group showed significant improvement in the checked outcomes, such as WOMAC, KOOS, VAS, 6-MWT, and get-up-and-go test. On the other hand, only one study [43] reported no differences between the rehabilitation group and the control group in any outcome measure. When analyzing sports, such as Tai Chi, Yoga, or Baduanjin, all the studies presented significant improvements in pain, physical function, stiffness, and quality of life after the treatment. The quality of the RCTs was determined by the Cochrane Risk of Bias Tool. 18 out of 22 studies presented an unclear or high risk of bias, and it was caused by the inability of blinding personnel and participants when performing physical activity interventions, even more, if control groups underwent no intervention. In fact, the blinding tool of Cochrane Risk of Bias was inadequate or unclear in all the studies selected. Two case series [29,50] were evaluated using the MINORS score. They presented an average score of 11.5 points on a maximum of 24, influenced by the fact that they were non-comparative studies, thus resulting in 0 points in 4 of 12 items. Dong et al. [52] presented no significant difference for pain relief and physical function between aquatic exercise and land-based exercise for patients with knee OA, for both short- and long-term interventions. Goh et al. [53] studied the relative efficacy of different exercises for patients with knee and hip OA. In their systematic review, pain, function, and performance were significantly better with all types of exercise than usual care. Aerobic was the most beneficial exercise for pain and performance, whereas mind-body was also the best for pain and function. Moreover, strengthening and flexibility exercises improved multiple outcomes at a moderate level, while mixed exercise was the least effective for all outcomes, superior only to usual care. Bartels et al. [22] proved that aquatic exercise produced a small short-term advancement compared to no intervention in pain, disability, and quality of life for people with knee or hip OA. In a systematic review and meta-analysis by Lauche et al. [54], participants with knee osteoarthritis training Tai Chi presented an increase of pain, physical function and stiffness with moderate evidence and an increase of quality of life with strong evidence. Cheung et al. [51] demonstrated the effectiveness of yoga to reduce pain, stiffness, and swelling, even if, in their review, the results on physical function were inconclusive because of a variety of outcome measures being used. Another limitation of this review was due to the heterogeneity of the included studies, which presented different scores with various primary and secondary outcomes, different protocols—especially for aquatic and land-based exercise—with distinct types of exercise, different timings of follow-up with variable duration of the single session and the entire program. Therefore, it was not possible to clearly compare the obtained results of the different study groups, although it was evident the efficacy of every type of physical activity compared to the control groups. Furthermore, adherence to physical activity was reported by 14 of the included studies. In these studies, the adherence to the programs was high, with an attendance of about 80% at the rehabilitation sessions, without significant differences between land-based and aquatic exercise and sport, although that attendance was higher in hydrotherapy when compared with other intervention groups [30,37,38]. The adherence to a physical exercise regimen is essential in order to improve physical performance and function and reduce pain, especially in older patients. Van Gool et al. [55] proved that higher exercise adherence leads to improvements in physical performance and self-reported disability in older adults with knee OA. All the included studies presented the details of dropouts. Twelve studies reported the adverse events that happened over the treatment period. In 4 studies no side effects, complications, or injuries were reported during the physical program [33,34,41,45]. Muscle soreness, increased foot and knee pain, and low back pain after exercise were the most common adverse effect, while they were recorded in a few patients [31,35,36,39,42,49]. Arnold et al. [42] described one moderate adverse effect, that consisted of spinal pain due to a fall. In a study by Fransen et al. [30], 11 participants presented a serious adverse, which were not related to the intervention. Lund et al. reported [38] 11 adverse effects in the land-based group and three adverse effects in the aquatic group ($p = 0.012$).

5. Conclusions

This review and meta-analysis show that all active exercise and sport are an effective conservative treatment for elderly people with OA, in order to improve pain and physical function. The meta-analysis reported no significant differences in improvements in pain, physical function, and QOL between aquatic and land-based exercise. Compared to controls, the aquatic exercise showed significant differences for pain reduction and increase of physical function, quality of live and dynamic balance, land-based exercise presented significant differences for physical function, Tai Chi and Yoga demonstrated significant differences in improvements in pain, physical function, and stiffness. However, the number of studies in this research area is still too few to establish which physical activity leads to better improvement in pain, physical function, stiffness, and quality of life. More high-quality studies with a lower risk of bias are needed in order to support these results, and they should be designed as RCTs comparing aquatic exercise with land-based exercise and sport. Moreover, in future studies aquatic and land-based exercise should be standardized, with the creation of an exercise protocol explaining the program, the frequency and the duration of the exercise's sessions and with the use of similar scores, in order to produce comparable data, to avoid dropouts and to increase the adherence to the programs.

Author Contributions: Conceptualization, R.P. and V.D.; methodology, G.F.P., and B.Z.; writing—original draft preparation, G.F.P. and B.Z.; writing—review and editing, S.C., S.V., and F.V.; supervision, C.F. and G.T.; funding acquisition, R.P. All authors have read and agreed to the published version of the manuscript.

References

1.　Glyn-Jones, S.; Palmer, A.J.R.; Agricola, R.; Price, A.J.; Vincent, T.L.; Weinans, H.; Carr, A.J. Osteoarthritis. *Lancet* **2015**, *386*, 376–387. [CrossRef]

2.　van Dijk, G.M.; Dekker, J.; Veenhof, C.; van den Ende, C.H.M. Carpa Study Group Course of functional status and pain in osteoarthritis of the hip or knee: A systematic review of the literature. *Arthritis Rheum.* **2006**, *55*, 779–785. [CrossRef] [PubMed]

3.　Ojoawo, A.O.; Olaogun, M.O.B.; Hassan, M.A. Comparative effects of proprioceptive and isometric exercises on pain intensity and difficulty in patients with knee osteoarthritis: A randomised control study. *Technol. Health Care* **2016**, *24*, 853–863. [CrossRef] [PubMed]

4. Clynes, M.A.; Jameson, K.A.; Edwards, M.H.; Cooper, C.; Dennison, E.M. Impact of osteoarthritis on activities of daily living: Does joint site matter? *Aging Clin. Exp. Res.* **2019**, *31*, 1049–1056. [CrossRef] [PubMed]

5. Johnson, V.L.; Hunter, D.J. The epidemiology of osteoarthritis. *Best Pract. Res. Clin. Rheumatol.* **2014**, *28*, 5–15. [CrossRef]

6. Segal, N.A.; Glass, N.A.; Teran-Yengle, P.; Singh, B.; Wallace, R.B.; Yack, H.J. Intensive Gait Training for Older Adults with Symptomatic Knee Osteoarthritis. *Am. J. Phys. Med. Rehabil.* **2015**, *94*, 848–858. [CrossRef]

7. Papalia, R.; Zampogna, B.; Torre, G.; Lanotte, A.; Vasta, S.; Albo, E.; Tecame, A.; Denaro, V. Sarcopenia and its relationship with osteoarthritis: Risk factor or direct consequence? *Musculoskelet. Surg.* **2014**, *98*, 9–14. [CrossRef]

8. Litwic, A.; Edwards, M.H.; Dennison, E.M.; Cooper, C. Epidemiology and burden of osteoarthritis. *Br. Med. Bull.* **2013**, *105*, 185–199. [CrossRef]

9. Kamaruzaman, H.; Kinghorn, P.; Oppong, R. Cost-effectiveness of surgical interventions for the management of osteoarthritis: A systematic review of the literature. *BMC Musculoskelet. Disord.* **2017**, *18*, 183. [CrossRef]

10. Rodriguez-Merchan, E.C. Conservative treatment of acute knee osteoarthritis: A review of the Cochrane Library. *J. Acute Dis.* **2016**, *5*, 190–193. [CrossRef]

11. Vaishya, R.; Pariyo, G.B.; Agarwal, A.K.; Vijay, V. Non-operative management of osteoarthritis of the knee joint. *J. Clin. Orthop. Trauma* **2016**, *7*, 170–176. [CrossRef] [PubMed]

12. Papalia, R.; Zampogna, B.; Russo, F.; Torre, G.; De Salvatore, S.; Nobile, C.; Tirindelli, M.C.; Grasso, A.; Vadalà, G.; Denaro, V.; et al. The combined use of platelet rich plasma and hyaluronic acid: Prospective results for the treatment of knee osteoarthritis. *J. Biol. Regul. Homeost. Agents* **2019**, *33*, 21–28. [PubMed]

13. Wellsandt, E.; Golightly, Y. Exercise in the management of knee and hip osteoarthritis. *Curr. Opin. Rheumatol.* **2018**, *30*, 151–159. [CrossRef] [PubMed]

14. Fernandopulle, S.; Perry, M.; Manlapaz, D.; Jayakaran, P. Effect of Land-Based Generic Physical Activity Interventions on Pain, Physical Function, and Physical Performance in Hip and Knee Osteoarthritis. *Am. J. Phys. Med. Rehabil.* **2017**, *96*, 773–792. [CrossRef]

15. Kraus, V.B.; Sprow, K.; Powell, K.E.; Buchner, D.; Bloodgood, B.; Piercy, K.; George, S.M.; Kraus, W.E. Effects of Physical Activity in Knee and Hip Osteoarthritis: A Systematic Umbrella Review. *Med. Sci. Sports Exerc.* **2019**, *51*, 1324–1339. [CrossRef]

16. Gademan, M.G.J.; Hofstede, S.N.; Vliet Vlieland, T.P.M.; Nelissen, R.G.H.H.; Marang-van de Mheen, P.J. Indication criteria for total hip or knee arthroplasty in osteoarthritis: A state-of-the-science overview. *BMC Musculoskelet. Disord.* **2016**, *17*, 463. [CrossRef]

17. Van Ginckel, A.; Hall, M.; Dobson, F.; Calders, P. Effects of long-term exercise therapy on knee joint structure in people with knee osteoarthritis: A systematic review and meta-analysis. *Semin. Arthritis Rheum.* **2018**, *48*, 941–949. [CrossRef]

18. Bartholdy, C.; Juhl, C.; Christensen, R.; Lund, H.; Zhang, W.; Henriksen, M. The role of muscle strengthening in exercise therapy for knee osteoarthritis: A systematic review and meta-regression analysis of randomized trials. *Semin. Arthritis Rheum.* **2017**, *47*, 9–21. [CrossRef]

19. Ageberg, E.; Roos, E.M. Neuromuscular Exercise as Treatment of Degenerative Knee Disease. *Exerc. Sport Sci. Rev.* **2015**, *43*, 14–22. [CrossRef]

20. Hurley, M.V.; Mitchell, H.L.; Walsh, N. In Osteoarthritis, the Psychosocial Benefits of Exercise Are as Important as Physiological Improvements. *Exerc. Sport Sci. Rev.* **2003**, *31*, 138–143. [CrossRef]

21. Wang, T.-J.; Belza, B.; Elaine Thompson, F.; Whitney, J.D.; Bennett, K. Effects of aquatic exercise on flexibility, strength and aerobic fitness in adults with osteoarthritis of the hip or knee. *J. Adv. Nurs.* **2007**, *57*, 141–152. [CrossRef] [PubMed]

22. Bartels, E.M.; Juhl, C.B.; Christensen, R.; Hagen, K.B.; Danneskiold-Samsøe, B.; Dagfinrud, H.; Lund, H. Aquatic exercise for the treatment of knee and hip osteoarthritis. *Cochrane Database Syst. Rev.* **2016**. [CrossRef] [PubMed]

23. Molloy, M.G.; Molloy, C.B. Contact sport and osteoarthritis. *Br. J. Sports Med.* **2011**, *45*, 275–277. [CrossRef] [PubMed]

24. Valderrabano, V.; Steiger, C. Treatment and Prevention of Osteoarthritis through Exercise and Sports. *J. Aging Res.* **2011**, *2011*, 1–6. [CrossRef]

25. Moher, D.; Liberati, A.; Tetzlaff, J.; Altman, D.G. Preferred Reporting Items for Systematic Reviews and Meta-Analyses: The PRISMA Statement. *PLoS Med.* **2009**, *6*, 7. [CrossRef]

26.   Armijo-Olivo, S.; Stiles, C.R.; Hagen, N.A.; Biondo, P.D.; Cummings, G.G. Assessment of study quality for systematic reviews: A comparison of the Cochrane Collaboration Risk of Bias Tool and the Effective Public Health Practice Project Quality Assessment Tool: Methodological research: Quality assessment for systematic reviews. *J. Eval. Clin. Pract.* **2012**, *18*, 12–18. [CrossRef]

27.   Slim, K.; Nini, E.; Forestier, D.; Kwiatkowski, F.; Panis, Y.; Chipponi, J. Methodological Index for Non-Randomized Studies (Minors): Development And Validation of A New Instrument. *ANZ J. Surg.* **2003**, *73*, 712–716. [CrossRef]

28.   Gopalakrishna, G.; Mustafa, R.A.; Davenport, C.; Scholten, R.J.P.M.; Hyde, C.; Brozek, J.; Schünemann, H.J.; Bossuyt, P.M.M.; Leeflang, M.M.G.; Langendam, M.W. Applying Grading of Recommendations Assessment, Development and Evaluation (GRADE) to diagnostic tests was challenging but doable. *J. Clin. Epidemiol.* **2014**, *67*, 760–768. [CrossRef]

29.   Bove, A.M.; Baker, N.; Livengood, H.; King, V.; Mancino, J.; Popchak, A.; Fitzgerald, G.K. Task-Specific Training for Adults With Chronic Knee Pain: A Case Series. *J. Orthop. Sports Phys. Ther.* **2017**, *47*, 548–556. [CrossRef]

30.   Fransen, M.; Nairn, L.; Winstanley, J.; Lam, P.; Edmonds, J. Physical activity for osteoarthritis management: A randomized controlled clinical trial evaluating hydrotherapy or Tai Chi classes. *Arthritis Rheum.* **2007**, *57*, 407–414. [CrossRef]

31.   Brismée, J.-M.; Paige, R.L.; Chyu, M.-C.; Boatright, J.D.; Hagar, J.M.; McCaleb, J.A.; Quintela, M.M.; Feng, D.; Xu, K.T.; Shen, C.-L. Group and home-based tai chi in elderly subjects with knee osteoarthritis: A randomized controlled trial. *Clin. Rehabil.* **2007**, *21*, 99–111. [CrossRef] [PubMed]

32.   Lee, H.-J.; Park, H.-J.; Chae, Y.; Kim, S.-Y.; Kim, S.-N.; Kim, S.-T.; Kim, J.-H.; Yin, C.-S.; Lee, H. Tai Chi Qigong for the quality of life of patients with knee osteoarthritis: A pilot, randomized, waiting list controlled trial. *Clin. Rehabil.* **2009**, *23*, 504–511. [CrossRef] [PubMed]

33.   Tsai, P.-F.; Chang, J.Y.; Beck, C.; Kuo, Y.-F.; Keefe, F.J. A Pilot Cluster-Randomized Trial of a 20-Week Tai Chi Program in Elders With Cognitive Impairment and Osteoarthritic Knee: Effects on Pain and Other Health Outcomes. *J. Pain Symptom Manag.* **2013**, *45*, 660–669. [CrossRef] [PubMed]

34.   Cheung, C.; Wyman, J.F.; Resnick, B.; Savik, K. Yoga for managing knee osteoarthritis in older women: A pilot randomized controlled trial. *BMC Complementary Altern. Med.* **2014**, *14*, 160. [CrossRef] [PubMed]

35.   Cheung, C.; Wyman, J.F.; Bronas, U.; McCarthy, T.; Rudser, K.; Mathiason, M.A. Managing knee osteoarthritis with yoga or aerobic/strengthening exercise programs in older adults: A pilot randomized controlled trial. *Rheumatol. Int.* **2017**, *37*, 389–398. [CrossRef] [PubMed]

36.   Wang, T.-J.; Lee, S.-C.; Liang, S.-Y.; Tung, H.-H.; Wu, S.-F.V.; Lin, Y.-P. Comparing the efficacy of aquatic exercises and land-based exercises for patients with knee osteoarthritis: Efficacy of aquatic vs. land exercises for knee OA. *J. Clin. Nurs.* **2011**, *20*, 2609–2622. [CrossRef]

37.   Foley, A. Does hydrotherapy improve strength and physical function in patients with osteoarthritis—a randomised controlled trial comparing a gym based and a hydrotherapy based strengthening programme. *Ann. Rheum. Dis.* **2003**, *62*, 1162–1167. [CrossRef]

38.   Lund, H.; Weile, U.; Christensen, R.; Rostock, B.; Downey, A.; Bartels, E.; Danneskiold-Samsøe, B.; Bliddal, H. A randomized controlled trial of aquatic and land-based exercise in patients with knee osteoarthritis. *J. Rehabil. Med.* **2008**, *40*, 137–144. [CrossRef]

39.   Hale, L.A.; Waters, D.; Herbison, P. A Randomized Controlled Trial to Investigate the Effects of Water-Based Exercise to Improve Falls Risk and Physical Function in Older Adults With Lower-Extremity Osteoarthritis. *Arch. Phys. Med. Rehabil.* **2012**, *93*, 27–34. [CrossRef]

40.   Casilda-López, J.; Valenza, M.C.; Cabrera-Martos, I.; Díaz-Pelegrina, A.; Moreno-Ramírez, M.P.; Valenza-Demet, G. Effects of a dance-based aquatic exercise program in obese postmenopausal women with knee osteoarthritis: A randomized controlled trial. *Menopause* **2017**, *24*, 768–773. [CrossRef]

41.   Taglietti, M.; Facci, L.M.; Trelha, C.S.; de Melo, F.C.; da Silva, D.W.; Sawczuk, G.; Ruivo, T.M.; de Souza, T.B.; Sforza, C.; Cardoso, J.R. Effectiveness of aquatic exercises compared to patient-education on health status in individuals with knee osteoarthritis: A randomized controlled trial. *Clin. Rehabil.* **2018**, *32*, 766–776. [CrossRef] [PubMed]

42.   Arnold, C.M.; Faulkner, R.A. The Effect of Aquatic Exercise and Education on Lowering Fall Risk in Older Adults With Hip Osteoarthritis. *J. Aging Phys. Act.* **2010**, *18*, 245–260. [CrossRef] [PubMed]

43. Bearne, L.M.; Walsh, N.E.; Jessep, S.; Hurley, M.V. Feasibility of an Exercise-Based Rehabilitation Programme for Chronic Hip Pain: Exercise-Based Rehabilitation for Chronic Hip Pain. *Musculoskelet. Care* **2011**, *9*, 160–168. [CrossRef] [PubMed]

44. Bezalel, T.; Carmeli, E.; Katz-Leurer, M. The effect of a group education programme on pain and function through knowledge acquisition and home-based exercise among patients with knee osteoarthritis: A parallel randomised single-blind clinical trial. *Physiotherapy* **2010**, *96*, 137–143. [CrossRef]

45. Huang, L.; Guo, B.; Xu, F.; Zhao, J. Effects of quadriceps functional exercise with isometric contraction in the treatment of knee osteoarthritis. *Int. J. Rheum. Dis.* **2018**, *21*, 952–959. [CrossRef]

46. Doi, T.; Akai, M.; Fujino, K.; Iwaya, T.; Kurosawa, H.; Hayashi, K.; Marui, E. Effect of Home Exercise of Quadriceps on Knee Osteoarthritis Compared with Nonsteroidal Antiinflammatory Drugs: A Randomized Controlled Trial. *Am. J. Phys. Med. Rehabil.* **2008**, *87*, 258–269. [CrossRef]

47. Marconcin, P.; Espanha, M.; Teles, J.; Bento, P.; Campos, P.; André, R.; Yázigi, F. A randomized controlled trial of a combined self-management and exercise intervention for elderly people with osteoarthritis of the knee: The PLE [2] NO program. *Clin. Rehabil.* **2018**, *32*, 223–232. [CrossRef]

48. Hurley, M.V.; Walsh, N.E.; Mitchell, H.L.; Pimm, T.J.; Patel, A.; Williamson, E.; Jones, R.H.; Dieppe, P.A.; Reeves, B.C. Clinical effectiveness of a rehabilitation program integrating exercise, self-management, and active coping strategies for chronic knee pain: A cluster randomized trial. *Arthritis Rheum.* **2007**, *57*, 1211–1219. [CrossRef]

49. Takacs, J.; Krowchuk, N.M.; Garland, S.J.; Carpenter, M.G.; Hunt, M.A. Dynamic Balance Training Improves Physical Function in Individuals With Knee Osteoarthritis: A Pilot Randomized Controlled Trial. *Arch. Phys. Med. Rehabil.* **2017**, *98*, 1586–1593. [CrossRef]

50. An, B.; Wang, Y.; Jiang, X.; Lu, H.; Fang, Z.; Wang, Y.; Dai, K. Effects of Baduanjin exercise on knee osteoarthritis: A one-year study. *Chin. J. Integr. Med.* **2013**, *19*, 143–148. [CrossRef]

51. Cheung, C.; Park, J.; Wyman, J.F. Effects of Yoga on Symptoms, Physical Function, and Psychosocial Outcomes in Adults with Osteoarthritis: A Focused Review. *Am. J. Phys. Med. Rehabil.* **2016**, *95*, 139–151. [CrossRef] [PubMed]

52. Dong, R.; Wu, Y.; Xu, S.; Zhang, L.; Ying, J.; Jin, H.; Wang, P.; Xiao, L.; Tong, P. Is aquatic exercise more effective than land-based exercise for knee osteoarthritis? *Medicine* **2018**, *97*, e13823. [CrossRef] [PubMed]

53. Goh, S.-L.; Persson, M.S.M.; Stocks, J.; Hou, Y.; Welton, N.J.; Lin, J.; Hall, M.C.; Doherty, M.; Zhang, W. Relative Efficacy of Different Exercises for Pain, Function, Performance and Quality of Life in Knee and Hip Osteoarthritis: Systematic Review and Network Meta-Analysis. *Sports Med.* **2019**, *49*, 743–761. [CrossRef]

54. Lauche, R.; Langhorst, J.; Dobos, G.; Cramer, H. A systematic review and meta-analysis of Tai Chi for osteoarthritis of the knee. *Complementary Ther. Med.* **2013**, *21*, 396–406. [CrossRef]

55. van Gool, C.H.; Penninx, B.W.J.H.; Kempen, G.I.J.M.; Rejeski, W.J.; Miller, G.D.; van Eijk, J.T.M.; Pahor, M.; Messier, S.P. Effects of exercise adherence on physical function among overweight older adults with knee osteoarthritis. *Arthritis Rheum.* **2005**, *53*, 24–32. [CrossRef]

8

The Role of Physical Activity and Rehabilitation Following Hip and Knee Arthroplasty in the Elderly

Rocco Papalia [1], Stefano Campi [1], Ferruccio Vorini [1], Biagio Zampogna [1], Sebastiano Vasta [1], Giuseppe Papalia [1], Chiara Fossati [2], Guglielmo Torre [1,*] and Vincenzo Denaro [1]

[1] Department of Orthopaedic and Trauma Surgery, Campus Bio-Medico University of Rome, 00128 Rome, Italy; r.papalia@unicampus.it (R.P.); s.campi@unicampus.it (S.C.); f.vorini@unicampus.it (F.V.); b.zampogna@unicampus.it (B.Z.); s.vasta@unicampus.it (S.V.); g.papalia@unicampus.it (G.P.); denaro@unicampus.it (V.D.)

[2] Department of Movement, Human and Health Sciences, University of Rome "Foro Italico", 00135 Rome, Italy; chiara.fossati@uniroma4.it

* Correspondence: g.torre@unicampus.it

Abstract: Hip and knee replacement is an effective treatment for symptomatic, end-stage hip and knee osteoarthritis, aiming to relieve pain and restore joint function. Several postoperative rehabilitation protocols and physical activities are proposed in routine clinical practice. However, their effect on clinical outcome and implant revision in patients undergoing joint replacement is still unclear. A systematic review of the literature was performed through a comprehensive search on online databases including Pubmed-Medline, Cochrane central, and Google scholar. We included all the available studies on postoperative physical activity and rehabilitation protocols after total knee and total hip arthroplasty in patients older than 65 years. The primary endpoint was to evaluate the effect of physical activity and rehabilitation on clinical outcome; the secondary outcome was to determine the effect on patients' quality of life (QoL) and implant survival. Although the heterogeneity of the rehabilitation protocols and outcome measures did not allow to draw definitive conclusions, most studies suggested that aquatic therapy, ergometer cycling, and fast-track protocols have a beneficial effect on muscle strength, gait speed, and main clinical scores after total hip arthroplasty. Similarly, enhanced rehabilitation protocols produced an improvement in primary and secondary outcomes after total knee arthroplasty.

Keywords: hip arthroplasty; knee arthroplasty; elderly; physical activity; rehabilitation; physiotherapy

1. Introduction

Osteoarthritis (OA) is a major cause of disability in elderly patients. The prevalence of hip and knee OA has been growing over the last decades, being around 25% in the population between 65 and 85 years of age [1]. OA has a considerable impact on patients' quality of life (QoL), activities of daily living, and general health status. Due to the large number of patients suffering from this condition and the considerable cost of care, OA represents a significant economic burden for healthcare systems [2].

Joint replacement is the only definitive treatment for symptomatic end-stage hip and knee OA, aiming to relieve the pain and restore joint function. Total hip arthroplasty (THA) and total knee arthroplasty (TKA) are usually followed by an intense rehabilitation program focused on muscle strengthening, stretching, range of motion (ROM) recovery, gait rehabilitation, neuromuscular function, and proprioception recovery.

Nowadays, there is an increasing number of elderly people practicing sports and physical activity, whether low-impact (such as cycling, aquafit, golf, swimming) or medium-/high-impact (skiing, running, tennis, dancing, Nordic walking, etc.). Often, patients undergoing hip and knee arthroplasty aim to return to their previous activity level. However, the effect of such activities on the clinical outcome and survival of the implant is still unclear.

Numerous postoperative interventions have been studied, including in-hospital rehabilitation, inpatient rehabilitation, home exercises, tele-rehabilitation, aquatic therapy, and fast-track protocols, but it is still unclear which of these interventions is the most effective following hip and knee arthroplasty in order to achieve a complete functional recovery. Moreover, there is poor evidence about what type of physical activity can be allowed or encouraged without affecting implant survival.

The primary endpoint of this systematic review was to evaluate the impact of physical activity and rehabilitation on clinical objective and subjective outcomes, after TKA and THA. The secondary outcome was to establish the effect of these activities on patients' QoL and on implant revision rates.

2. Materials and Methods

The present systematic review was performed in accordance to the PRISMA guidelines [3] and followed the Cochrane methodology for systematic reviews [4]. The MINORS (methodological index for non-randomized studies) score was used to assess the methodological quality of non-randomized studies [5].

2.1. Primary Outcomes

The primary endpoint was to assess the effect of physical activity and rehabilitation on clinical outcome, measured by validated joint-specific objective and subjective clinical measurements. When reported, the considered outcome measures for THA were the WOMAC (Western Ontario and Mc Master University) index, hip abductor strength, Harris Hip Score (HHS), gait speed, UCLA score, Lequesne Hip/Knee score. The considered outcome measures for TKA were the WOMAC index, Lequesne Hip/Knee score, 10 min walking test, walking speed, stair ascending time, knee extensor and flexor power, thigh muscle cross-sectional area, 6 min walking test (6MWT), Knee Society score (KSS), range of motion (ROM), modified gait efficacy scale (mGES), timed up and go (TUG).

2.2. Secondary Outcomes

The secondary endpoint was to assess the effect of physical activity and rehabilitation on implant revision rates and self-reported quality of life, using questionnaires.

2.3. Search Methods for Identification of the Studies

Online databases, including Pubmed-Medline and Google Scholar, were searched for relevant articles. The search string used was the following: ("sports"(MeSH Terms) OR "sports"(All Fields) OR "sport"(All Fields)) AND ("exercise"(MeSH Terms) OR "exercise"(All Fields) OR ("physical"(All Fields) AND "activity"(All Fields)) OR "physical activity"(All Fields)) AND after(All Fields) AND ("arthroplasty"(MeSH Terms) OR "arthroplasty"(All Fields)) AND ("aged"(MeSH Terms) OR "aged" (All Fields) OR "elderly"(All Fields)).

The studies retrieved were firstly screened by title, and if relevant, the whole abstract was red. After a first selection and exclusion of nonrelevant papers, the full text of the potentially eligible articles was retrieved and red by two reviewers, for possible inclusion. Discordant opinions were solved through the consultation of a third reviewer. After the electronic search was completed, the bibliography of the included relevant articles was screened manually to identify further papers, potentially missed in the electronic search. The search process is summarized in the flow diagram in Figure 1.

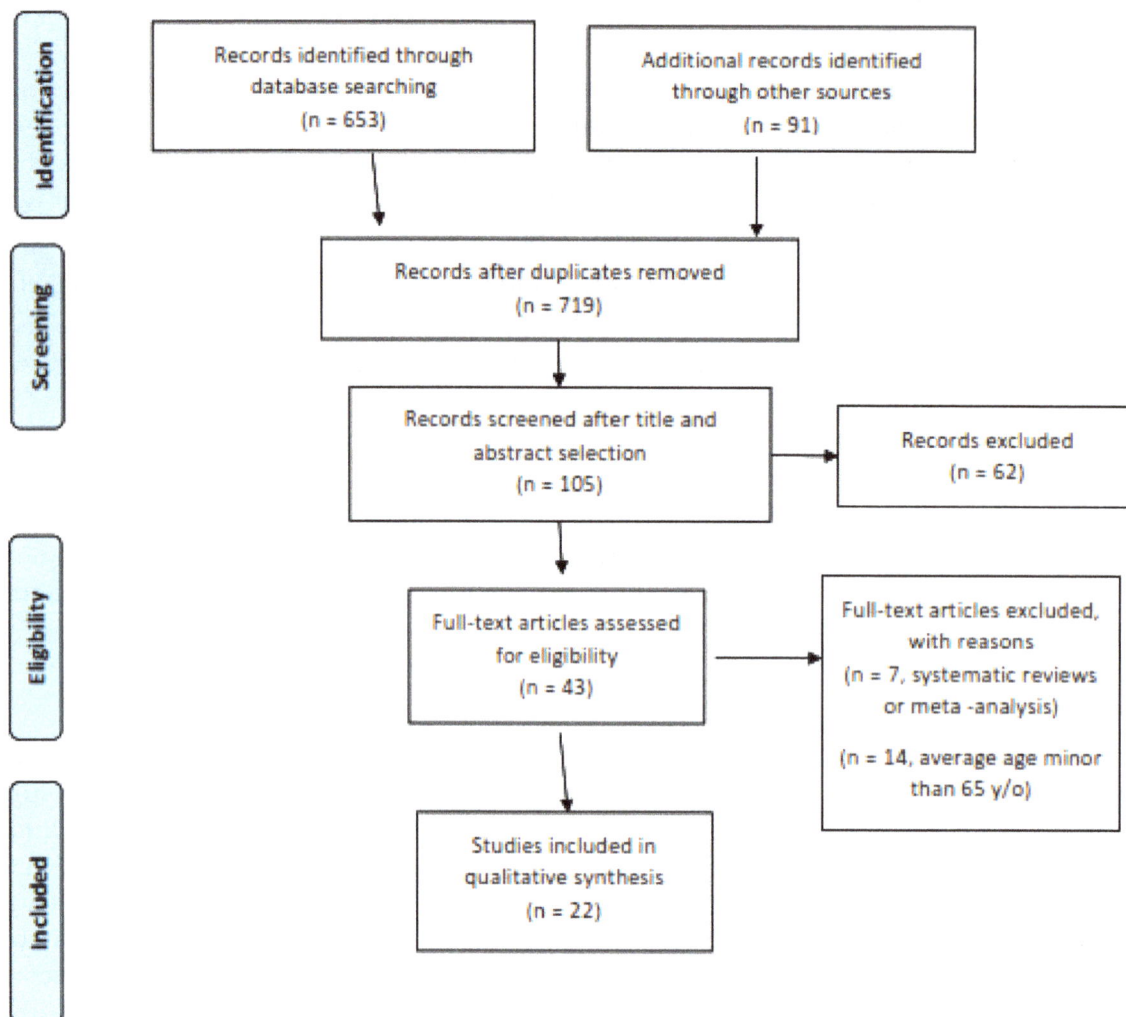

Figure 1. Flow chart of the study inclusion process.

2.4. Inclusion and Exclusion Criteria

The studies considered for inclusion were randomized controlled trials (RCT), prospective cohort studies (PCS), retrospective and prospective case–control studies (CCS), longitudinal studies (LS), and cross-sectional studies (CSS). Case reports, reviews, and meta-analyses were excluded. Studies had to report on the postoperative physical activity (intended as early and late physiotherapy, aquatic therapy, and sport activity) in elderly patients who underwent THA and/or TKA. According to the definition of elderly of the WHO, only studies where the average age of the cohorts was superior to 65 years were considered. Studies reporting on both THA and TKA patients needed to present the results of the two groups separately.

2.5. Data Collection and Analysis

Data were extracted from the included articles, according to the primary and secondary outcomes considered for the aim of this review. After extraction, generic data concerning the paper were reported in Table 1. For an appropriate presentation of the data, the results were divided on the basis of the type of surgery (TKA or THA).

Table 1. Details of the included studies.

Study	Type of study, Level of Evidence	Number of Patients	Mean Age (y)	Type of Surgery	Type of Physiotherapy–Exercise–Sport Activity
Gschwend N, et al. Acta Orthop Scand. 2000 [6]	Retrospective clinical study–LOE III	100	65 GROUP A; 65 GROUP B	THA	Group A: alpine/cross-country skiing, summer sports (trekking, biking, swimming) Group B: no winter sports
Lavernia CJ et al., J Arthroplasty 2001 [7]	Retrospective	28	68 at the time of surgery	TKA	Physical activity level assessed with UCLA activity score and Charnley class
Jones DL et al. J Rheumatol. 2004 [8]	CCS–LOE III	52	cases 70.5; controls 75	TKA	Leisure and occupational historical/high-intensity activity, measured as MET (metabolic equivalent of task) -hours/wk
Mont MA et al. J Arthroplasty. 2008 [9]	Retrospective CCS–LOE III	148	High-Impact cohort: 66; High-activity cohort: 69; Sedentary cohort: 71	TKA	High-activity: baseball and basketball, gymnastics, hockey; High-impact: aerobics, ice/roller skating, jogging, martial arts, racquetball/squash, rock climbing, skiing (downhill), soccer, tennis (singles)
Giaquinto S et al. Arch Gerontol Geriatr. 2010 [10]	RCT–LOE I	64	Group A: 70.6; Group B: 70.1	THA	Group A: conventional gyms (no-hydrotherapy group) Group B: hydrotherapy group
Giaquinto S et al. Arch Gerontol Geriatr. 2010 [11]	RCT–LOE I	58	Geriatric population, groups matched by age, gender, and body mass index (BMI)	TKA	Group A: conventional gym treatment Group B: hydrotherapy
Liebs TR et al. J Bone Joint Surg Am. 2010 [12]	RCT–LOE I	203 THA; 159 TKA	THA Group A: 67.2; Group B 67.2; TKA Group A: 69.9; Group B 69.7	TKA and THA	Group A: No ergometer cycling Group B: ergometer cycling
Liebs TR et al., Arch Phys Med Rehabil. 2012 [13]	RCT–LOE I	280 THA; 185 TKA	THA Group A: 66.7; Group B 69.1; TKA Group A: 68.5; Group B 70.9	TKA and THA	Group A: aquatic therapy (pool exercises aimed at training of proprioception, coordination, and strengthening) from the 6th day after surgery Group B: aquatic therapy from the 14th day after surgery
Mayr HO et al., J Arthroplasty. 2015 [14]	Retrospective CCS–LOE III	81	71.8 ± 5.4	TKA	High-impact: alpine skiing, rock climbing, dancing, tennis; Medium-impact: hiking, cross-country skiing, Nordic walking, fitness; Low-impact: aqua fit, golf, cycling, swimming

Table 1. *Cont.*

Study	Type of study, Level of Evidence	Number of Patients	Mean Age (y)	Type of Surgery	Type of Physiotherapy–Exercise–Sport Activity
Winther SB et al. Acta Orthop. 2015 [15]	Retrospective cohort study–LOE III	585 THA 335 TKA	65–66 for THA/TKA primary surgery, 68/67 for revision surgery	TKA and THA	Fast-track (treatment chain)
Heiberg KE et al., Arthritis Care Res. 2016 [16]	RCT–LOE I	60	Training group 70.2 Control group 70.6	THA	Case group: walking skill training program 3–5 months after surgery Control group: usual training
Paxton EW et al., Acta Orthop. 2016 [17]	Prospective comparative study–LOE II	5.678 THA; 11.084 TKA	THA: 68 TKA: 67	THA and TKA	Self-reported minutes of physical activity/week
Taniguchi M et al. J Arthroplasty. 2016 [18]	PCS–LOE II	81	72.1	TKA	Passive knee range of motion (ROM) exercises, strengthening, gait and ADL (activities of daily living) training, cycling with a stationary bicycle
Hiyama Y et al., J Knee Surg. 2017 [19]	Prospective cohort study–LOE II	59	71.7	TKA	standardized rehabilitation program, targeting knee range of motion, pain control, and quadriceps strength
Mitrovic D et al., Clin Rehabil. 2017 [20]	RCT–LOE I	70	Study group: 69.2 Control group: 68.1	THA	Supplementary arm and upper body exercise program to be compared with the standard-rehabilitation program group (upper limb flexibility, range of motion, and muscle strength, along with regular, deep breathing exercises)
Valle C et al., Sportverletz Sportschaden Organ Ges Orthopadisch–Traumatol Sportmed. 2017 [21]	Retrospective CCS–LOE III	130	69.2	TKA	Sport group: trekking, swimming, golf, Nordic walking, skiing No-sport group: without any sport activity
Mikkelsen LR et al., Physiother Res Int J Res Clin Phys Ther. 2012 [22]	RCT–LOE I	44	Intervention group 67.7 Control group 66.8	THA	Fast-track group: rubber band resistance (Thera-Band) and step exercises. Address the muscle groups mostly affected after THA Control group: standard rehabilitation consisting of exercises without external resistance and progression
Rahmann AE et al., Arch Phys Med Rehabil. 2009 [23]	RCT–LOE I	65	Group 1: 70.4 Group 2: 69.4 Group 3: 69	TKA and THA	Group 1: ward physiotherapy treatment each day, following the standard orthopedic clinical pathway; Group 2: aquatic physiotherapy program (30% body weight (BW)); Group 3: water exercise program (10%BW).

Table 1. *Cont.*

Study	Type of study, Level of Evidence	Number of Patients	Mean Age (y)	Type of Surgery	Type of Physiotherapy–Exercise–Sport Activity
Moffet H et al., Arch Phys Med Rehabil. 2004 [24]	RCT–LOE I	77	Standard physiotherapy 68.7 Intensive physiotherapy 66.7	TKA	STANDARD: simple exercises to retrain lower-limb strength (quadriceps, hamstrings, hip abductors, and extensors) and to increase knee mobility, as well as some advice about knee positioning, ice application, and gait retraining; INTENSIVE: 5 components: warm-up, specific strengthening exercises, functional task-oriented exercises, endurance exercises, and cool-down
Valtonen A et al., Arch Phys Med Rehabil. 2010 [25]	RCT–LOE I	50	Training Group 66.2 Control Group 65.7	TKA	Training group: 12-week progressive aquatic resistance training; Control: no intervention
Valtonen A et al., Arch Phys Med Rehabil. 2011 [26]	RCT–LOE I Follow up	42	Training Group 66.2 Control Group 65.7	TKA	Training group: 12-week progressive aquatic resistance training; Control: no intervention
Bauman S et al., Clin J Sport Med. 2007 [27]	Retrospective case series–LOE IV	170 THA 184 TKA	THA 66.4 TKA 68.9	TKA and THA	Physical activity assessed by UCLA activity score

TKA: total knee arthroplasty, THA: total hip arthroplasty, LOE: Level of evidence, CCS: case–control studies, RCT: randomized controlled trials, PCS: prospective cohort studies.

2.6. Risk of Bias Assessment

Given the heterogeneity of the included studies, two different critical appraisal tools were used. For randomized clinical trials, the Cochrane risk of bias assessment tool was applied, providing a grade of risk (low and high risk) of bias for the index study in five elements of the study design (sequence generation, allocation concealment, blinding, incomplete data addressment, and selective reporting). The MINORS score was used for non-randomized studies.

3. Results

3.1. Results of the Search

From the electronic and manual search, a total of 744 papers were identified. After the selection process, 43 papers where considered eligible to be included in the study. Fourteen papers were excluded because the average age of the cohort was below 65 years; 7 further papers were excluded for being reviews or meta-analyses. Twenty-two papers (11 RCT, 3 PCS, 6 retrospective CCS, one retrospective CS) were eventually included in the study (Figure 1).

The results of risk of bias assessment are presented in Appendices A and B.

The included studies reported data on a total of 20,139 patients: 12,818 underwent TKA, while 7321 underwent THA. The average age ranged from 65 to 72.1 years.

3.2. Total Hip Arthroplasty

Six studies reported the results of THA alone and five studies the results of both THA and TKA. Seven studies were RCT, two were retrospective CCS, one was a PCS, and one was a retrospective case series.

The risk of bias assessment revealed that six of the seven RCT had one or more major methodology flaws, therefore the risk of bias within a single trial was present for these studies (Appendix A). Among non-randomized studies, some showed major limitations, especially concerning patient allocation, blinding, and data collection. The mean MINORS score was 13, indicating a moderate risk of bias (Appendix B). Only one study specified the surgical approach (posterior) [16].

The most frequent primary outcome reported was the WOMAC index, mentioned in four papers [7–10]. All the included studies showed an improvement in the three subscales (function, pain, and stiffness), with mean values of 13.7, 9.3, and 18.5, respectively. Different types of physical activity and physiotherapy (early and late hydrotherapy [10,13], ergometer cycling [12], intensive physiotherapy addressing specific muscle groups [22]) had a beneficial effect after THA, as measured by the WOMAC score.

Other studies reported heterogeneous patient-related outcome measures and physical test measures. An improvement in Hip disability and Osteoarthritis Outcome Score – Physical Function Shortform (HOOS-PS) was reported by Winther et al. [15] and by Heiberg et al. [16], after an intensive fast-track treatment and after a walking skill training program, respectively. Two papers reported an increase in HHS values [11,12]. Regarding the physical tests, improvements in hip abductor strength, gait speed, one-legged stance, and 6MWT were reported after intensive aquatic therapy [23] and fast-track gym treatment [22].

Considering the effect of physical activity on quality of life, three papers reported a significant increase of it using the SF-36 questionnaire (mean value 55.6 three months after surgery) [12,13,20]; other authors reported an improvement using the health-related (HR)QoL and EQ-5D questionnaires after fast-track intensive treatment [15,22]. Poor evidence is available about the effect of physical activity on revision rates: Gschwend et al. reported an inferior rate of implant loosening and revisions in active patients [6], while Bauman et al. reported no signs of wear or loosening in patients with high UCLA score 40 months after surgery [27].

The included studies reported on a vast and heterogeneous group of postoperative activities, ranging from high- and low-impact sport activity, to enhanced physiotherapic protocols and early and late hydrotherapy (Table 2). Aquatic therapy, fast-track treatmen,t and leisure physical activity were the most frequently reported activities.

Table 2. Types of activity and number of studies in which they were reported.

TYPE OF ACTIVITIES	THA (n° of studies)	TKA (n° of studies)
Hydrotherapy	3 [1–3]	5 [2–6]
Ergometer cycling	1 [7]	2 [7,8]
Intensive physiotherapy		3 [8–10]
Fast-track treatment	2 [11,12]	1 [11]
Walking skill training	1 [13]	
Arm/upper body exercise	1 [14]	
Leisure activity (MET-hours/week, minutes/week)	2 [15,16]	4 [15–18]
Winter sports (alpine skiing, cross-country skiing)	1 [19]	3 [18,20,21]
Summer sports (trekking, hiking, biking, swimming)	1 [19]	3 [18,20,21]
High-impact physical activity (baseball, gymnastics, hockey, basketball, martial arts, football, tennis)		2 [18,20]
Low-impact physical activity (aquafit, golf, cycling, swimming)		2 [18,20]

3.3. Total Knee Arthroplasty

Nine studies reported the effect of physical activities on TKA alone, and five on both THA and TKA. Out of these, six were RCT, four were retrospective CCS, three were PCS, and one was a retrospective case series. The risk of bias assessment showed that three of the six RCT had one or more major methodological flaws, therefore the risk of bias within a single trial was present for these studies (Appendix A). Among non-randomized studies, some also showed major limitations, especially concerning patient allocation, blinding, and data collection. The mean MINORS score for TKA studies was 13.4, indicating a moderate risk of bias (Appendix B).

Similar to THA, the most frequently reported measure of primary outcome was the WOMAC index, mentioned by six studies [11–14,24,25]. Differently from the data presented on THA, only four of six studies showed an improvement in the WOMAC index. Only in two of these, the difference was statistically significant. The study by Liebs et al. did not corroborate the use of a cycloergometer after TKA [12]. An early start of hydrotherapy after TKA led to an improved WOMAC at three and six months of follow-up [11,13], but after one year the difference with respect to the control groups disappeared [13,25,26]. In a retrospective CCS by Mayr et al., a significant correlation between sport activity level (high-, medium-, and low-impact) and WOMAC index was reported.

Other patient-related outcome measures analyzed in the reported studies were the Knee injury and Osteoarthritis Outcome Score (KOOS) – Physical Function Shortform (KOOS-PS), KSS, Lequesne Hip/Knee score, and Oxford Knee Score (OKS). An improvement in KSS, KOOS, and OKS was reported after fast-track treatment [15] in patients performing high-activity and high-impact sports [9,14] (though no difference was shown in clinical outcome between these subgroups) [21], after a rehabilitation program targeting quadriceps strength and range of motion [19], and in patients accomplishing moderate-to-high physical activity (UCLA > 6) [27]. Moreover, a wide range of physical tests were reported, including the 6MWT, TUG, sit-to-stand time, knee flexor and extensor power, mGES, gait speed, and thigh muscle cross-sectional area. Aquatic therapy, gait training, muscular strengthening, and enhanced rehabilitation programs had a beneficial effect on these parameters [18,19,24,25], even at long-term follow-up [20].

Considering the effect of physical activity on quality of life, ergometer cycling did not produce significant improvement evaluated with the SF-36 questionnaire [12]. In contrast, early-phase aquatic therapy, enhanced physiotherapic protocols, and fast-track treatment induced beneficial effects according to the SF-36 and EQ-5D questionnaires [9,11,18,21].

Considering revision rates and prosthetic wear or loosening, Jones et al. showed that leisure, occupational, and high-intensity activity, measured as MET-hours/week, did increase the risk for revision [8]. Mont et al. reported that high-impact and high-activity sports are not a cause of implant failure (considering clinical and radiographical criteria of the Knee Society rating system), at 4 years of mean follow-up [9]. Similarly, Mayr et al. reported no evidence of wear or loosening, as well as similar revision rates, in patients performing high-impact activity vs. those performing medium- or low- impact activities [14]. Finally, comparing a sportive patient group with an inactive patient group, Valle et al. showed a reduced revision rate in the sport group (15.2% vs. 23.8%) at 12 years of follow-up [25].

4. Discussion

THA and TKA are extremely common surgical procedures. However, there is no consensus about the most effective postoperative physiotherapy and physical activities allowing an optimal recovery. The aim of this systematic review was to analyze the current evidence on the role of physical activity and rehabilitation in patients' clinical outcome after hip and knee arthroplasty.

Aquatic therapy resulted beneficial after THA, with improvements in terms of muscle strength, gait speed, main clinical scores (WOMAC, Lequesne Hip/Knee score, HOOS, HHS), patient satisfaction, and QoL (SF-36, EQ-5D questionnaires). However, an early start of hydrotherapy (6 vs. 14 days after surgery) did not produce further advantages [10,13,23]. Both ergometer cycling and intensified exercise programs resulted beneficial in terms of patient QoL, maximal gait speed, hip abductor muscle strength, and WOMAC index [12]. Interestingly, a supplementary arm and upper body exercise program produced a significant improvement in functional abilities [20]. In general, all protocol focusing on intensified exercises and additional activities and the practice of an adequate sport activity produced a beneficial effect on early and late postoperative recovery and limb function. However, it is unclear whether the same advantages are relevant in term of durability of the prosthetic implant, though it has been reported that a moderate or active lifestyle do not affect implant survival [14,15,26]. Nonetheless, more than 50% of patients undergoing total joint arthroplasty (TJA) do not respect the physical activity guidelines, suggesting that patient education should be improved [17].

It has been demonstrated that fast-track THA protocols are effective in terms of reduced length of stay, patient satisfaction and function [15,28]. However, fast-track is a complex approach, requiring patient preoperative optimization, anesthesia management, systemic pain treatment (nonsteroidal anti-inflammatory drugs (NSAIDs), acetaminophen, short-acting opioids), early mobilization, and physiotherapy [11,27–30]. It can be really challenging to set up this process in some institutions or for patients with severe comorbidities [31].

Aquatic therapy produced a beneficial effect on the clinical outcome after TKA. The WOMAC index improved in four out of six studies, similarly to SF-36 score, Lequesne Hip/Knee score, and patient satisfaction score [9,13,16,19,20]. Furthermore, also the use of early hydrotherapy (6 days after surgery) showed a beneficial effect similar to the use of NSAIDs [8]. Aquatic therapy improved quadriceps strength, walking speed, stair ascending time. The results of the cycle ergometer are controversial, and this practice is not supported for TKA recovery [12]. It has been suggested that ergometer cycling produces an improvement in strength and proprioception after TKA but that the overload on the knee may induce soft tissue edema and joint effusion, jeopardizing the positive effects [12].

In general, enhanced rehabilitation protocols and fast-track surgery after TKA produced an improvement in primary and secondary outcomes, thus indicating that an early recovery of muscular function and joint proprioception is essential.

The practice of high-impact and high-activity sports is often discouraged by surgeons because of the risk of mobilization and wear of implants' components. However, the current evidence shows that this practice leads to improved clinical outcomes in elderly patients in term of ROM, KOOS scores, WOMAC index, KSS, pain, and rate of revision [9,14]. Several authors reported that physical activity does not increase the risk of revision. One study suggested that moderate sport activity can improve osteointegration, with a decrease in osteolytic changes and prosthetic loosening [21]. On the basis of these findings, orthopedic surgeons should recommend exercising and participation in moderate and high-level sport activities after joint replacement. However, these data are limited, and there is a need for well-designed studies to draw definitive conclusions on these aspects.

This review has some limitations. First of all, the heterogeneity of the postoperative rehabilitation protocols and activities and the variety of outcome measures reported do not allow to pool the results and perform a statistical analysis. In addition, only one study reported about the surgical technique used and operation details. Nowadays, there are several surgical approaches and different implants that can significantly influence patients' recovery. However, there is scarce evidence suggesting consistent advantages of one technique over the others on medium- to long-term outcome.

To limit the risk of bias, all papers were evaluated through Cochrane Risk of Bias Assessment and MINORS score, thus enlightening how all RCT were well structured, showing only some incongruity in allocation concealment and blinding. Nevertheless, this seemed not to compromise the quality and the relevance of the results.

5. Conclusions

Although the heterogeneity of the rehabilitation protocols and outcome measures do not allow to draw definitive conclusions, most studies suggest that patients over 65 years of age benefit from enhanced physiotherapy protocols, aquatic therapy, and physical activity after knee and hip arthroplasty. The effect of physical activity on implant revision rate and survival remains controversial.

Author Contributions: Conceptualization, R.P., V.D., S.C.; F.V., G.T., B.Z., C.F., and S.V.; methodology, R.P., S.C.; F.V.; validation, S.C., G.T., and F.V.; formal analysis, F.V. and S.C.; investigation, F.V.; resources, F.V.; data curation, F.V and G.T.; writing—original draft preparation, F.V.; writing—review and editing, S.C., G.P.; visualization, S.C. and R.P.; supervision, S.C.; project administration, C.F., S.C., R.P. and V.D. All authors have read and agreed to the published version of the manuscript.

Appendix A. Cochrane Risk of Bias Assessment. Low risk (L), High risk (H), Unclear (U)

Study	Sequence Generation	Allocation Concealment	Blinding	Incomplete Data Addressed	Free of Selective Reporting	Free of Other Bias
Giaquinto et al. [7]	U	L	U	L	L	L
Giaquinto et al. [16]	L	L	L	L	L	L
Liebs et al. [8]	L	L	H	L	L	L
Liebs et al. [9]	L	L	L	L	L	L
Heiberg et al. [6]	H	H	L	L	L	H
Mitrovic et al. [12]	L	L	L	L	L	L
Mikkelsen et al. [10]	U	U	H	U	L	H
Rahmann et al. [13]	L	L	L	L	L	H
Moffet et al. [24]	L	L	L	L	L	L
Valtonen et al. [25]	U	L	H	L	L	L

Appendix B. MINORS score. The Ideal Scores for Non-Randomized Studies are 16 for Non-Comparative Studies and 24 for Comparative Studies

Study	SCORE
Gschwend et al. [6]	19
Jones et al. [8]	20
Mont et al. [9]	12
Mayr et al. [14]	17
Winther et al. [11]	11
Paxton et al. [17]	12
Taniguchi et al. [18]	15
Hiyama et al. [19]	15
Valle et al. [21]	11
Valtonen et al. [26]	11
Bauman et al. [15]	10

References

1.   Zambon, A.; Bertocco, S.; Vitturi, N.; Polentarutti, V.; Vianello, D.; Crepaldi, G. Relevance of hepatic lipase to the metabolism of triacylglycerol-rich lipoproteins. *Biochem. Soc. Trans.* **2003**, *31*, 1070–1074. [CrossRef] [PubMed]

2.   Cross, M.; Smith, E.; Hoy, D.; Nolte, S.; Ackerman, I.; Fransen, M.; Bridgett, L.; Williams, S.; Guillemin, F.; Hill, C.L.; et al. The global burden of hip and knee osteoarthritis: Estimates from the Global Burden of Disease 2010 study. *Ann. Rheum. Dis.* **2014**, *73*, 1323–1330. [CrossRef] [PubMed]

3.   Moher, D.; Liberati, A.; Tetzlaff, J.; Altman, D.G. PRISMA Group Preferred reporting items for systematic reviews and meta-analyses: The PRISMA statement. *PLoS Med.* **2009**, *6*, e1000097. [CrossRef] [PubMed]

4.   Higgins, J.P.T.; Altman, D.G.; Gøtzsche, P.C.; Jüni, P.; Moher, D.; Oxman, A.D.; Savovic, J.; Schulz, K.F.; Weeks, L.; Sterne, J.A.C.; et al. The Cochrane Collaboration's tool for assessing risk of bias in randomised trials. *BMJ* **2011**, *343*, d5928. [CrossRef]

5.   Slim, K.; Nini, E.; Forestier, D.; Kwiatkowski, F.; Panis, Y.; Chipponi, J. Methodological index for non-randomized studies (minors): Development and validation of a new instrument. *Anz J. Surg.* **2003**, *73*, 712–716. [CrossRef]

6.   Gschwend, N.; Frei, T.; Morscher, E.; Nigg, B.; Loehr, J. Alpine and cross-country skiing after total hip replacement: 2 cohorts of 50 patients each, one active, the other inactive in skiing, followed for 5-10 years. *Acta Orthop. Scand.* **2000**, *71*, 243–249. [CrossRef]

7.   Lavernia, C.J.; Sierra, R.J.; Hungerford, D.S.; Krackow, K. Activity level and wear in total knee arthroplasty: a study of autopsy retrieved specimens. *J. Arthroplasty* **2001**, *16*, 446–453. [CrossRef]

8.   Jones, D.L.; Cauley, J.A.; Kriska, A.M.; Wisniewski, S.R.; Irrgang, J.J.; Heck, D.A.; Kwoh, C.K.; Crossett, L.S. Physical activity and risk of revision total knee arthroplasty in individuals with knee osteoarthritis: A matched case-control study. *J. Rheumatol.* **2004**, *31*, 1384–1390.

9.   Mont, M.A.; Marker, D.R.; Seyler, T.M.; Jones, L.C.; Kolisek, F.R.; Hungerford, D.S. High-impact sports after total knee arthroplasty. *J. Arthroplasty* **2008**, *23*, 80–84. [CrossRef]

10. Giaquinto, S.; Ciotola, E.; Dall'armi, V.; Margutti, F. Hydrotherapy after total hip arthroplasty: a follow-up study. *Arch. Gerontol. Geriatr.* **2010**, *50*, 92–95. [CrossRef]

11. Giaquinto, S.; Ciotola, E.; Dall'Armi, V.; Margutti, F. Hydrotherapy after total knee arthroplasty. A follow-up study. *Arch. Gerontol. Geriatr.* **2010**, *51*, 59–63. [CrossRef] [PubMed]

12. Liebs, T.R.; Herzberg, W.; Rüther, W.; Haasters, J.; Russlies, M.; Hassenpflug, J. Ergometer cycling after hip or knee replacement surgery: a randomized controlled trial. *J. Bone Joint Surg. Am.* **2010**, *92*, 814–822. [CrossRef] [PubMed]

13. Liebs, T.R.; Herzberg, W.; Rüther, W.; Haasters, J.; Russlies, M.; Hassenpflug, J. Multicenter Arthroplasty Aftercare Project Multicenter randomized controlled trial comparing early versus late aquatic therapy after total hip or knee arthroplasty. *Arch. Phys. Med. Rehabil.* **2012**, *93*, 192–199. [CrossRef]

14. Mayr, H.O.; Reinhold, M.; Bernstein, A.; Suedkamp, N.P.; Stoehr, A. Sports activity following total knee arthroplasty in patients older than 60 years. *J. Arthroplasty* **2015**, *30*, 46–49. [CrossRef] [PubMed]

15. Winther, S.B.; Foss, O.A.; Wik, T.S.; Davis, S.P.; Engdal, M.; Jessen, V.; Husby, O.S. 1-year follow-up of 920 hip and knee arthroplasty patients after implementing fast-track. *Acta Orthop.* **2015**, *86*, 78–85. [CrossRef]

16. Heiberg, K.E.; Figved, W. Physical Functioning and Prediction of Physical Activity After Total Hip Arthroplasty: Five-Year Followup of a Randomized Controlled Trial. *Arthritis Care Res.* **2016**, *68*, 454–462. [CrossRef]

17. Paxton, E.W.; Torres, A.; Love, R.M.; Barber, T.C.; Sheth, D.S.; Inacio, M.C.S. Total joint replacement: A multiple risk factor analysis of physical activity level 1-2 years postoperatively. *Acta Orthop.* **2016**, *87 Suppl 1*, 44–49. [CrossRef]

18. Taniguchi, M.; Sawano, S.; Kugo, M.; Maegawa, S.; Kawasaki, T.; Ichihashi, N. Physical Activity Promotes Gait Improvement in Patients With Total Knee Arthroplasty. *J. Arthroplasty* **2016**, *31*, 984–988. [CrossRef]

19. Hiyama, Y.; Wada, O.; Nakakita, S.; Mizuno, K. Factors Affecting Mobility after Knee Arthroplasty. *J. Knee Surg.* **2017**, *30*, 304–308.

20. Mitrovic, D.; Davidovic, M.; Erceg, P.; Marinkovic, J. The effectiveness of supplementary arm and upper body exercises following total hip arthroplasty for osteoarthritis in the elderly: a randomized controlled trial. *Clin. Rehabil.* **2017**, *31*, 881–890. [CrossRef]

21. Valle, C.; Sperr, M.; Lemhöfer, C.; Bartel, K.E.; Schmitt-Sody, M. [Does Sports Activity Influence Total Knee Arthroplasty Durability? Analysis with a Follow-Up of 12 Years]. *Sportverletz. Sportschaden Organ Ges. Orthopadisch-Traumatol. Sportmed.* **2017**, *31*, 111–115.

22. Mikkelsen, L.R.; Mikkelsen, S.S.; Christensen, F.B. Early, intensified home-based exercise after total hip replacement–a pilot study. *Physiother. Res. Int. J. Res. Clin. Phys. Ther.* **2012**, *17*, 214–226. [CrossRef] [PubMed]

23. Rahmann, A.E.; Brauer, S.G.; Nitz, J.C. A specific inpatient aquatic physiotherapy program improves strength after total hip or knee replacement surgery: a randomized controlled trial. *Arch. Phys. Med. Rehabil.* **2009**, *90*, 745–755. [CrossRef] [PubMed]

24. Moffet, H.; Collet, J.-P.; Shapiro, S.H.; Paradis, G.; Marquis, F.; Roy, L. Effectiveness of intensive rehabilitation on functional ability and quality of life after first total knee arthroplasty: A single-blind randomized controlled trial. *Arch. Phys. Med. Rehabil.* **2004**, *85*, 546–556. [CrossRef] [PubMed]

25. Valtonen, A.; Pöyhönen, T.; Sipilä, S.; Heinonen, A. Effects of aquatic resistance training on mobility limitation and lower-limb impairments after knee replacement. *Arch. Phys. Med. Rehabil.* **2010**, *91*, 833–839. [CrossRef] [PubMed]

26. Valtonen, A.; Pöyhönen, T.; Sipilä, S.; Heinonen, A. Maintenance of aquatic training-induced benefits on mobility and lower-extremity muscles among persons with unilateral knee replacement. *Arch. Phys. Med. Rehabil.* **2011**, *92*, 1944–1950. [CrossRef] [PubMed]

27. Bauman, S.; Williams, D.; Petruccelli, D.; Elliott, W.; Beer, J. de Physical Activity After Total Joint Replacement: A Cross-Sectional Survey. *Clin. J. Sport Med.* **2007**, *17*, 104–108. [CrossRef]

28. Bandholm, T.; Wainwright, T.W.; Kehlet, H. Rehabilitation strategies for optimisation of functional recovery after major joint replacement. *J. Exp. Orthop.* **2018**, *5*, 44. [CrossRef]

29. Berg, U.; Berg, M.; Rolfson, O.; Erichsen-Andersson, A. Fast-track program of elective joint replacement in hip and knee-patients' experiences of the clinical pathway and care process. *J. Orthop. Surg.* **2019**, *14*, 186. [CrossRef]

30. Petersen, P.B.; Jørgensen, C.C.; Kehlet, H. Fast-track hip and knee arthroplasty in older adults-a prospective cohort of 1,427 procedures in patients ≥85 years. *Age Ageing* **2019**, *49*, 425–431. [CrossRef]

31. Hansen, T.B. Fast track in hip arthroplasty. *EFORT Open Rev.* **2017**, *2*, 179–188. [CrossRef] [PubMed]

9

Common Musculoskeletal Disorders in the Elderly: The Star Triad

Marco Alessandro Minetto [1], Alessandro Giannini [1], Rebecca McConnell [1], Chiara Busso [1], Guglielmo Torre [2,*] and Giuseppe Massazza [1]

[1] Division of Physical Medicine and Rehabilitation, Department of Surgical Sciences, University of Turin, 10126 Turin, Italy; marco.minetto@unito.it (M.A.M.); alessandro.giannini@unito.it (A.G.); 2rebeccamcconnell@gmail.com (R.M.); chiara.busso@unito.it (C.B.); giuseppe.massazza@unito.it (G.M.)

[2] Department of Orthopaedic And Trauma Surgery, Campus Bio-Medico University of Rome, 00128 Rome, Italy

* Correspondence: g.torre@unicampus.it

Abstract: Musculoskeletal disorders are debilitating conditions that significantly impair the state of health, especially in elderly subjects. A pathological triad of inter-related disorders that are highly prevalent in the elderly consists of the following main "components": sarcopenia, tendinopathies, and arthritis. The aim of this review is to critically appraise the literature relative to the different disorders of this triad, in order to highlight the pathophysiological common denominator and propose strategies for personalized clinical management of patients presenting with this combination of musculoskeletal disorders. Their pathophysiological common denominator is represented by progressive loss of (focal or generalized) neuromuscular performance with a risk of adverse outcomes such as pain, mobility disorders, increased risk of falls and fractures, and impaired ability or disability to perform activities of daily living. The precise management of these disorders requires not only the use of available tools and recently proposed operational definitions, but also the development of new tools and approaches for prediction, diagnosis, monitoring, and prognosis of the three disorders and their combination.

Keywords: aging; osteoarthritis; sarcopenia; tendinopathies

1. Introduction

Musculoskeletal disorders are debilitating conditions that significantly impair the state of health, especially in elderly subjects, since they are associated with pain, mobility disorders, increased risk of falls and fractures, and impaired ability or disability to perform activities of daily living. A pathological triad of inter-related disorders that are highly prevalent in elderly subjects consists of the following main "components": sarcopenia, tendinopathies, and arthritis (the acronym "STAR" will be henceforth adopted).

Interdependency within the different components of the triad fuels an accelerating disease progression that culminates in motor impairment, reduced quality of life, and increased risks of disability, morbidity, and mortality. Clinical and experimental findings show the interdependency within the three disorders. In fact, quadriceps weakness increases the risk of knee and hip osteoarthritis and also increases disease- and treatment-related complications [1,2]. Similarly, poor abductor hip function and low physical performance are known risk factors for gluteal tendinopathy [3,4]. Recent studies also showed that motor impairments (that are common in patients with both lower limb tendinopathies and hip or knee osteoarthritis) may predispose to sarcopenia and contribute to its progression [5]. Furthermore, age-related comorbidities, such as chronic obstructive pulmonary disease and congestive heart failure, can limit mobility resulting in decreased muscle and tendon function, thus propagating changes already occurring in the musculoskeletal system [6]. Although common pathways have been implicated in the pathogenesis of the different components of the triad [6], these diseases are rarely evaluated in a comprehensive manner [6] and, to the best of our knowledge, no previous study has investigated the frequency of comorbidity of sarcopenia, tendinopathies, and arthritis.

An example of a clinical case that is commonly seen in daily practice, highlighting the possible interdependency of the STAR triad's musculoskeletal disorders is as follows. A 70-year-old female presents to her general practitioner with complaints of difficulty in moving and pain. She reports that it is becoming difficult to rise from a chair and she sometimes loses her balance when walking on uneven surfaces. Reaching cups on the high kitchen shelves causes shoulder pain, and her knees, which used to ache only in the morning, now hurt all the time. Though she had multiple minor musculoskeletal injuries in her youth and worked in a factory for twenty years, she had only a few medical concerns during adulthood. After she retired, however, her activity level declined, and controlling her weight gain and diabetes has been difficult. Her doctor is concerned that multiple musculoskeletal disorders are affecting her independence and quality of life.

The aim of this narrative review is to critically appraise the literature relative to the different disorders of this "STAR" triad, in order to highlight the pathophysiological common denominators and propose strategies for personalized clinical management of patients presenting with this combination of musculoskeletal disorders. Literature research was performed, including all relevant studies up to January 2020 by searching the Medline/PubMed database and Web of Science using the following search terms: arthritis, muscle weakness, musculoskeletal pain, osteoarthritis, physical frailty, sarcopenia, tendinopathy, tendon injury, and healing.

2. Sarcopenia

2.1. Definition

Sarcopenia is the loss of skeletal muscle mass and function that occurs during the aging process (primary sarcopenia) or due to the presence of an underlying disease or medication (secondary sarcopenia). While secondary sarcopenia relies on the diagnosis and treatment for the underlying causation, primary sarcopenia has been more challenging to characterize. The European Working Group on Sarcopenia in Older People described sarcopenia as "a syndrome characterized by progressive and generalized loss of skeletal muscle mass and strength with a risk of adverse outcomes such as physical disability, poor quality of life, and death" [7].

2.2. Epidemiology

Epidemiological studies showed that from the second to the eighth decade of life, whole body and appendicular lean mass decline by about 20% in men and 30% in women [8,9]. Sarcopenia, therefore, is prevalent in older adults, especially women, and presents substantial variations depending on age and geographic area. A 2014 systematic review reported the following sarcopenia prevalence data within different healthcare settings: 1%–29% in the community, 10% in acute hospital care, and 14%–33% in long-term care setting [10].

2.3. Pathophysiology

From a pathophysiologic perspective, sarcopenia can be considered as an organ failure: Correa-de-Araujo and Hadley [11] proposed the concept of "skeletal muscle function deficit", while Marzetti et al. [12] proposed the pathophysiologic construct of "muscle insufficiency".

This organ failure can develop chronically (more often) or acutely (e.g., during immobilization) and results from a combination of neural and muscular adaptations [13,14]. The former adaptations consist of neuropathic processes leading to motor unit denervation and preferential loss of fast motor units. The latter adaptations consist of a loss of muscle mass that is due to a decrease in muscle fiber number (hypoplasia) and size (atrophy), which particularly affects type 2 fibers (that are more vulnerable to atrophy than type 1 fibers). Given the abovementioned preferential loss of fast motor units (containing fast type 2 fibers), the muscular adaptations could also imply a fast-to-slow transition of fiber types (i.e., a change of the myosin heavy chain (MHC) isoform expression toward the slower phenotype) [13]. However, MHC expression is also affected by the level of neuromuscular activity: disuse favors the expression of fast MHC isoforms, while physical activity leads to either a fast-to-slow (glycolytic-to-oxidative) phenotype transition or a shift toward the slower population of fast fibers (i.e., a bidirectional transformation from MHC-1 and MHC-2X isoforms toward MHC-2A isoform) [13–15]. This variability in muscle adaptations to physical activity is a function of the pre-training MHC phenotype, training history, and training type. Hence, an MHC phenotype characteristic of aging does not exist since it is the result of the complex interaction between age-related neurodegenerative changes and physical activity status, which varies across different individuals.

2.4. Clinical Presentation

The European Working Group on Sarcopenia in Older People proposed in 2010 an operational definition of sarcopenia based on the co-occurrence of low muscle mass and low muscle function (strength or performance) [7]. This operational definition has recently been updated as follows: (1) low muscle strength is identified as a key characteristic and a primary indicator of probable sarcopenia; (2) sarcopenia diagnosis is confirmed by the presence of low muscle quantity or quality; and (3) detection of low physical performance predicts adverse outcomes, so such measures are thus used to identify the severity of sarcopenia. Therefore, when low muscle strength, low muscle quantity/quality, and low physical performance are all detected, sarcopenia is considered to be severe [16].

Other consensus groups (International Working Group on Sarcopenia (IWGS), Society of Sarcopenia, Cachexia and Wasting Disorders (SSCWD), Foundation for the National Institutes of Health Sarcopenia Project, and Asian Working Group on Sarcopenia) agree that the diagnosis of sarcopenia should incorporate a muscle mass evaluation with the assessment of strength and/or physical performance [17–20].

Therefore, the reduction in muscle size and strength and neuromuscular performance impairment must be considered as core clinical presentations of sarcopenia: a critical mass of these phenotypic components identifies and evaluates the severity of the syndrome. This operationalization of the sarcopenic syndrome resembles the definition of the frailty phenotype previously proposed by Fried et al. [21] that is based on the co-occurrence of (three or more of) the following criteria: unintentional weight loss, self-reported exhaustion, muscle weakness (low grip strength), slow walking speed, and low physical activity. Most of these criteria are the same required for the diagnosis of sarcopenia. Consistently, sarcopenia must be considered as a key component of frailty [22].

In addition to the formal clinical presentation framework, a recent stated-preference study performed in community dwelling, elderly, sarcopenic patients provided insights on the clinical features of sarcopenia that are relevant from the patients' perspective, including mobility impairment, inability to manage domestic activities, increased risk of falls, fatigue, and reduced quality of life [23].

Therefore, treatment interventions for sarcopenic patients should be performed to address not only the core phenotypic components of the syndrome (the impairments of muscle mass and function), but also the associated negative health outcomes.

2.5. Management

Understanding the pathophysiology and core clinical characteristics of sarcopenia is key to developing effective interventions, and translational research in this area is rapidly increasing [24]. Current management strategies include non-pharmacological and pharmacological approaches. Physical exercise, alone or in combination with nutritional interventions, is the non-pharmacological approach currently recommended as the primary treatment of sarcopenia [25]. In fact, physical exercise, most notably high-intensity resistance training, improves the strength and mass of skeletal muscles and counteracts the age-related decline in muscle size and function [24–26]. It is, however, worth noting that the feasibility, sustainability, and safety of resistance training in individuals with sarcopenia deserve further investigation [26], especially because high-intensity resistance exercises increase the risk of muscle and tendon injuries and can also produce post-exercise muscle soreness and persistent fatigue. These symptoms (that also represent the core clinical characteristics of overtraining syndrome) [27] should be avoided in elderly subjects as they can be associated with reduced motor performance, mood changes, and poor quality of life. As older individuals seem to prefer easy and accessible training regimens that are easy to perform in any setting, body weight-based exercise programs for strength training may be preferable to programs involving gym equipment [28]. Current recommendations for physical exercise prescription in sarcopenic and frail older people include a balanced program of both endurance and strength exercises, performed on a regular schedule [29,30].

The effects of exercise may be enhanced by a wide variety of other treatments, including patient education (patients must be instructed to progressively increase training load and to train at a high intensity) [26] and nutritional supplements providing an adequate intake of protein, vitamin D, antioxidant nutrients, and long-chain polyunsaturated fatty acids [31].

Furthermore, evidence for the benefits of different physical therapies in improving muscle strength and mass individually is compelling, and evidence for their benefit in sarcopenia is growing. For example, neuromuscular electrical stimulation (i.e., the application of high-intensity and intermittent electrical stimuli to the skin above the muscles, with the main objective to generate involuntary muscle contractions, most often in isometric tetanic conditions) [32], whole body vibration (i.e., the use of a vertical or rotary oscillating platform as an exercise stimulus, while the individual engages in sustained static positioning or dynamic movements) [33], and focal muscle vibration (i.e., the application of pneumatic stimuli to the skin above the muscles, with the main objective to stimulate cutaneous and subcutaneous receptors without triggering visible muscle contractions) [34] proved to be effective in sarcopenic patients. However, the heterogeneity of the data regarding the adopted stimulation paradigms and training protocols does not yet allow firm conclusions to guide clinical recommendations for physical therapy prescription in sarcopenic patients.

Regarding pharmacological approaches, it is worth highlighting that no drugs have been approved yet for the treatment of sarcopenia. A recent umbrella review of systematic reviews and meta-analyses reported that only vitamin D, especially in older women, and testosterone in older men with low testosterone levels and muscle weakness can be justified in daily clinical practice to improve muscle mass and function in sarcopenic patients [35].

3. Tendinopathies

3.1. Definition

Tendinopathy is a musculoskeletal disorder characterized by tendon pain during an activity, tendon swelling and localized tenderness upon palpation, and loss of function [36]. Different medical terms are frequently used to define this disorder [37] and this ambiguity reflects the controversy that surrounds pathogenesis of tendinopathy. The traditional assumption was that tendon injury may result from repetitive mechanical loads and subsequent inflammatory responses (hence the term "tendinitis") [38]. However, histopathological findings were unable to consistently find "classical" inflammatory cells. Instead, light microscopy investigation of samples of pathological tendons showed collagen degeneration, increased mucoid ground substance, and increased tenocytes with myofibroblastic differentiation (tendon repair cells) [39]. For this reason, "tendinosis" became the preferred term over "tendinitis" to avoid the implication of inflammation. Modern molecular techniques, however, have clearly shown the increased presence of macrophages and mast cells in tendinopathic tissues [40]. Therefore, chronic, low-grade inflammation may still be part of the pathogenesis [41,42]. For all the reasons mentioned above, tendon experts recommend the use of "tendinopathy", a term that does not imply the presence of a particular pathological or biochemical process [36,43,44].

3.2. Epidemiology

The most common tendinopathies in the elderly involve two tendons (i.e., subscapularis and supraspinatus) of the rotator cuff of the shoulder [45,46] and the gluteal tendons of the hip [47]. Rotator cuff tendinopathy prevalence in the elderly population ranges from 5% to 7% [45,46], and a recent study investigating tendinopathies in a Dutch general practice found gluteal tendinopathy to have the highest prevalence (4.22 per 1000 person years) and incidence (3.29 per 1000 person years) of all lower limb tendinopathies [48]. Therefore, the following sections will focus on the pathophysiology, clinical characteristics, and management strategies for degenerative rotator cuff tendinopathy and gluteal tendinopathy (also known as "greater trochanteric pain syndrome").

3.3. Pathophysiology

Despite the progress achieved over the last decades, there is still great uncertainty over the factors causing this pathology and controlling its progression. A widely accepted concept for explaining the origin and development of tendinopathy is the generation of excessive tensile loads within the tendon over time. If a rapid increase in the magnitude, duration, or frequency of loading occurs, tensile strength might be exceeded locally causing a micro-injury. The mechanisms underlying the progression of this micro-injury are currently not established, but it has been hypothesized that repetitive overloading of the tendon may overwhelm the tissue's healing capacity causing a more severe injury [43,44]. This concept identifies excessive tensile load to be the key factor in tendinopathy origin and development. However, a number of other findings indicated that there is more into the etiology and pathophysiology of tendinopathy than just excessive tensile load. For example, it has been shown in recent in vivo studies that human tendons may undergo non-uniform displacements during passive or active force application, with deeper tissue layers deforming more than superficial ones [49]. Therefore, not only excessive tensile stress, but also excessive compressive stress as well as "stress-shielding" (i.e., the lack of adequate local stress producing understimulation of the tendon cells), could lead to tensile weakening and degeneration over time [50,51]. For greater trochanteric pain syndrome, the role of compression seems to be clear: the gluteus medius and minimus tendons compress against the greater trochanter in positions of hip adduction [52]. Similarly, the deep fibers of the supraspinatus tendon are exposed to high compressive loads against the humeral insertion [53]. High levels of tendon compression and the associated tissue hypoxia stimulate the fibrocartilaginous metaplasia of tenocytes that differentiate into hypertrophic chondrocyte-like cells to produce calcium deposits (predominantly hydroxyapatite) [54,55]. The clinical sequela is a condition known as calcific tendinopathy [56]. The negative effects of the excess or lack of adequate local stress on the tendon can also be amplified by systemic factors such as metabolic alterations related to aging (i.e., obesity and type 2 diabetes) [57]. Therefore, age-related tendinopathies could be viewed as the result of a degenerative process underlain by local and systemic factors. However, neither the "failed healing model" nor the "degenerative model" of tendinopathy fully explains the heterogeneity of its presentation. The "continuum model" of tendon pathology was proposed in 2009 and revisited in 2016 by Cook et al. [58,59] to overcome the limitations of previous models. This model assumes that tendons may have discrete regions that are in different stages (normal, reactive, or degenerative) at one time. This model also assumes that regardless of the initiating event (overstimulation or understimulation of resident tenocytes, collagen disruption or micro-injury, or inflammation), tendon pathology is characterized by a significant cell response to injury. Therefore, a tendon cell-based response could occur in a structurally normal (to conventional imaging modalities at least) tendon portion that may drift in and out of a reactive response. Although the exact mechanisms responsible for tendon pain remain to be clarified [60], the "continuum model" also suggests that paracrine signaling by tenocytes could represent one of the drivers of nociception. In fact, cytokines released by tenocytes (and/or infiltrating immune cells) could sensitize peripheral mechanoreceptors near or in the paratenon (that could also be irritated by the increased tendon size) as well as nociceptor terminals, ultimately resulting in the stimulation of the peripheral nerve. However, mechanisms for tendon pain should extend beyond local tissue changes and include increased axonal sprouting from repeated injury as well as peripheral and central mechanisms of nociception modulation [60].

3.4. Clinical Presentation

Core clinical characteristics of rotator cuff degenerative tendinopathy include old age, focal night pain, weakness of shoulder muscles, and movement restriction [61,62]. Shoulder pain generally radiates to the deltoid and the middle part of the upper arm. Weakness, movement restriction, or both, especially in active external rotation, are found in half of radiologically confirmed rotator cuff tears [62]. Movement testing helps to distinguish rotator cuff degenerative tendinopathy from frozen shoulder (adhesive capsulitis). Frozen shoulder is an idiopathic and self-limiting condition in which movement of the shoulder becomes restricted in both active and passive external rotation [63].

Calcific tendinopathy is another important, self-limiting differential diagnosis for patients presenting with shoulder pain, especially in middle-aged patients. It is a condition in which calcium deposits develop in the supraspinatus (80% of cases), infraspinatus (15% of cases), and subscapularis (5% of cases) tendons [55,56]. Calcific tendinopathy can be diagnosed through imaging of calcium deposits and may respond differently to treatments compared to degenerative tendinopathies [55,56].

Like shoulder tendinopathy, low-grade pain (with or without movement restriction) is characteristic of gluteal tendinopathy. This pain presents in the lateral hip and is aggravated with activities (such as walking and other weight-bearing activities) and side-lying on the affected side [52]. Further core clinical characteristics of gluteal tendinopathy include old age, female gender, comorbidities such as pain generated from the back and hip joint, overweight/obesity, poor abductor hip function, altered gait parameters, and psychological distress [3,4].

3.5. Management

The best approaches for clinical management of rotator cuff and gluteal tendinopathies have yet to be elucidated. Careful analysis of the medical history and symptoms must guide clinical decision making. Studied interventions include exercise, interventional approaches (i.e., corticosteroid or platelet-rich plasma injections), physical therapy modalities (radial pressure wave treatment and focused shock wave therapy), and topical glyceryl nitrate application.

Positioning and exercise therapy seem to be effective in both rotator cuff tendinopathy and greater trochanteric pain syndrome; however, it is unclear what protocol is the best. Overuse may be managed by reducing loads and improving biomechanics. Reducing compression must be evaluated carefully in static and dynamic positioning. In greater trochanteric pain syndrome, it is probably useful to advise patients to avoid hip-adducted positions, such as standing with "hanging on one hip" or standing with crossed legs. In the same way, patients with rotator cuff tendinopathy should avoid sustained work positions where the shoulder is unsupported in abduction. Exercises commonly start with isometric contractions because they are easy to perform, well-tolerated, and may have analgesic benefits [64]. Once pain is more tolerable, then a restorative exercise program with an early and gradually progressive tensile loading may improve the tendon's architecture and function. Increased loading improves the load-bearing capacity, and low-velocity, high-tensile load exercises benefit the tendon structure [65]. Eccentric exercises provide additional strain that transmit higher forces through the joint [66]. As the symptoms continue to improve, more functional exercises, such as jumping, running, and throwing, can be added progressively. More detailed exercise programs for both shoulder tendinopathies and greater trochanteric pain syndrome can be found in the literature [67,68].

For both gluteal tendinopathy and degenerative rotator cuff tendinopathy, peritendinous corticosteroid injection provides moderate pain relief, but only for a short time (less than 4 weeks) [69,70]. Recent preliminary evidence suggests that platelet-rich plasma injections may also clinically benefit patients with gluteal tendinopathy [71–73].

However, a physiotherapy-led education and exercise program performs better than corticosteroid injection in the long-term follow-up of gluteal tendinopathy patients and should be considered as first-line treatment [67]. Similar to the previous findings, Korakakis et al. [74] observed that corticosteroid injection is superior to radial pressure wave treatment in the short-term (1 month), but that physical therapy is superior to corticosteroid injection at mid-term (4 months) and long-term (>12 months) follow-up in gluteal tendinopathy patients. Moreover, focused shock wave therapy was effective in reducing lateral hip pain, both in the short-term (2 months) and mid-term (6 months) follow-up [75]. Given that the gluteal tendon insertion on the greater trochanter has variable depth to the skin surface, especially in female patients presenting a gynoid fat distribution [4,52], it is generally assumed that focused shock wave therapy is more effective compared with radial pressure wave treatment [76]. However, no previous study has compared these two modalities in the management of gluteal tendinopathy.

Regarding rotator cuff tendinopathy, there is consistent evidence that both focused shock wave therapy and radial pressure wave treatment reduce pain and improve shoulder function when degenerative tendinopathy is present [76,77]. Conversely, extracorporeal shock wave therapies may be less effective for calcific rotator cuff tendinopathy, while ultrasound-guided percutaneous irrigation treatment [55,78–80], also known as ultrasound-guided lavage [80], seems to be more effective than physical therapies or corticosteroid injection [80].

Experiments suggest that nitric oxide, a free radical produced by different enzymes, enhances new tissue synthesis through several processes. A randomized control trial showed significant improvement in tendinopathy-induced shoulder pain and function at 12 and 24 weeks with glyceryl trinitrate (1.25 mg/24 h) compared to placebo [81]. No studies are available about the effect of the glyceryl trinitrate in greater trochanteric pain syndrome.

4. Arthritis

4.1. Definition

Arthritis is a disease of articular joints that alters the joints biochemically, structurally, and physiologically. There are many classifications for arthritis since it is a heterogeneous, degenerative disorder with multiple etiologies and presentations [82]. Primary or idiopathic arthritis is without a specific or known antecedent and primarily affects the hands, hips, knees, and spine. Secondary arthritis has an underlying cause such as acute trauma or a rheumatologic, metabolic, or infectious disease. This historical categorization has continuously been challenged by our continued understanding of this widespread disease [83]. Therefore, multiple descriptive categories have been proposed for joint size, local or generalized joint involvement, and clinical, biochemical, and radiological presentations [82]. In practice, the terms "arthritis" and "osteoarthritis" most commonly refer to the primary, degenerative "wear and tear" of chronic joint use and exclude autoimmune subtypes (e.g., psoriatic arthritis, rheumatoid arthritis, and spondyloarthritis) and acute secondary causes (e.g., gout and infection). This has remained the practical definition even though we continue to find overlaps in pathological processes [84,85].

4.2. Epidemiology

Osteoarthritis is a leading cause of pain and disability around the world [86]. Utilizing the 2010 Global Burden of Disease study, the WHO states that 10% of men and 20% of women over the age of 60 have symptomatic osteoarthritis [87]. The Johnston arthritis study found the lifetime risk of symptomatic knee osteoarthritis to be "nearly 1 in 2 overall" and "more than 2 in 3" for obese people [88]. Based on the United Nations' population predictions, the WHO suspects that 130 million people will have symptomatic osteoarthritis by 2050 [89].

4.3. Pathophysiology

The main reason cited for the increasing prevalence and disability of osteoarthritis is our aging population. Biochemical and mechanical changes associated with aging are the greatest non-modifiable risk factors for osteoarthritis development and progression [90]. Women have a higher prevalence and severity of osteoarthritis, especially in the hands, hips, and knees. However, results suggesting that estrogen plays a role in incidence and progression have been conflicting [91]. Joint-specific variations are seen in different ethnic and racial groups, but osteoarthritis exists across all populations [92]. Multiple osteoarthritis genetic loci on genome-wide scans have been identified that may help to elucidate the pathophysiology and associated phenotypes in the future [93].

Osteoarthritis starts as a biochemical process affecting the synovium, cartilage, or subchondral bone and progresses to biochemical and anatomical abnormalities of the entire joint complex, culminating in illness [82,89,92]. The initial phases of this biochemical process consist of joint inflammation, as documented by Driban et al. through synovial fluid protein concentration analyses [94]. The joint inflammation could be initiated by mechanical trauma, metabolic changes, aging, or a combination of these factors. Obesity is thought to induce a local, mechanical trauma, especially on the knees. One unit of weight loss leads to a 4-unit reduction in knee load per step [95]. Obesity also contributes to osteoarthritis in non-weight-bearing joints of the hand, supporting the pathophysiological contribution of systemic metabolic inflammation to osteoarthritis incidence and progression [96]. Likewise, alcohol and nicotine both contribute to systemic inflammation and could potentiate pro-inflammatory mediators in the joint complex. Trauma, whether related to a major joint injury or occupational microtrauma, destabilizes and deforms the joint, worsening the mechanical forces affecting the cartilage and subchondral bone. Ligament laxity, sarcopenia (especially related to quadriceps weakness in knee osteoarthritis), and osteoporosis also contribute to the progression of osteoarthritis [1,2,92].

The synovium can be the source of multiple pro-inflammatory mediators that lead to pain and changes to the synovial fluid. The synovial fluid nourishes the avascular, aneural cartilage as well as produces hyaluronic acid (HA) and lubricin to reduce friction during movement. An increase in pro-inflammatory and catabolic products decrease the concentrations of cartilage-protecting factors and increase the production of cartilage degradation factors. There are also changes to the molecular weight of HA and a decrease in the concentration of lubricin [97].

The cartilage is also protected from mechanical stress and nourished by the subchondral bone. Early osteoarthritis bone remodeling could occur through different mechanisms: cellular signaling leading to bone remodeling and resorption and vascular invasion leading to cartilage degeneration and diminished mechanical integrity. As osteoarthritis progresses, there is a net increase in remodeled bone formation, leading to the characteristic osteophytes, sclerosis, and joint deformity seen in advanced disease [89,92].

When an imbalance exists in the structure or functioning of the extracellular matrix of the cartilage, additional inflammatory mediators and mechanical stress create a "vicious cycle" of cartilage degeneration. Over time this "low-grade" inflammation and mechanical stress limit chondrocyte production of functional collagen (collagen type I), reduce space-occupying proteoglycans, and increase inflammatory mediators. While mechanical stress can occur over time and increase with age, there is likely an inherent age-associated change in the chondrocyte phenotype that also impairs cartilage homeostasis [89,92]. This change leads to multiple molecular events and consequences (including altered gene expression related to senescence, DNA and telomere dysfunction, altered protein secretion, oxidative damage, decreased growth factor response, and apoptosis), precipitating cartilage destruction and susceptibility for osteoarthritis in the elderly [90,98].

4.4. Clinical Presentation

Patients with osteoarthritis can be identified through a range of common phenotypes, the presence of risk factors, clinical signs, and symptoms [99].

Patients presenting with osteoarthritis complain of short-lived (<30 min) pain and joint stiffness at the beginning of movement, especially in the morning. As osteoarthritis worsens, pain can be present after a period of activity or become continuous. Pain and stiffness create a functional limitation in movement, affecting the ability to perform activities of daily living. Primary physical exam findings can include crepitus, restricted movement, and bony enlargement (Heberden, Bouchard, and Luschka's joint). There is no or only minimal palpable warmth, redness, or effusion in joints affected by osteoarthritis. Through the progressive increase in pain and loss of mobility, reduction in fitness and social isolation can be common [89,92]. Consistently, previous studies suggested that chronic pain and reduced fitness, common in patients with osteoarthritis, contribute to depression, obesity, cardiovascular disease, and decreased quality of life—potentiating the risk of overall morbidity and mortality [89,92].

Radiography is considered as the "gold standard" for osteoarthritis diagnosis and is commonly used to identify the severity and to monitor the progression of joint disease in symptomatic patients [89,92]. Kellgren and Lawrence [100] proposed a prominent system to classify radiographic osteoarthritis changes and look for osteophytes, joint space narrowing, subchondral sclerosis, and deformity. The absence of radiological evidence of osteoarthritis does not eliminate the possibility of disease, and the presence of radiological evidence does not directly correlate to patient symptoms. Therefore, nearly all leading osteoarthritis groups state that an appropriate diagnosis can be made on clinical presentation alone in a symptomatic elderly adult [89,92,101], though radiographs likely add diagnostic specificity [102]. Additional imaging (e.g., magnetic resonance) and laboratory findings (e.g., synovial fluid and serum analyses) rule out other causes of joint pain, assist in research advances, or prepare for surgical intervention. Furthermore, the abovementioned clinical variables, alone or in combination with radiological variables, can also be useful for patient stratification [103]. For example, a stratification based on the severity of symptoms distinguishes between asymptomatic and symptomatic arthritis sufferers, while a stratification based on imaging findings distinguishes between diffuse disorder and joint-specific disorder. Driban et al. [104] have provided recent evidence that age, glucose concentrations, body mass index, and static alignment are the most important variables for classifying individuals with incident accelerated knee arthritis. Stratification techniques based on clinical and radiological variables may be the key to developing disease-modifying interventions for subsets of patients within this heterogeneous disease [103].

4.5. Management

Multiple protocols for therapeutic management of osteoarthritis exist, including those from the European League Against Rheumatism (EULAR) [101], European Society for Clinical and Economic Aspects of Osteoporosis, Osteoarthritis and Musculoskeletal Diseases (ESCEO) [105,106], Osteoarthritis Research Society International (OARSI) [107], and American College of Rheumatology (ACR) [108,109]. Treatment algorithms from these organizations and others can roughly be broken into three, stepwise segments: (1) lifestyle treatments, (2) pharmacologic treatments, and (3) interventional treatments.

First, all osteoarthritis organizations support patient information and education about their condition to promote mechanical and metabolic improvements. These include self-management, weight loss, and an exercise program to strengthen the joint and supporting structures. Additionally, a psychosocial assessment is likely beneficial for patients with chronic pain. Weight loss and obesity treatment is a universal recommendation, though many recognize the difficulty of achieving success [92]. ESCEO's comprehensive recommendations in 2014 highlighted the need for weight loss and included an endorsement of 5% weight reduction in 6 months with the goal of 10% weight loss to achieve significant symptom benefit [105]; however, ESCEO's 2019 update admitted to a lack of evidence-based treatment regarding weight management and physical exercise [106]. Exercise programs vary in their specific recommendations and generally encourage both cardiovascular and strength training (specifically quadriceps strengthening) [110]. Physical therapy and supervised, progressive exercise programs are encouraged, especially if they successfully transition into a self-administered home program [111]. Aquatic exercises are useful, especially if land-based activities are too painful [108]. A walking cane can help with functional movement when pain is present [106,108]. Braces, splints, and taping can be used for comfort or to provide mechanical support of a deformity depending on the location of the offending joint [110]. Recommendations for wedged insoles are mixed, but generally negative due to limited improvement and possible side effects [110]. Guidelines are also mixed regarding the most common physical therapy modalities, including thermal (heat/cold) application, manual therapy, acupuncture, and electrotherapies [112].

Pharmacologic treatment recommendations vary depending on the joints affected and patient comorbidities. The most common initial treatment recommendation is acetaminophen (paracetamol) due to its favorable side-effect profile [110]. ESCEO diverges from this recommendation (due to paracetamol's minimal benefit and possible side effects) and recommends the use of symptomatic slow-acting drugs for osteoarthritis (SYSADOAs) with prescription grade-only crystalline glucosamine sulfate or chondroitin sulfate as a first-line pharmacologic treatment of symptomatic osteoarthritis [106]. This was not supported by neither the 2012 nor the updated 2019 ACR recommendations [108,109], but it should be noted that prescription-grade SYSADOAs are not available in the United States. Capsaicin is a topical agent with mixed support that could be used if tolerated [107]. If the patient is still symptomatic, NSAIDs are considered by all osteoarthritis treatment algorithms [110]. Due to bleeding, renal, and cardiovascular risks, topical NSAIDs should be considered first for superficially located joints [106,107,110]. COX-2 inhibitors with a proton-pump inhibitor should be considered in the setting of gastrointestinal risk. However, COX-2 inhibitors should be avoided in patients with known cardiovascular risks. Patients with glomerular filtration rate < 30 cc/min should avoid all NSAIDs [106]. Opioids, especially tramadol, are recommended for severe pain, but should be used with caution due to concerns of addiction, abuse, and diversion [106–109]. OARSI, ESCEO, and ACR additionally support duloxetine for patients with multiple symptomatic joints and signs of central sensitization [106–109].

Interventions for osteoarthritis typically begin with intraarticular injections and can escalate to total joint replacement. Corticosteroid injections can temporarily help with pain (<3 weeks) and are generally recommended when there are additional signs of inflammation like breakthrough pain or a mild effusion, but not on a continuous basis [106,107,109,110]. Intra-articular hyaluronate (viscosupplementation) can also improve pain and joint inflammation and is a popular alternative to steroids. Formal recommendations, however, remain controversial due to mixed research results, cost, and availability; the most recent guidelines (by ESCEO and ACR) offer no to low-strength recommendations for its use in the hip and knee [106,109,110]. With our aging population, total joint replacements are becoming more prevalent [113]. Surgical intervention remains reserved for patients with daily pain despite conservative treatment to ensure the benefits outweigh the risks [89,92].

5. Conclusions

We reviewed the literature relative to three inter-related musculoskeletal disorders (i.e., sarcopenia, tendinopathies, and arthritis) that are highly prevalent in elderly subjects, in order to highlight the pathophysiological common denominator and propose strategies for personalized clinical management of patients presenting with this combination of disorders. Even though their clinical presentation can be different (loss of skeletal muscle mass and function in sarcopenia, persistent tendon pain and loss of function in tendinopathies, and persistent joint pain and stiffness in arthritis) [7,36,89,92], the three disorders have common pathophysiological and clinical characteristics. On the basis of the general content of this article, we report in the following a non-comprehensive list of highlights relative to the common pathophysiological and clinical characteristics of the three disorders.

1. The progressive loss of (focal or generalized) neuromuscular performance is the pathophysiological denominator common to the three disorders [7,13,22,24].

2. The three disorders increase the risk of adverse outcomes such as pain, motor impairment, increased risk of falls and fractures, impaired ability or disability to perform activities of daily living, and reduced quality of life [13,59,89,92].

3. The three disorders have a heterogeneous clinical presentation: patient stratification based on clinical and imaging variables may be the key to developing disease-modifying interventions for different subsets of patients [103,104].

4. The precise management of the three disorders requires not only the use of available tools and recently proposed operational definitions, but also the development of new tools and approaches for prediction, diagnosis, monitoring, and prognosis of the three disorders and their combination.

5. Physical exercise, alone or in combination with nutritional interventions, is the approach currently recommended as the primary treatment of the three disorders [24,25,49,67,107].

Author Contributions: Conceptualization, M.A.M. and G.M.; data acquisition (literature search and study selection), A.G. and R.M.; analysis and interpretation of data (literature), A.G. and R.M.; drafting of the manuscript, A.G., R.M., and C.B.; writing—review and editing the manuscript, M.A.M., R.M., G.T., and G.M. All authors have read and agreed to the published version of the manuscript.

References

1. Godziuk, K.; Prado, C.M.; Woodhouse, L.J.; Forhan, M. The impact of sarcopenic obesity on knee and hip osteoarthritis: A scoping review. *BMC Musculoskelet. Disord.* **2018**, *19*, 271. [CrossRef] [PubMed]

2. Vlietstra, L.; Stebbings, S.; Meredith-Jones, K.; Abbott, J.; Treharne, G.J.; Waters, D.L. Sarcopenia in osteoarthritis and rheumatoid arthritis: The association with self-reported fatigue, physical function and obesity. *PLoS ONE* **2019**, *14*, e0217462. [CrossRef] [PubMed]

3. Fearon, A.M.; Ganderton, C.; Scarvell, J.; Smith, P.; Neeman, T.; Nash, C.; Cook, J. Development and validation of a VISA tendinopathy questionnaire for greater trochanteric pain syndrome, the VISA-G. *Man. Ther.* **2015**, *20*, 805–813. [CrossRef] [PubMed]

4. Plinsinga, M.L.; Ross, M.H.; Coombes, B.K.; Vicenzino, B.T. Physical findings differ between individuals with greater trochanteric pain syndrome and healthy controls: A systematic review with meta-analysis. *Musculoskelet. Sci. Pr.* **2019**, *43*, 83–90. [CrossRef]

5. Yoshimura, N.; Muraki, S.; Iidaka, T.; Oka, H.; Horii, C.; Kawaguchi, H.; Akune, T.; Nakamura, K.; Tanaka, S. Prevalence and co-existence of locomotive syndrome, sarcopenia, and frailty: The third survey of Research on Osteoarthritis/Osteoporosis Against Disability (ROAD) study. *J. Bone Miner. Metab.* **2019**, *37*, 1058–1066. [CrossRef]

6. Grote, C.; Reinhardt, D.; Zhang, M.; Wang, J. Regulatory mechanisms and clinical manifestations of musculoskeletal aging. *J. Orthop. Res.* **2019**, *37*, 1475–1488. [CrossRef]

7. Cruz-Jentoft, A.J.; Baeyens, J.P.; Bauer, J.M.; Boirie, Y.; Cederholm, T.; Landi, F.; Martin, F.C.; Michel, J.-P.; Rolland, Y.; Schneider, S.M.; et al. Sarcopenia: European consensus on definition and diagnosis: Report of the European Working Group on Sarcopenia in Older People. *Age Ageing* **2010**, *39*, 412–423. [CrossRef]

8. Janssen, I.; Heymsfield, S.B.; Wang, Z.; Ross, R. Skeletal muscle mass and distribution in 468 men and women aged 18–88 yr. *J. Appl. Physiol.* **2000**, *89*, 81–88. [CrossRef]

9. Kelly, T.L.; Wilson, K.E.; Heymsfield, S.B. Dual Energy X-Ray Absorptiometry Body Composition Reference Values from NHANES. *PLoS ONE* **2009**, *4*, e7038. [CrossRef]

10. Cruz-Jentoft, A.J.; Landi, F.; Schneider, S.M.; Zúñiga, C.; Arai, H.; Boirie, Y.; Chen, L.-K.; Fielding, R.A.; Martin, F.C.; Michel, J.-P.; et al. Prevalence of and interventions for sarcopenia in ageing adults: A systematic review. Report of the International Sarcopenia Initiative (EWGSOP and IWGS). *Age Ageing* **2014**, *43*, 748–759. [CrossRef]

11. Correa-De-Araujo, R.; Hadley, E. Skeletal Muscle Function Deficit: A New Terminology to Embrace the Evolving Concepts of Sarcopenia and Age-Related Muscle Dysfunction. *J. Gerontol. Ser. A Boil. Sci. Med. Sci.* **2014**, *69*, 591–594. [CrossRef] [PubMed]

12. Marzetti, E.; Calvani, R.; Tosato, M.; Cesari, M.; Di Bari, M.; Cherubini, A.; Collamati, A.; D'Angelo, E.; Pahor, M.; Bernabei, R.; et al. Sarcopenia: An overview. *Aging Clin. Exp. Res.* **2017**, *29*, 11–17. [CrossRef] [PubMed]

13. Narici, M.V.; Maffulli, N. Sarcopenia: Characteristics, mechanisms and functional significance. *Br. Med. Bull.* **2010**, *95*, 139–159. [CrossRef] [PubMed]

14. Borzuola, R.; Giombini, A.; Torre, G.; Campi, S.; Albo, E.; Bravi, M.; Borrione, P.; Fossati, C.; Macaluso, A. Central and Peripheral Neuromuscular Adaptations to Ageing. *J. Clin. Med.* **2020**, *9*, 741. [CrossRef]

15. Minetto, M.A.; Botter, A.; Bottinelli, O.; Miotti, D.; Bottinelli, R.; D'Antona, G. Variability in Muscle Adaptation to Electrical Stimulation. *Int. J. Sports Med.* **2013**, *34*, 544–553. [CrossRef]

16. Cruz-Jentoft, A.J.; Bahat, G.; Bauer, J.; Boirie, Y.; Bruyère, O.; Cederholm, T.; Cooper, C.; Landi, F.; Rolland, Y.; Sayer, A.A.; et al. Sarcopenia: Revised European consensus on definition and diagnosis. *Age Ageing* **2019**, *48*, 16–31. [CrossRef]

17. Fielding, R.A.; Vellas, B.; Evans, W.J.; Bhasin, S.; Morley, J.E.; Newman, A.B.; Van Kan, G.A.; Andrieu, S.; Bauer, J.; Breuillé, D.; et al. Sarcopenia: An Undiagnosed Condition in Older Adults. Current Consensus Definition: Prevalence, Etiology, and Consequences. International Working Group on Sarcopenia. *J. Am. Med. Dir. Assoc.* **2011**, *12*, 249–256. [CrossRef]

18. Morley, J.E.; Abbatecola, A.M.; Argilés, J.M.; Baracos, V.; Bauer, J.; Bhasin, S.; Cederholm, T.; Coats, A.J.S.; Cummings, S.R.; Evans, W.J.; et al. Sarcopenia with limited mobility: An international consensus. *J. Am. Med. Dir. Assoc.* **2011**, *12*, 403–409. [CrossRef]

19. Studenski, S.; Peters, K.W.; Alley, D.E.; Cawthon, P.M.; McLean, R.R.; Harris, T.B.; Ferrucci, L.; Guralnik, J.M.; Fragala, M.S.; Kenny, A.M.; et al. The FNIH sarcopenia project: Rationale, study description, conference recommendations, and final estimates. *J. Gerontol. Ser. A Boil. Sci. Med. Sci.* **2014**, *69*, 547–558. [CrossRef]

20. Chen, L.-K.; Liu, L.-K.; Woo, J.; Assantachai, P.; Auyeung, T.-W.; Bahyah, K.S.; Chou, M.-Y.; Chen, L.-Y.; Hsu, P.-S.; Krairit, O.; et al. Sarcopenia in Asia: Consensus Report of the Asian Working Group for Sarcopenia. *J. Am. Med. Dir. Assoc.* **2014**, *15*, 95–101. [CrossRef]

21. Fried, L.P.; Tangen, C.M.; Walston, J.; Newman, A.B.; Hirsch, C.; Gottdiener, J.; Seeman, T.; Tracy, R.; Kop, W.J.; Burke, G.; et al. Frailty in older adults: Evidence for a phenotype. *J. Gerontol. Ser. A Boil. Sci. Med. Sci.* **2001**, *56*, M146–M157. [CrossRef] [PubMed]

22. Clegg, A.; Young, J.; Iliffe, S.; Rikkert, M.O.; Rockwood, K.; Iliffe, S. Frailty in elderly people. *Lancet* **2013**, *381*, 752–762. [CrossRef]

23. Hiligsmann, M.; Beaudart, C.; Bruyère, O.; Biver, E.; Bauer, J.; Cruz-Jentoft, A.J.; Gesmundo, A.; Goisser, S.; Landi, F.; Locquet, M.; et al. Outcome Priorities for Older Persons With Sarcopenia. *J. Am. Med. Dir. Assoc.* **2020**, *21*, 267–271. [CrossRef]

24. Cruz-Jentoft, A.J.; A Sayer, A. Sarcopenia. *Lancet* **2019**, *393*, 2636–2646. [CrossRef]

25. Dent, E.; Morley, J.E.; Cruz-Jentoft, A.J.; Arai, H.; Kritchevsky, S.B.; Guralnik, J.; Bauer, J.M.; Pahor, M.; Clark, B.C.; Cesari, M.; et al. International Clinical Practice Guidelines for Sarcopenia (ICFSR): Screening, Diagnosis and Management. *J. Nutr. Heal. Aging* **2018**, *22*, 1148–1161. [CrossRef] [PubMed]

26. Vikberg, S.; Sörlén, N.; Brandén, L.; Johansson, J.; Nordström, A.; Hult, A.; Nordström, P. Effects of Resistance Training on Functional Strength and Muscle Mass in 70-Year-Old Individuals With Pre-sarcopenia: A Randomized Controlled Trial. *J. Am. Med. Dir. Assoc.* **2019**, *20*, 28–34. [CrossRef]

27. Hawley, C.J.; Schoene, R.B. Overtraining syndrome: A guide to diagnosis, treatment, and prevention. *Physician Sportsmed.* **2003**, *31*, 25–31. [CrossRef]

28. Borde, R.; Hortobágyi, T.; Granacher, U. Dose-Response Relationships of Resistance Training in Healthy Old Adults: A Systematic Review and Meta-Analysis. *Sports Med.* **2015**, *45*, 1693–1720. [CrossRef]

29. Landi, F.; Marzetti, E.; Martone, A.M.; Bernabei, R.; Onder, G. Exercise as a remedy for sarcopenia. *Curr. Opin. Clin. Nutr. Metab. Care* **2013**, *17*, 1. [CrossRef]

30. Marzetti, E.; Calvani, R.; Tosato, M.; Cesari, M.; Di Bari, M.; Cherubini, A.; Broccatelli, M.; Savera, G.; D'Elia, M.; Pahor, M.; et al. Physical activity and exercise as countermeasures to physical frailty and sarcopenia. *Aging Clin. Exp. Res.* **2017**, *29*, 35–42. [CrossRef]

31. Robinson, S.M.; Reginster, J.; Rizzoli, R.; Shaw, S.; Kanis, J.; Bautmans, I.; Bischoff-Ferrari, H.; Bruyère, O.; Cesari, M.; Dawson-Hughes, B.; et al. Does nutrition play a role in the prevention and management of sarcopenia? *Clin. Nutr.* **2017**, *37*, 1121–1132. [CrossRef] [PubMed]

32. Maffiuletti, N.A.; Gondin, J.; Place, N.; Stevens-Lapsley, J.; Vivodtzev, I.; Minetto, M.A. Clinical Use of Neuromuscular Electrical Stimulation for Neuromuscular Rehabilitation: What Are We Overlooking? *Arch. Phys. Med. Rehabil.* **2018**, *99*, 806–812. [CrossRef] [PubMed]

33. Wei, N.; Pang, M.Y.C.; Ng, S.S.; Ng, G.Y. Optimal frequency/time combination of whole body vibration training for developing physical performance of people with sarcopenia: A randomized controlled trial. *Clin. Rehabil.* **2017**, *31*, 1313–1321. [CrossRef] [PubMed]

34. Pietrangelo, T.; Mancinelli, R.; Toniolo, L.; Cancellara, L.; Paoli, A.; Puglielli, C.; Iodice, P.; Doria, C.; Bosco, G.; D'Amelio, L.; et al. Effects of local vibrations on skeletal muscle trophism in elderly people: Mechanical, cellular, and molecular events. *Int. J. Mol. Med.* **2009**, *24*, 503–512. [CrossRef]

35. De Spiegeleer, A.; The Sarcopenia Guidelines Development Group of the Belgian Society of Gerontology and Geriatrics (BSGG); Beckwée, D.; Bautmans, I.; Petrovic, M. Pharmacological Interventions to Improve Muscle Mass, Muscle Strength and Physical Performance in Older People: An Umbrella Review of Systematic Reviews and Meta-analyses. *Drugs Aging* **2018**, *35*, 719–734. [CrossRef]

36. Scott, A.; Squier, K.; Alfredson, H.; Bahr, R.; Cook, J.L.; Coombes, B.; De Vos, R.-J.; Fu, S.N.; Grimaldi, A.; Lewis, J.S.; et al. ICON 2019: International Scientific Tendinopathy Symposium Consensus: Clinical Terminology. *Br. J. Sports Med.* **2019**, *54*, 260–262. [CrossRef]

37. Maffulli, N.; Wong, J.; Almekinders, L.C. Types and epidemiology of tendinopathy. *Clin. Sports Med.* **2003**, *22*, 675–692. [CrossRef]

38. Almekinders, L.C.; Temple, J.D. Etiology, diagnosis, and treatment of tendonitis: An analysis of the literature. *Med. Sci. Sports Exerc.* **1998**, *30*, 1183–1190. [CrossRef]

39. Khan, K.M.; Cook, J.L.; Bonar, F.; Harcourt, P.; Astrom, M. Histopathology of common tendinopathies. Update and implications for clinical management. *Sports Med.* **1999**, *27*, 393–408. [CrossRef]

40. Dean, B.J.F.; Gettings, P.; Dakin, S.G.; Carr, A.J. Are inflammatory cells increased in painful human tendinopathy? A systematic review. *Br. J. Sports Med.* **2015**, *50*, 216–220. [CrossRef]

41. Del Buono, A.; Battery, L.; Denaro, V.; Maccauro, G.; Maffulli, N. Tendinopathy and Inflammation: Some Truths. *Int. J. Immunopathol. Pharmacol.* **2011**, *24*, 45–50. [CrossRef] [PubMed]

42. Gao, H.G.L.; Fisher, P.W.; Lambi, A.G.; Wade, C.K.; Barr-Gillespie, A.E.; Popoff, S.N.; Barbe, M. Increased Serum and Musculotendinous Fibrogenic Proteins following Persistent Low-Grade Inflammation in a Rat Model of Long-Term Upper Extremity Overuse. *PLoS ONE* **2013**, *8*, e71875. [CrossRef] [PubMed]

43. Sharma, P.; Maffulli, N. Tendon injury and tendinopathy: Healing and repair. *J. Bone Joint. Surg. Am.* **2005**, *87*, 187–202. [PubMed]

44. Sharma, P.; Maffulli, N. Biology of tendon injury: Healing, modeling and remodeling. *J. Musculoskelet. Neuronal Interact.* **2006**, *6*, 181–190.

45. Hopkins, C.; Fu, S.C.; Chua, E.; Hu, X.; Rolf, C.; Mattila, V.M.; Qin, L.; Yung, P.S.-H.; Chan, K.-M. Critical review on the socio-economic impact of tendinopathy. *Asia Pacific J. Sports Med. Arthrosc. Rehabil. Technol.* **2016**, *4*, 9–20. [CrossRef]

46. Minagawa, H.; Yamamoto, N.; Abe, H.; Fukuda, M.; Seki, N.; Kikuchi, K.; Kijima, H.; Itoi, E. Prevalence of symptomatic and asymptomatic rotator cuff tears in the general population: From mass-screening in one village. *J. Orthop.* **2013**, *10*, 8–12. [CrossRef]

47. Stephens, G.; O'Neill, S.; Clifford, C.; Cuff, A.; Forte, F.; Hawthorn, C.; Littlewood, C. Greater trochanteric pain syndrome in the UK National Health Service: A multicentre service evaluation. *Musculoskelet. Care* **2019**, *17*, 390–398. [CrossRef]

48. Albers, S.; Zwerver, J.; Diercks, R.L.; Dekker, J.H.; Akker-Scheek, I.V.D. Incidence and prevalence of lower extremity tendinopathy in a Dutch general practice population: A cross sectional study. *BMC Musculoskelet. Disord.* **2016**, *17*, 16. [CrossRef]

49. Maganaris, C.N.; Chatzistergos, P.; Reeves, N.; Narici, M.V. Quantification of Internal Stress-Strain Fields in Human Tendon: Unraveling the Mechanisms that Underlie Regional Tendon Adaptations and Mal-Adaptations to Mechanical Loading and the Effectiveness of Therapeutic Eccentric Exercise. *Front. Physiol.* **2017**, *8*, 55. [CrossRef]

50. Almekinders, L.C.; Weinhold, P.; Maffulli, N. Compression etiology in tendinopathy. *Clin. Sports Med.* **2003**, *22*, 703–710. [CrossRef]

51. Maganaris, C.N.; Narici, M.; Almekinders, L.C.; Maffulli, N. Biomechanics and pathophysiology of overuse tendon injuries: Ideas on insertional tendinopathy. *Sports Med.* **2004**, *34*, 1005–1017. [CrossRef] [PubMed]

52. Grimaldi, A.; Mellor, R.; Hodges, P.W.; Bennell, K.L.; Wajswelner, H.; Vicenzino, B.T. Gluteal Tendinopathy: A Review of Mechanisms, Assessment and Management. *Sports Med.* **2015**, *45*, 1107–1119. [CrossRef] [PubMed]

53. Bey, M.J.; Song, H.K.; Wehrli, F.W.; Soslowsky, L.J. Intratendinous strain fields of the intact supraspinatus tendon: The effect of glenohumeral joint position and tendon region. *J. Orthop. Res.* **2002**, *20*, 869–874. [CrossRef]

54. Oliva, F.; Via, A.D.E.G.; Maffulli, N. Physiopathology of intratendinous calcific deposition. *BMC Med.* **2012,** *10,* 95. [CrossRef] [PubMed]

55. Serafini, G.; Sconfienza, L.M.; Lacelli, F.; Silvestri, E.; Aliprandi, A.; Sardanelli, F. Rotator Cuff Calcific Tendonitis: Short-term and 10-year Outcomes after Two-Needle US-guided Percutaneous Treatment— Nonrandomized Controlled Trial. *Radiology* **2009,** *252,* 157–164. [CrossRef] [PubMed]

56. Chianca, V.; Albano, D.; Messina, C.; Midiri, F.; Mauri, G.; Aliprandi, A.; Catapano, M.; Pescatori, L.C.; Monaco, C.G.; Gitto, S.; et al. Rotator cuff calcific tendinopathy: From diagnosis to treatment. *Acta Biomed.* **2018,** *89,* 186–196.

57. Oliva, F.; Misiti, S.; Maffulli, N. Metabolic diseases and tendinopathies: The missing link. *Muscle Ligaments Tendons J.* **2014,** *4,* 273–274. [CrossRef]

58. Cook, J.L.; Purdam, C.R. Is tendon pathology a continuum? A pathology model to explain the clinical presentation of load-induced tendinopathy. *Br. J. Sports Med.* **2009,** *43,* 409–416. [CrossRef]

59. Cook, J.; Rio, E.; Purdam, C.R.; Docking, S. Revisiting the continuum model of tendon pathology: What is its merit in clinical practice and research? *Br. J. Sports Med.* **2016,** *50,* 1187–1191. [CrossRef]

60. Rio, E.; Moseley, G.L.; Purdam, C.; Samiric, T.; Kidgell, D.J.; Pearce, A.J.; Jaberzadeh, S.; Cook, J. The Pain of Tendinopathy: Physiological or Pathophysiological? *Sports Med.* **2013,** *44,* 9–23. [CrossRef]

61. Hegedus, E.J.; Cook, C.; Lewis, J.; Wright, A.; Park, J.-Y. Combining orthopedic special tests to improve diagnosis of shoulder pathology. *Phys. Ther. Sport* **2015,** *16,* 87–92. [CrossRef] [PubMed]

62. Van Kampen, D.A.; Berg, T.V.D.; Van Der Woude, H.J.; Castelein, R.M.; Ab Scholtes, V.; Terwee, C.B.; Willems, W.J. The diagnostic value of the combination of patient characteristics, history, and clinical shoulder tests for the diagnosis of rotator cuff tear. *J. Orthop. Surg. Res.* **2014,** *9,* 70. [CrossRef] [PubMed]

63. Lewis, J. Frozen shoulder contracture syndrome—Aetiology, diagnosis and management. *Man. Ther.* **2015,** *20,* 2–9. [CrossRef] [PubMed]

64. Naugle, K.M.; Fillingim, R.B.; Riley, J.L. A meta-analytic review of the hypoalgesic effects of exercise. *J. Pain* **2012,** *13,* 1139–1150. [CrossRef]

65. Kongsgaard, M.; Qvortrup, K.; Larsen, J.; Aagaard, P.; Døssing, S.; Hansen, P.; Kjaer, M.; Magnusson, P. Fibril Morphology and Tendon Mechanical Properties in Patellar Tendinopathy. *Am. J. Sports Med.* **2010,** *38,* 749–756. [CrossRef]

66. Ryschon, T.W.; Fowler, M.D.; Wysong, R.E.; Anthony, A.-R.; Balaban, R.S. Efficiency of human skeletal muscle in vivo: Comparison of isometric, concentric, and eccentric muscle action. *J. Appl. Physiol.* **1997,** *83,* 867–874. [CrossRef]

67. Mellor, R.; Bennell, K.; Grimaldi, A.; Nicolson, P.; Kasza, J.; Hodges, P.; Wajswelner, H.; Vicenzino, B. Education plus exercise versus corticosteroid injection use versus a wait and see approach on global outcome and pain from gluteal tendinopathy: Prospective, single blinded, randomised clinical trial. *Br. J. Sports Med.* **2018,** *52,* 1464–1472. [CrossRef]

68. Lombardi, I.; Magri Ângela, G.; Fleury, A.M.; Da Silva, A.C.; Natour, J. Progressive resistance training in patients with shoulder impingement syndrome: A randomized controlled trial. *Arthritis Rheum.* **2008,** *59,* 615–622. [CrossRef]

69. Brinks, A.; Van Rijn, R.M.; Willemsen, S.P.; Bohnen, A.M.; Verhaar, J.; Koes, B.W.; Bierma-Zeinstra, S.M.A. Corticosteroid Injections for Greater Trochanteric Pain Syndrome: A Randomized Controlled Trial in Primary Care. *Ann. Fam. Med.* **2011,** *9,* 226–234. [CrossRef] [PubMed]

70. Mohamadi, A.; Chan, J.J.; Claessen, F.M.A.P.; Ring, D.; Chen, N.C. Corticosteroid Injections Give Small and Transient Pain Relief in Rotator Cuff Tendinosis: A Meta-analysis. *Clin. Orthop. Relat. Res.* **2016,** *475,* 232–243. [CrossRef]

71. Jacobson, J.A.; Yablon, C.M.; Do, P.T.H.; Kazmers, I.S.; Urquhart, A.; Hallstrom, B.; Bedi, A.; Parameswaran, A.M.S. Greater Trochanteric Pain Syndrome. *J. Ultrasound Med.* **2016,** *35,* 2413–2420. [CrossRef]

72. Fitzpatrick, J.; Bulsara, M.K.; O'Donnell, J.; McCrory, P.; Zheng, M.H. The Effectiveness of Platelet-Rich Plasma Injections in Gluteal Tendinopathy: A Randomized, Double-Blind Controlled Trial Comparing a Single Platelet-Rich Plasma Injection With a Single Corticosteroid Injection. *Am. J. Sports Med.* **2018,** *46,* 933–939. [CrossRef] [PubMed]

73. Fitzpatrick, J.; Bulsara, M.K.; O'Donnell, J.; Zheng, M.H. Leucocyte-Rich Platelet-Rich Plasma Treatment of Gluteus Medius and Minimus Tendinopathy: A Double-Blind Randomized Controlled Trial With 2-Year Follow-up. *Am. J. Sports Med.* **2019**, *47*, 1130–1137. [CrossRef] [PubMed]

74. Korakakis, V.; Whiteley, R.; Tzavara, A.; Malliaropoulos, N. The effectiveness of extracorporeal shockwave therapy in common lower limb conditions: A systematic review including quantification of patient-rated pain reduction. *Br. J. Sports Med.* **2017**, *52*, 387–407. [CrossRef] [PubMed]

75. Carlisi, E.; Cecini, M.; Di Natali, G.; Manzoni, F.; Tinelli, C.; Lisi, C. Focused extracorporeal shock wave therapy for greater trochanteric pain syndrome with gluteal tendinopathy: A randomized controlled trial. *Clin. Rehabil.* **2018**, *33*, 670–680. [CrossRef]

76. Speed, C. A systematic review of shockwave therapies in soft tissue conditions: Focusing on the evidence. *Br. J. Sports Med.* **2013**, *48*, 1538–1542. [CrossRef]

77. Malliaropoulos, N.; Thompson, D.; Meke, M.; Pyne, D.; Alaseirlis, D.; Atkinson, H.; Korakakis, V.; Lohrer, H. Individualised radial extracorporeal shock wave therapy (rESWT) for symptomatic calcific shoulder tendinopathy: A retrospective clinical study. *BMC Musculoskelet. Disord.* **2017**, *18*, 513. [CrossRef]

78. Sconfienza, L.M.; Viganò, S.; Martini, C.; Aliprandi, A.; Randelli, P.; Serafini, G.; Sardanelli, F. Double-needle ultrasound-guided percutaneous treatment of rotator cuff calcific tendinitis: Tips & tricks. *Skelet. Radiol.* **2012**, *42*, 19–24. [CrossRef]

79. Lanza, E.; Banfi, G.; Serafini, G.; Lacelli, F.; Orlandi, D.; Bandirali, M.; Sardanelli, F.; Sconfienza, L.M. Ultrasound-guided percutaneous irrigation in rotator cuff calcific tendinopathy: What is the evidence? A systematic review with proposals for future reporting. *Eur. Radiol.* **2015**, *25*, 2176–2183. [CrossRef]

80. Lafrance, S.; Doiron-Cadrin, P.; Saulnier, M.; Lamontagne, M.; Bureau, N.J.; Dyer, J.-O.; Roy, J.-S.; Desmeules, F. Is ultrasound-guided lavage an effective intervention for rotator cuff calcific tendinopathy? A systematic review with a meta-analysis of randomised controlled trials. *BMJ Open Sport Exerc. Med.* **2019**, *5*, e000506. [CrossRef]

81. Paoloni, J.A.; Appleyard, R.; Nelson, J.; Murrell, G.A.C. Topical Glyceryl Trinitrate Application in the Treatment of Chronic Supraspinatus Tendinopathy. *Am. J. Sports Med.* **2005**, *33*, 806–813. [CrossRef] [PubMed]

82. Kraus, V.B.; Blanco, F.J.; Englund, M.; Karsdal, M.A.; Lohmander, L.S. Call for standardized definitions of osteoarthritis and risk stratification for clinical trials and clinical use. *Osteoarthr. Cartil.* **2015**, *23*, 1233–1241. [CrossRef] [PubMed]

83. Solomon, L. Patterns of osteoarthritis of the hip. *J. Bone Jt. Surg. Br. Vol.* **1976**, *58*, 176–183. [CrossRef]

84. McGonagle, D.; Hermann, K.G.A.; Tan, A.L. Differentiation between osteoarthritis and psoriatic arthritis: Implications for pathogenesis and treatment in the biologic therapy era. *Rheumatology (Oxford)* **2014**, *54*, 29–38. [CrossRef]

85. Ma, C.A.; Leung, Y.Y. Exploring the Link between Uric Acid and Osteoarthritis. *Front. Med.* **2017**, *4*, 225. [CrossRef]

86. Blackburn, S.; Research User Group; Rhodes, C.; Higginbottom, A.; Dziedzic, K. The OARSI standardised definition of osteoarthritis: A lay version. *Osteoarthr. Cartil.* **2016**, *24*, S192. [CrossRef]

87. Cross, M.; Smith, E.; Hoy, D.G.; Nolte, S.; Ackerman, I.N.; Fransen, M.; Bridgett, L.; Williams, S.; Guillemin, F.; Hill, C.L.; et al. The global burden of hip and knee osteoarthritis: Estimates from the Global Burden of Disease 2010 study. *Ann. Rheum. Dis.* **2014**, *73*, 1323–1330. [CrossRef]

88. Murphy, L.B.; A Schwartz, T.; Helmick, C.G.; Renner, J.B.; Tudor, G.; Koch, G.; Dragomir, A.; Kalsbeek, W.D.; Luta, G.; Jordan, J.M. Lifetime risk of symptomatic knee osteoarthritis. *Arthritis Rheum.* **2008**, *59*, 1207–1213. [CrossRef]

89. Wittenauer, R.; Smith, L.; Aden, K. *Background Paper 6.12—Osteoarthritis*; World Health Organization: Geneva, Switzerland, 2013.

90. Valdes, A.M.; Stocks, J. Osteoarthritis and ageing. *Eur. Med. J.* **2018**, *3*, 116–123.

91. Neogi, T.; Zhang, Y. Epidemiology of osteoarthritis. *Rheum. Dis. Clin. North Am.* **2012**, *39*, 1–19. [CrossRef]

92. Arden, N.; Blanco, F.J.; Bruyère, O.; Cooper, C.; Guermazi, A.; Hayashi, D.; Hunter, D.; Kassim Javaid, M.; Rannou, F.; Reginster, J.Y.; et al. *Atlas of Osteoarthritis*, 2nd ed.; Springer Healthcare Ltd.: London, UK, 2018.

93. Warner, S.C.; Valdes, A.M. Genetic association studies in osteoarthritis. *Curr. Opin. Rheumatol.* **2017**, *29*, 103–109. [CrossRef] [PubMed]

94. Driban, J.B.; Balasubramanian, E.; Amin, M.; Sitler, M.R.; Ziskin, M.C.; Barbe, M. The potential of multiple synovial-fluid protein-concentration analyses in the assessment of knee osteoarthritis. *J. Sport Rehabil.* **2010**, *19*, 411–421. [CrossRef] [PubMed]

95. Messier, S.; Gutekunst, D.; Davis, C.; DeVita, P. Weight loss reduces knee-joint loads in overweight and obese older adults with knee osteoarthritis. *Arthritis Rheum.* **2005**, *52*, 2026–2032. [CrossRef] [PubMed]

96. Oliveria, S.A.; Felson, D.; Cirillo, P.A.; Reed, J.I.; Walker, A.M. Body Weight, Body Mass Index, and Incident Symptomatic Osteoarthritis of the Hand, Hip, and Knee. *Epidemiology* **1999**, *10*, 161–166. [CrossRef] [PubMed]

97. Scanzello, C.R.; Goldring, S.R. The role of synovitis in osteoarthritis pathogenesis. *Bone* **2012**, *51*, 249–257. [CrossRef] [PubMed]

98. Leong, D.J.; Sun, H. Events in Articular Chondrocytes with Aging. *Curr. Osteoporos. Rep.* **2011**, *9*, 196–201. [CrossRef]

99. Zhang, W.; Doherty, M.; Peat, G.; Bierma-Zeinstra, M.A.; Arden, N.K.; Bresnihan, B.; Herrero-Beaumont, G.; Kirschner, S.; Leeb, B.F.; Lohmander, L.S.; et al. EULAR evidence-based recommendations for the diagnosis of knee osteoarthritis. *Ann. Rheum. Dis.* **2009**, *69*, 483–489. [CrossRef]

100. Kellgren, J.H.; Lawrence, J.S. Radiological Assessment of Osteo-Arthrosis. *Ann. Rheum. Dis.* **1957**, *16*, 494–502. [CrossRef]

101. Sakellariou, G.; Conaghan, P.G.; Zhang, W.; Bijlsma, J.W.J.; Boyesen, P.; D'Agostino, M.A.; Doherty, M.; Fodor, D.; Kloppenburg, M.; Miese, F.; et al. EULAR recommendations for the use of imaging in the clinical management of peripheral joint osteoarthritis. *Ann. Rheum. Dis.* **2017**, *76*, 1484–1494. [CrossRef]

102. Altman, R.; Alarcon, G.; Appelrouth, D.; Bloch, D.; Borenstein, D.; Brandt, K.; Brown, C.; Cooke, T.D.; Daniel, W.; Feldman, D.; et al. The American College of Rheumatology criteria for the classification and reporting of osteoarthritis of the hip. *Arthritis Rheum.* **1991**, *34*, 505–514. [CrossRef]

103. Driban, J.B.; Sitler, M.R.; Barbe, M.; Balasubramanian, E. Is osteoarthritis a heterogeneous disease that can be stratified into subsets? *Clin. Rheumatol.* **2009**, *29*, 123–131. [CrossRef]

104. Driban, J.B.; Eaton, C.B.; Lo, G.H.; Price, L.L.; Lu, B.; Barbe, M.; McAlindon, T.E. Overweight older adults, particularly after an injury, are at high risk for accelerated knee osteoarthritis: Data from the Osteoarthritis Initiative. *Clin. Rheumatol.* **2015**, *35*, 1071–1076. [CrossRef]

105. Bruyère, O.; Cooper, C.; Pelletier, J.-P.; Branco, J.; Brandi, M.L.; Guillemin, F.; Hochberg, M.C.; Kanis, J.A.; Kvien, T.K.; Martel-Pelletier, J.; et al. An algorithm recommendation for the management of knee osteoarthritis in Europe and internationally: A report from a task force of the European Society for Clinical and Economic Aspects of Osteoporosis and Osteoarthritis (ESCEO). *Semin. Arthritis Rheum.* **2014**, *44*, 253–263. [CrossRef]

106. Bruyère, O.; Honvo, G.; Veronese, N.; Arden, N.K.; Branco, J.; Curtis, E.M.; Al-Daghri, N.M.; Herrero-Beaumont, G.; Martel-Pelletier, J.; Pelletier, J.-P.; et al. An updated algorithm recommendation for the management of knee osteoarthritis from the European Society for Clinical and Economic Aspects of Osteoporosis, Osteoarthritis and Musculoskeletal Diseases (ESCEO). *Semin. Arthritis Rheum.* **2019**, *49*, 337–350. [CrossRef]

107. McAlindon, T.E.; Bannuru, R.R.; Sullivan, M.C.; Arden, N.K.; Berenbaum, F.; Bierma-Zeinstra, S.; Hawker, G.; Henrotin, Y.; Hunter, D.J.; Kawaguchi, H.; et al. OARSI guidelines for the non-surgical management of knee osteoarthritis. *Osteoarthr. Cartil.* **2014**, *22*, 363–388. [CrossRef] [PubMed]

108. Hochberg, M.C.; Altman, R.D.; April, K.T.; Benkhalti, M.; Guyatt, G.; McGowan, J.; Towheed, T.; Welch, V.; Wells, G.; Tugwell, P. American College of Rheumatology 2012 recommendations for the use of nonpharmacologic and pharmacologic therapies in osteoarthritis of the hand, hip, and knee. *Arthritis Rheum.* **2012**, *64*, 465–474. [CrossRef] [PubMed]

109. Kolasinski, S.L.; Neogi, T.; Hochberg, M.C.; Oatis, C.; Guyatt, G.; Block, J.; Callahan, L.; Copenhaver, C.; Dodge, C.; Felson, D.; et al. 2019 American College of Rheumatology/Arthritis Foundation Guideline for the Management of Osteoarthritis of the Hand, Hip, and Knee. *Arthritis Rheum.* **2020**, *72*, 149–162. [CrossRef]

110. Nelson, A.E.; Allen, K.D.; Golightly, Y.M.; Goode, A.P.; Jordan, J.M. A systematic review of recommendations and guidelines for the management of osteoarthritis: The Chronic Osteoarthritis Management Initiative of the U.S. Bone and Joint Initiative. *Semin. Arthritis Rheum.* **2014**, *43*, 701–712. [CrossRef] [PubMed]

111. Fernandes, L.; Hagen, K.B.; Bijlsma, J.W.J.; Andreassen, O.; Christensen, P.; Conaghan, P.G.; Doherty, M.; Geenen, R.; Hammond, A.; Kjeken, I.; et al. EULAR recommendations for the non-pharmacological core management of hip and knee osteoarthritis. *Ann. Rheum. Dis.* **2013**, *72*, 1125–1135. [CrossRef] [PubMed]

112. Rice, D.; McNair, P.J.; Huysmans, E.; Letzen, J.E.; Finan, P.H. Best Evidence Rehabilitation for Chronic Pain Part 5: Osteoarthritis. *J. Clin. Med.* **2019**, *8*, 1769. [CrossRef] [PubMed]

113. Ackerman, I.N.; Bohensky, M.; De Steiger, R.N.; Brand, C.; Eskelinen, A.; Fenstad, A.M.; Furnes, O.; Garellick, G.; Graves, S.; Haapakoski, J.; et al. Substantial rise in the lifetime risk of primary total knee replacement surgery for osteoarthritis from 2003 to 2013: An international, population-level analysis. *Osteoarthr. Cartil.* **2017**, *25*, 455–461. [CrossRef] [PubMed]

10

Return to Sport after Anatomic and Reverse Total Shoulder Arthroplasty in Elderly Patients

Rocco Papalia [1], Mauro Ciuffreda [1], Erika Albo [1,*], Chiara De Andreis [1],
Lorenzo Alirio Diaz Balzani [1], Anna Maria Alifano [1], Chiara Fossati [2],
Andrea Macaluso [2], Riccardo Borzuola [2], Antonio De Vincentis [1] and Vincenzo Denaro [1]

[1] Department of Orthopaedic and Trauma Surgery, Campus Bio-Medico University of Rome,
    00128 Rome, Italy; r.papalia@unicampus.it (R.P.); m.ciuffreda@unicampus.it (M.C.);
    c.deandreis@unicampus.it (C.D.A.); l.diaz@unicampus.it (L.A.D.B.); a.alifano@unicampus.it (A.M.A.);
    a.devincentis@unicampus.it (A.D.V.); v.denaro@unicampus.it (V.D.)
[2] Department of Movement, Human and Health Sciences, University of Rome "Foro Italico",
    00135 Rome, Italy; chiara.fossati@uniroma4.it (C.F.); andrea.macaluso@uniroma4.it (A.M.);
    r.borzuola@studenti.uniroma4.it (R.B.)
*   Correspondence: e.albo@unicampus.it

Abstract: The aim of this systematic review and meta-analysis was to evaluate the rate of return to sport in elderly patients who underwent anatomic (ATSA) and reverse (RTSA) total shoulder arthroplasty, to assess postoperative pain and functional outcomes and to give an overview of postoperative rehabilitation protocols. A systematic search in Pubmed-Medline, Cochrane Library, and Google Scholar was carried out to identify eligible randomized clinical trials, observational studies, or case series that evaluated the rate of return to sport after RTSA or ATSA. Six retrospective studies, five case series, and one prospective cohort study were included in this review. The overall rate of return to sport was 82% (95% CI 0.76–0.88, $p < 0.01$). Patients undergoing ATSA returned at a higher rate (90%) (95% CI 0.80–0.99, $p < 0.01$) compared to RTSA (77%) (95% CI 0.69–0.85, $p < 0.01$). Moreover, the results showed that patients returned to sport at the same or a higher level in 75% of cases. Swimming had the highest rate of return (84%), followed by fitness (77%), golf (77%), and tennis (69%). Thus, RTSA and ATSA are effective to guarantee a significative rate of return to sport in elderly patients. A slightly higher rate was found for the anatomic implant.

Keywords: shoulder; arthroplasty; replacement; return to sport; elderly; systematic review; meta-analysis

1. Introduction

Total shoulder arthroplasty (TSA) is the third most common replacement procedure after hip and knee arthroplasty and is considered the elective treatment for patients affected by advanced shoulder pathology with loss of function and severe pain [1]. Indeed, the main indications for shoulder replacement are primary and secondary glenohumeral osteoarthritis, osteonecrosis, and fractures of the proximal epiphysis of the humerus or its sequelae [1–5].

Three main different designs of shoulder prostheses allow surgeons to decide which is the best option for each specific case, trying also to meet patients' health needs [6]. The reverse shoulder arthroplasty (RTSA) has a specific design that determines the medialization of the rotation center, permitting the recruitment of a large part of the deltoid muscle [7]. Thus, even if the rotator cuff is damaged, the arc of movement is preserved [7]. Conversely, the biomechanics of the anatomic total shoulder arthroplasty (ATSA) is based on rotator cuff integrity. The third implant option includes hemiarthroplasty (HHA) and humeral head resurfacing that differ from the above mentioned because they do not require glenoid replacement. Currently, these implants are more often indicated for the treatment of end-stage osteoarthritis as well as fractures of the humeral head in young patients [8]. As a consequence, the number of implanted HHAs has decreased in the last 15 years in favor of TSAs [1,9–11].

The constant increase of TSAs, in younger as well as older individuals, correlates with their good long-term outcomes and with the widening of surgical indications [1,2]. In this scenario, as life expectancy is increasing, older patients are also asking their surgeons for better outcomes in order to return to previous sports activities after surgery [3]. Return to sports activities at a preoperative level has widely been investigated for patients with hip and knee arthroplasties with satisfactory rates of return [4–6]. However, limited data exist regarding rates of return after TSA, even if this field is becoming of increasing interest. A recent multi-center international study, carried out by the American and European Society of Shoulder and Elbow Surgeons, stated that non-contact low-load activities with low risk of fall or collision were most frequently allowed by surgeons [7].

The TSA post-operative rehabilitation protocol plays an important role in active patients to achieve satisfactory post-operative clinical outcomes and range of motion (ROM) [8]. Despite the existence of a large number of studies about rehabilitation protocol after hip and knee replacement, there are still only a few papers focused on specific and standardized postoperative rehabilitation protocols for patients with TSA [9,10]. Current postoperative guidelines are usually based on the original protocol developed by Hughes and Neer [11]. This protocol contemplates different steps with a gradual mobilization of the arm, avoiding flexion and abduction movements until the fourth postoperative week, but it does not provide indications for rehabilitation finalized to the resumption of sports activities. Nevertheless, for these patients, a postoperative rehabilitation protocol with a specific exercise routine could be advisable [11–13].

The primary aim of this systematic review and meta-analysis is to evaluate the rate of return to sport in elderly patients after ATSA and RTSA. The secondary and tertiary endpoints focus on the assessment of postoperative pain and functional outcomes and to give an overview of current postoperative rehabilitation protocols.

2. Materials and Methods

The present systematic review and meta-analysis was performed according to the Preferred Reporting Items for Systematic reviews and Meta-Analyses (PRISMA) guidelines [14]. In this review, we included randomized clinical trials, observational studies, and case series, which evaluated the return to sport of cohorts with an average age greater than 65 years who underwent RTSA and ATSA.

2.1. Eligibility Criteria

According to the Oxford Centre of Evidence-Based Medicine, peer-reviewed studies of I to IV levels of evidence were considered for inclusion. Case reports, studies on animals, biomechanical reports, technical notes, letters to editors, instructional courses, cadaver or in vitro investigations, systematic reviews and meta-analyses, or studies without an abstract were excluded. According to the definition of the elderly by the WHO, the search was focused on papers reporting on return to sports of cohorts, with an average age greater than 65 years who underwent RTSA and ATSA. Only studies with a minimum of 10 patients and a minimum of one-year follow-up were included. Moreover, only articles in Italian, English, Spanish, and French were considered.

2.2. Study Outcomes

The primary outcome of the analysis was to establish the rate of return to sport of elderly patients after ATSA and RTSA. Among the included papers, the secondary endpoint was to assess the postoperative pain and functional outcomes, taking into account the reported standardized clinical scores. The tertiary endpoint of this systematic review was to give an overview of the proposed rehabilitation protocols.

2.3. Search Methods for Identification of Studies

A systematic literature search in Pubmed-Medline, the Cochrane Library and Google Scholar databases was carried out between September 2019 and April 2020. For Pubmed, the following search strategy was used: (((("Shoulder Joint"[Mesh] OR ("shoulder"[All Fields] AND "joint"[All Fields]) AND ("Arthroplasty"[Mesh] OR ("Arthroplasty"[All Fields]) OR ("Replacement"[All Fields])) AND ("Sports"[Mesh] OR ("return to sport" [All Fields] OR ("return" [All Fields] AND ("sport" [All Fields])) AND "Aged"[Mesh])). No time interval was set for publication date. Two independent reviewers (M.C. and C.D.A.) conducted the electronic search identifying the potentially relevant studies. Firstly, the retrieved articles were screened by title and, if relevant, by reading the abstract. After the exclusion of non-eligible studies, the full-text of the remaining articles was evaluated for eligibility. To minimize the risk of bias, the authors reviewed and discussed all the selected articles, the references, as well as the articles excluded from the study. If any disagreement between the reviewers was found, the senior investigator (R.P.) made the final decision. At the end of the process, further potentially missed studies were manually searched for among the reference lists of the included papers and the relevant systematic reviews.

2.4. Data Collection

All reviewers discussed the relevant items for data extraction before starting the process in order to avoid data omission. Data were independently extracted by two reviewers (M.C. and C.D.A.) and divergences were discussed with the third reviewer (R.P.) if necessary. All data related to primary, secondary and tertiary outcomes were summarized in standardized tables. Specifically, the following variables were recorded: authors, year of publication, type of study, level of evidence, number of participants, mean age, dominant or not-dominant limb, surgical approach, mean follow-up, complications, patients returned to sport and type of activity, secondary outcome measures, and rehabilitative protocols. Among the outcomes, we analyzed functional outcomes and severity of pain.

2.5. Risk of Bias Assessment

The quality of the included studies was independently evaluated by two reviewers (C.D.A. and M.C.) using the Methodological Index for Non-randomized Studies (MINORS) score [15]. The following domains were assessed: a clearly stated purpose, inclusion of consecutive subjects, prospective data collection, endpoints appropriate to the purpose of the study, unbiased assessment of the study endpoints, follow-up period appropriate for the study, loss to follow-up of less than 5%, prospective calculation of the study size, adequate control group, contemporary group, baseline group equivalence, and adequate statistical analysis. The last four items are specific to comparative studies. Each item was scored from 0 to 2 points, with a global ideal score of 16 points for non-comparative studies and 24 points for comparative studies.

2.6. Statistical Analysis

Meta-analysis was performed to determine the overall proportion of subjects returning to sport and the functional and pain level after shoulder arthroplasty across all the retrieved studies. Raw, i.e., untransformed, proportions and means were used to report the pooled proportions and means that were obtained with the inverse variance method. Heterogeneity was evaluated using Q statistic, expressed as the p value for the χ^2 test under the null hypothesis that the between-study variance (τ^2) equals 0, and I^2 test. All the conducted meta-analyses evidenced the presence of significant heterogeneity, defined as a $I^2 > 55\%$ and a Q statistic p value below 0.05. Accordingly, random effect models were applied. Finally, the likelihood of publication bias was estimated with a visual inspection of the funnel plot. All analyses were carried out using metaphor and meta-packages in R 3.6.1 software for Mac (R Foundation for Statistical Computing, Vienna, Austria).

3. Results

3.1. Study Selection

The initial database searches identified 235 potentially eligible papers. After reviewing title and abstract, 217 papers were excluded and 18 were selected for full-text evaluation. Out of these, eight papers were excluded for the following reasons: mean age of the cohort < 65 years ($n = 1$), German language ($n = 1$), return to sport not clearly stated ($n = 4$), and insufficient outcomes data ($n = 2$). One paper was added from hand search. At the end of the selection process, 11 studies were included in this systematic review and 11 papers were included in the meta-analysis [16–25]. The search process is summarized in the PRISMA flowchart (Figure 1) [14].

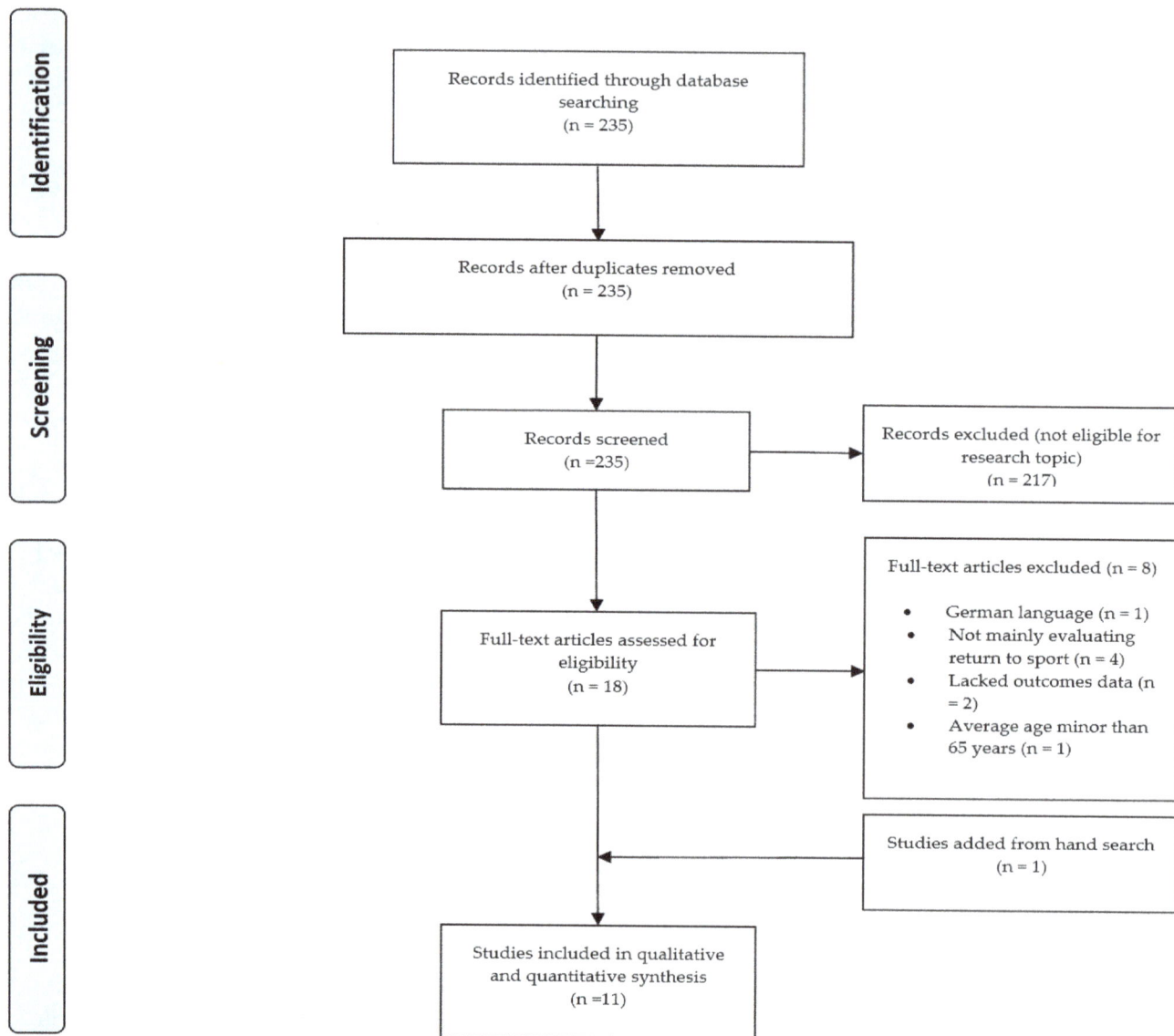

Figure 1. PRISMA flow-chart of included studies.

3.2. Study Characteristics and Demographic Details

Of the included studies, one was a single-center prospective cohort study (PCS) of level of evidence (LOE) III [19], four were retrospective studies (RS) of LOE III [18,20,23,25], one was a retrospective study of LOE IV [26], and five were case series of LOE IV [16,17,21,22,24]. All studies were published between 2010 [21] and 2018 [26]. The 11 included studies reported on 1254 shoulder arthroplasties in 1238 patients. Within the included studies, the number of subjects varied from 35 [24] to 276 [26]. The mean age of the cohorts was 72.5 years. The mean duration of follow-up was 3.7 years, ranging from 2.4 [26] to 6.2 years [17]. Four out of the 11 studies had a mean follow-up longer than four years [16,17,19,23]. The indications for surgery were several: rotator cuff arthropathy (522 patients), primary osteoarthritis (270 patients), fracture sequelae (37 patients), and rheumatoid arthritis (15 patients). Pre-operative diagnosis was not specified for 367 patients [19,22,23,26].

In total, 375 ATSA and 750 RTSA were implanted. The side of surgery was specified in 9 studies [16–23,25]. The dominant shoulder was involved in 544 patients, while the non-dominant shoulder was treated in 288 patients. Bilateral shoulder arthroplasty was performed in 17 patients [17,24]. The most frequent indication for ATSA was primary osteoarthritis without cuff disfunction [17,19,21,24]. Conversely, RTSA was performed in patients affected by primary osteoarthritis [16,20], cuff tear arthropathy [16,18,20,23,25], proximal humeral fractures [18,20,23], rheumatoid arthritis [18,20], and shoulder tumors [23]. Two studies did not specify surgical indications [22,26]. The main characteristics of the included papers are summarized in Table 1.

Table 1. Study characteristics, demographic details and Methodological Index for Non-randomized Studies (MINORS) score.

Authors	Year of Publication	Study Design	LOE	N° of Shoulders (N° of Patients)	Dominant/Not Dominant	Mean Age (Years)	Type of Implant	Mean Follow-Up (Years)	MINORS Score
Bulhoff et al. [17]	2015	CS	IV	170 (154)	103/51	72	ATSA	6.2	7/16
Bulhoff et al. [16]	2016	CS	IV	38 (38)	29/9	Group A: 76.2; Group B: 78.4	RTSA	4.8	14/24
Liu et al. [18]	2016	RS	III	102 (102)	58/44	72.3	RTSA	2.6	14/24
Kolling et al. [25]	2017	RS	III	271 (271)	203/68	77.1	RTSA	2.9	7/16
Schumann et al. [21]	2010	CS	IV	100 (100)	60/40	66.2	ATSA	2.8	8/16
Garcia et al. [19]	2016	PS	III	40 (40)	26/14	66.3	ATSA	5.1	9/16
Papaliodis et al. [24]	2015	CS	IV	36 (35)	NR	67.2	ATSA	3.2	8/16
Simovitch et al. [22]	2015	CS	IV	67 (67)	NR	73	RTSA	3.6	10/16
Barnes et al. [23]	2015	RS	III	78 (78)	48/30	75.3	RTSA	4.8	11/16
Garcia et al. [20]	2015	RS	III	76 (76)	46/30	74.8	RTSA	2.6	16/24
Kurowicki et al. [26]	2018	RS	IV	276 (276)	NR	RTSA: 75 ATSA: 69	RTSA ATSA	2.4	14/24

ATSA: anatomic shoulder arthroplasty; RTSA: reverse total shoulder arthroplasty; CS: case series; RS: retrospective study; PS: prospective study; LOE: level of evidence; NR: not reported. Group A: patients who practiced sports within the last 5 years prior to shoulder replacement surgery; Group B: patients that have never participated in sports activities.

3.3. Methodological Evaluation

The MINORS score ranged from 7 [17,25] to 11 [23] for non-comparative studies and from 14 [16,18] to 16 [20,26] for the comparative ones (Table 1). The mean value was 8.5 for non-comparative studies and 14.5 for comparative studies. All papers resulted at high risk of bias.

3.4. Return to Sport

The overall rate of return to sport for elderly patients was 82% (95% CI 0.76–0.88, $p < 0.01$) (Figure 2). Patients undergoing ATSA returned at a higher rate (90%) (95% CI 0.80–0.99, $p < 0.01$) compared to RTSA (77%) (95% CI 0.69–0.85, $p < 0.01$) (Figure 2). The time to resume sports was reported in five studies [18–21,24] with a mean period of seven months ranging from 5.3 [18,20] to 11 months [15,21]. The results [16–20,25] showed that patients returned to sports activities at the same or a higher level in 75% of cases (95% CI 0.61–0.89, $p < 0.01$) (Figure 3). Six out of 11 studies [16–20,25] (54.5%) reported sport-specific rates of return. When combined by meta-analysis according to a random-effects model, swimming had the highest rate of return (84%), followed by fitness (77%), golf (77%), and tennis (69%) (Figures 4–7). Regarding publication bias, the funnel chart was asymmetric, suggesting the presence of bias, particularly in smaller studies (Figure 8). The details of return to sport are reported in Table 2.

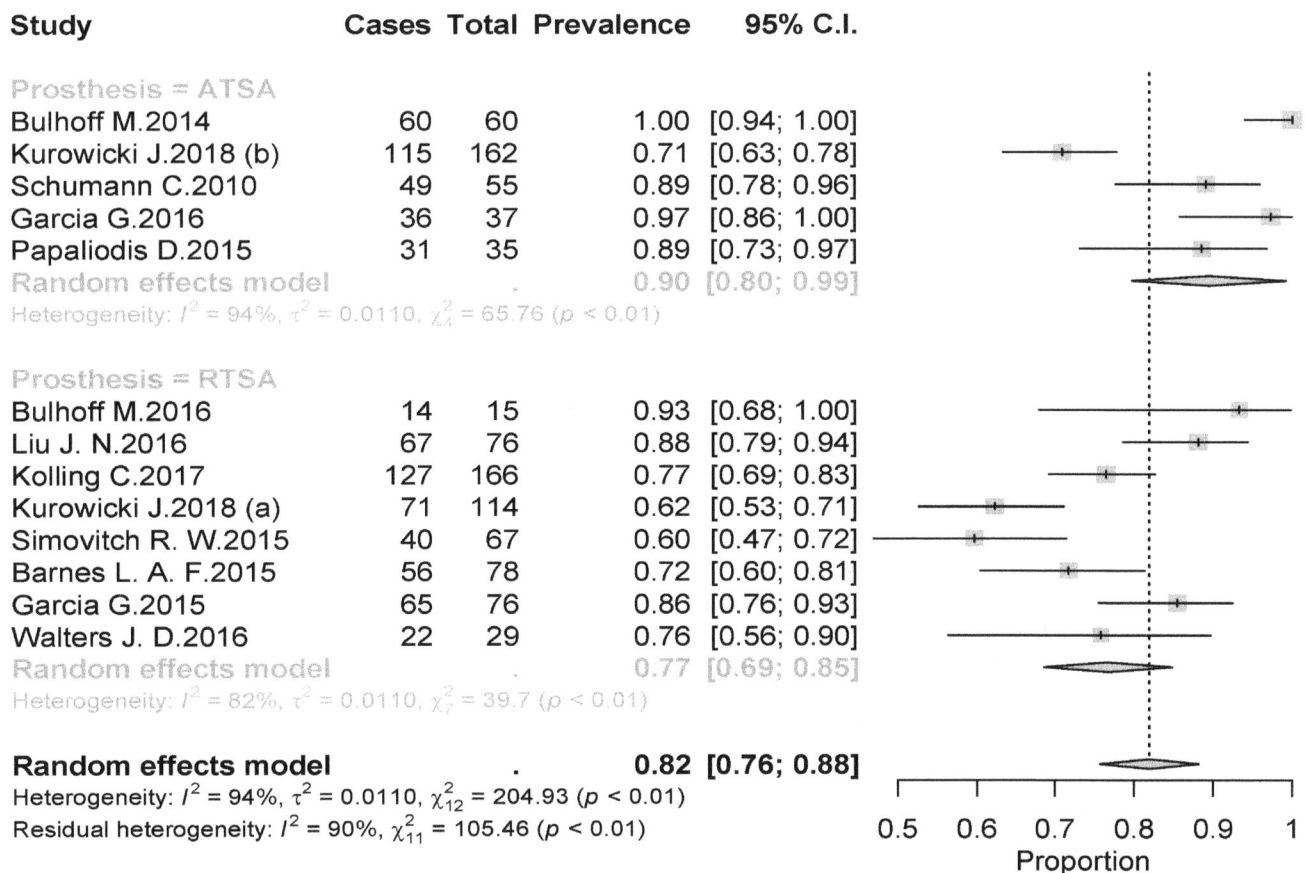

Study	Cases	Total	Prevalence	95% C.I.
Prosthesis = ATSA				
Bulhoff M.2014	60	60	1.00	[0.94; 1.00]
Kurowicki J.2018 (b)	115	162	0.71	[0.63; 0.78]
Schumann C.2010	49	55	0.89	[0.78; 0.96]
Garcia G.2016	36	37	0.97	[0.86; 1.00]
Papaliodis D.2015	31	35	0.89	[0.73; 0.97]
Random effects model			0.90	[0.80; 0.99]
Heterogeneity: $I^2 = 94\%$, $\tau^2 = 0.0110$, $\chi_4^2 = 65.76$ ($p < 0.01$)				
Prosthesis = RTSA				
Bulhoff M.2016	14	15	0.93	[0.68; 1.00]
Liu J. N.2016	67	76	0.88	[0.79; 0.94]
Kolling C.2017	127	166	0.77	[0.69; 0.83]
Kurowicki J.2018 (a)	71	114	0.62	[0.53; 0.71]
Simovitch R. W.2015	40	67	0.60	[0.47; 0.72]
Barnes L. A. F.2015	56	78	0.72	[0.60; 0.81]
Garcia G.2015	65	76	0.86	[0.76; 0.93]
Walters J. D.2016	22	29	0.76	[0.56; 0.90]
Random effects model			0.77	[0.69; 0.85]
Heterogeneity: $I^2 = 82\%$, $\tau^2 = 0.0110$, $\chi_7^2 = 39.7$ ($p < 0.01$)				
Random effects model			**0.82**	**[0.76; 0.88]**

Heterogeneity: $I^2 = 94\%$, $\tau^2 = 0.0110$, $\chi_{12}^2 = 204.93$ ($p < 0.01$)
Residual heterogeneity: $I^2 = 90\%$, $\chi_{11}^2 = 105.46$ ($p < 0.01$)

Figure 2. Forest plot chart of the combined rate of return to sports by meta-analysis with 95% confidence interval. ATSA, anatomic total shoulder arthroplasty; RTSA, reverse total shoulder arthroplasty.

Study	Cases	Total	Prevalence	95% C.I.
Bulhoff M. et al 2016	14	15	0.93	[0.81; 1.00]
Liu J. N. et al 2016	31	76	0.41	[0.30; 0.52]
Garcia G. et al 2016	34	40	0.85	[0.74; 0.96]
Simovitch R. W. Et al 2015	38	67	0.57	[0.45; 0.69]
Bulhoff M. et al 2014	51	60	0.85	[0.76; 0.94]
Kolling C. et al 2017	97	127	0.76	[0.69; 0.84]
Garcia G. et al 2015	57	65	0.88	[0.80; 0.96]
Random effects model			**0.75**	**[0.61; 0.89]**

Heterogeneity: $I^2 = 92\%$, $\tau^2 = 0.0330$, $\chi_6^2 = 70.84$ $(p < 0.01)$

0.3 0.4 0.5 0.6 0.7 0.8 0.9 1
Proportion

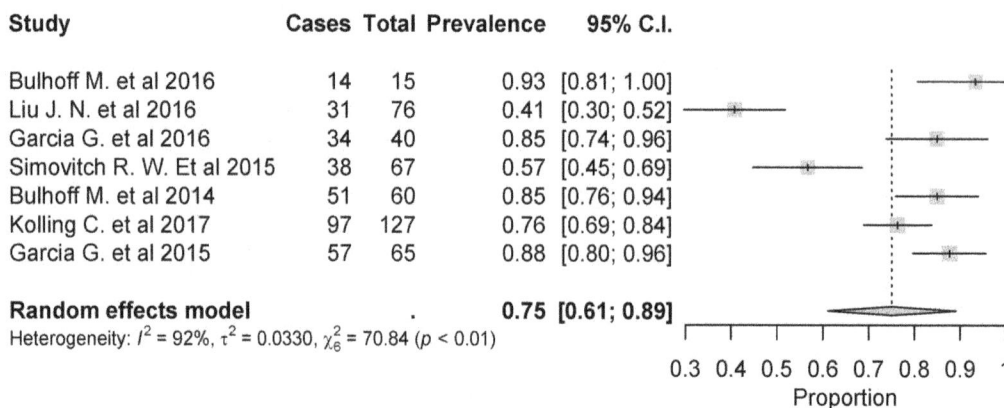

Figure 3. Forest plot chart of the rate of return to sports at the same or a higher level of play as before shoulder arthroplasty with 95% confidence interval.

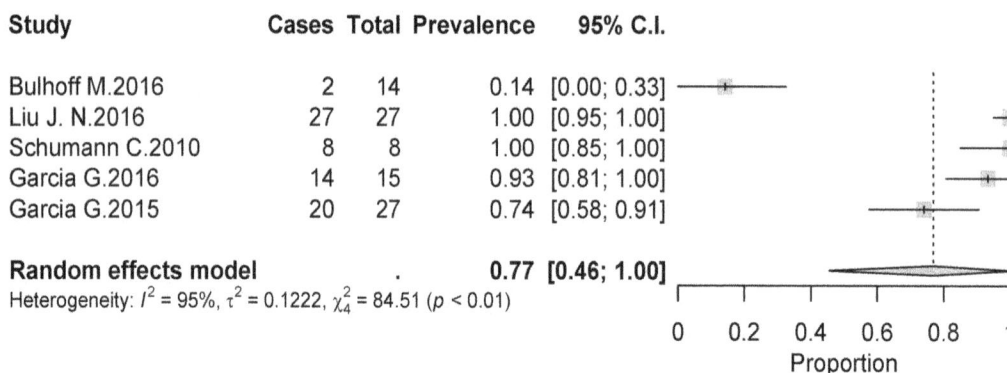

Study	Cases	Total	Prevalence	95% C.I.
Bulhoff M.2016	2	14	0.14	[0.00; 0.33]
Liu J. N.2016	27	27	1.00	[0.95; 1.00]
Schumann C.2010	8	8	1.00	[0.85; 1.00]
Garcia G.2016	14	15	0.93	[0.81; 1.00]
Garcia G.2015	20	27	0.74	[0.58; 0.91]
Random effects model			**0.77**	**[0.46; 1.00]**

Heterogeneity: $I^2 = 95\%$, $\tau^2 = 0.1222$, $\chi_4^2 = 84.51$ $(p < 0.01)$

0   0.2   0.4   0.6   0.8   1
Proportion

Figure 4. Forest plot chart of the rate of return to fitness after shoulder arthroplasty with 95% confidence interval.

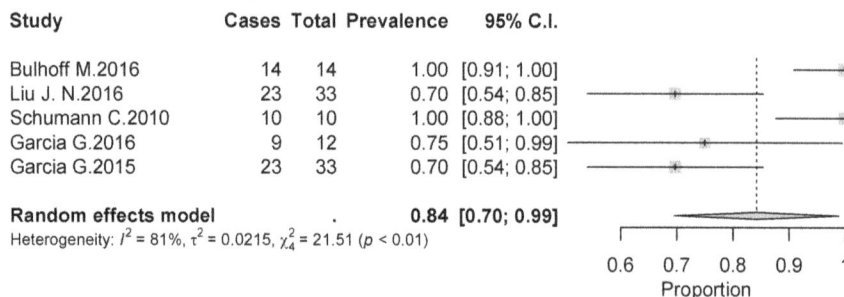

Study	Cases	Total	Prevalence	95% C.I.
Bulhoff M.2016	14	14	1.00	[0.91; 1.00]
Liu J. N.2016	23	33	0.70	[0.54; 0.85]
Schumann C.2010	10	10	1.00	[0.88; 1.00]
Garcia G.2016	9	12	0.75	[0.51; 0.99]
Garcia G.2015	23	33	0.70	[0.54; 0.85]
Random effects model			**0.84**	**[0.70; 0.99]**

Heterogeneity: $I^2 = 81\%$, $\tau^2 = 0.0215$, $\chi_4^2 = 21.51$ $(p < 0.01)$

0.6   0.7   0.8   0.9   1
Proportion

Figure 5. Forest plot chart of the rate of return to swimming after shoulder arthroplasty with 95% confidence interval.

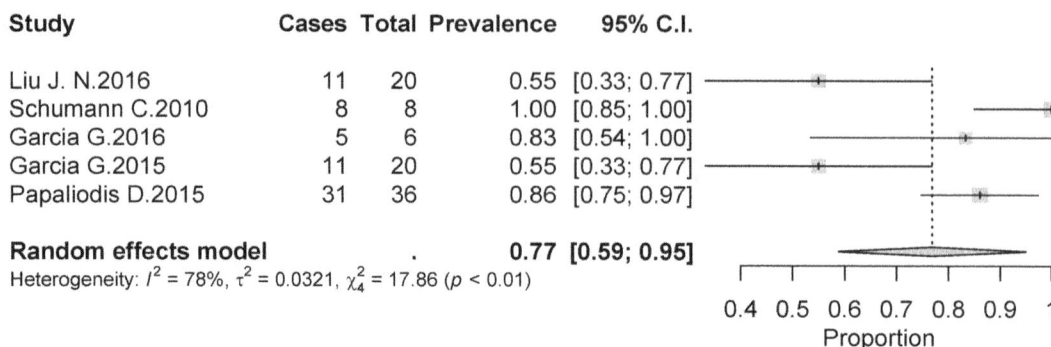

Study	Cases	Total	Prevalence	95% C.I.
Liu J. N.2016	11	20	0.55	[0.33; 0.77]
Schumann C.2010	8	8	1.00	[0.85; 1.00]
Garcia G.2016	5	6	0.83	[0.54; 1.00]
Garcia G.2015	11	20	0.55	[0.33; 0.77]
Papaliodis D.2015	31	36	0.86	[0.75; 0.97]
Random effects model			**0.77**	**[0.59; 0.95]**

Heterogeneity: $I^2 = 78\%$, $\tau^2 = 0.0321$, $\chi_4^2 = 17.86$ $(p < 0.01)$

0.4 0.5 0.6 0.7 0.8 0.9 1
Proportion

Figure 6. Forest plot chart of the rate of return to golf after shoulder arthroplasty with 95% confidence interval.

Study	Cases	Total	Prevalence	95% C.I.
Bulhoff M.2016	8	14	0.57	[0.31; 0.83]
Liu J. N.2016	7	20	0.35	[0.14; 0.56]
Schumann C.2010	3	3	1.00	[0.68; 1.00]
Garcia G.2016	8	9	0.89	[0.68; 1.00]
Garcia G.2015	8	12	0.67	[0.40; 0.93]
Random effects model		.	**0.69**	**[0.46; 0.91]**

Heterogeneity: $I^2 = 78\%$, $\tau^2 = 0.0506$, $\chi_4^2 = 17.90$ ($p < 0.01$)

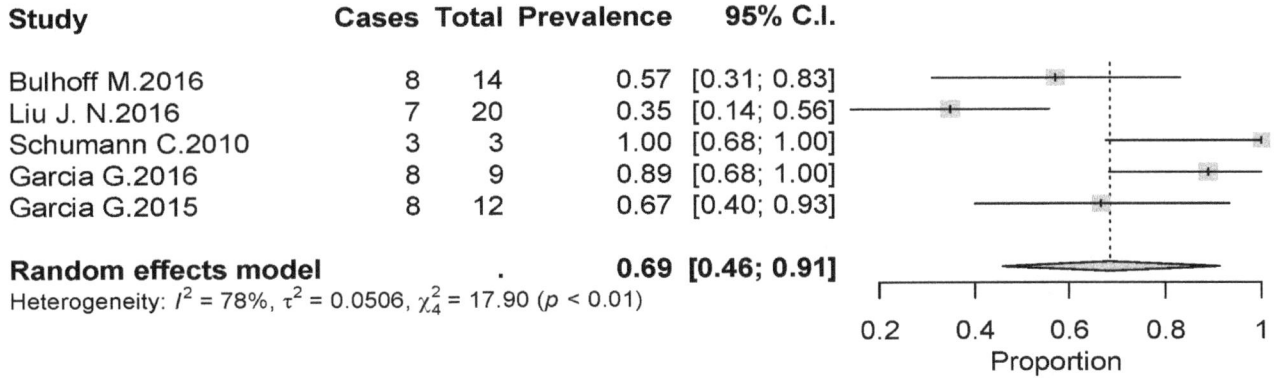

Figure 7. Forest plot chart of the rate of return to golf after shoulder arthroplasty with 95% confidence interval.

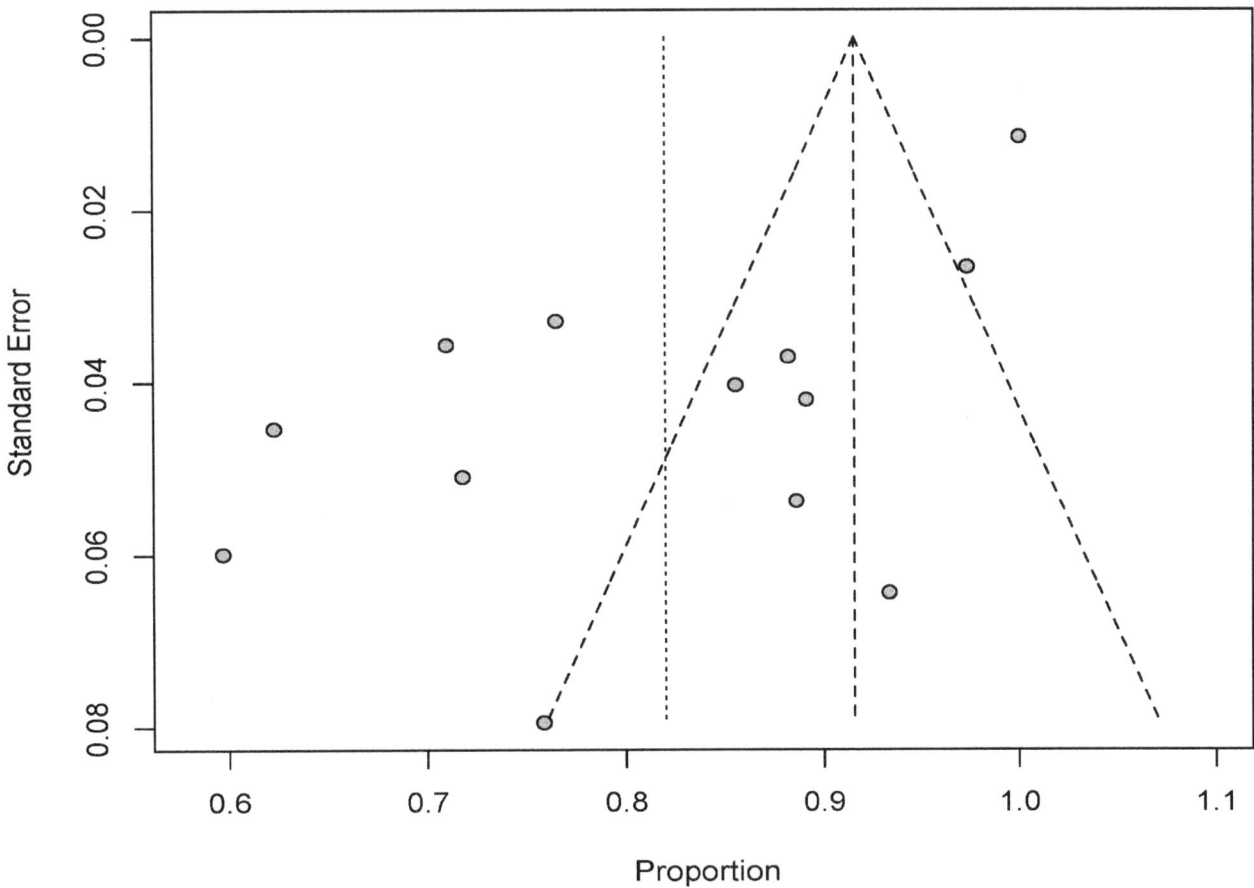

Figure 8. Funnel plot chart evaluating publication bias.

Table 2. Return to sport.

Study	Sports	Number of Patient Practicing Sport (%)	Number of Evaluated Patients	Rate of Return to Sport for Single Sport (%)	Overall Rate of Return to Sport (%)
Schumann et al. [21]	Swimming	10 (20.4%)	55	NR	49 (89%)
	Golf	8 (16.3%)			
	Cycling	8 (16.3%)			
	Fitness	8 (16.3%)			
	Other	21 (30.7%)			
Papaliodis et al. [24]	Golf	35 (100%)	35	NR	31 (88.57%)
Garcia et al., 2015 [20]	Fitness	27	76 (some patients practiced more than 1 sport)	22 (81.5%)	65 (85.5%)
	Swimming	33		22 (66.7%)	
	Golf	20		10 (50%)	
	Cycling	10		5 (50%)	
Bulhoff et al., 2015 [17]	Swimming		105	60 (57%)	60 (100%)
	Fitness including lower limb			42 (27%)	
	Skiing			31 (30%)	
	Gardening			29 (28%)	
	Bowling/skittles	60 (57%)		18 (17%)	
	Tennis			15 (14%)	
	Handball			6 (4%)	
	Athletics			4 (3%)	
	Volleyball			3 (2%)	
	Golf			2 (1%)	
	Other			26 (25%)	

Table 2. *Cont.*

Study	Sports	Number of Patient Practicing Sport (%)	Number of Evaluated Patients	Rate of Return to Sport for Single Sport (%)	Overall Rate of Return to Sport (%)
Bulhoff et al., 2016 [16]	Swimming	15 (71%)	22	14 (100%)	14 (93%)
	Fitness including lower limb			8 (57%)	
	Skiing			7 (50%)	
	Gardening			8 (57%)	
	Bowling			7 (50%)	
	Tennis			8 (57%)	
	Handball			2 (14%)	
Kolling et al. [25]	Calisthenics	166	305	28 (17%)	127 (77%)
	Hiking			28 (17%)	
	Swimming			26 (16%)	
	Alpine skiing			13 (8%)	
	Tennis			12 (7%)	
	Others			58 (35%)	
Liu et al. [18]	Single tennis	12 (12.2%)	102	4 (33%)	87 (85.9%)
	Double tennis	18 (18.3%)		3 (16.6%)	
	Baseball	1 (1.02%)		1 (100%)	
	Swimming	33 (33.66%)		23 (70%)	
	Fitness	27 (27.54%)		27 (100%)	
	Golf	20 (20.4%)		11 (55%)	
	Cycling	12 (12.2%)		8 (67%)	
	Fishing	4 (4.8%)		1 (25%)	
	Rowing	1 (1.02%)		1 (100%)	
	Running	7 (7.14%)		5 (71.4%)	
	Skiing	7 (7.14%)		2 (29%)	
	Dancing	2 (2.04%)		1 (50%)	
	Horseback riding	2 (2.04%)		1 (50%)	
	Basketball	1 (1.02%)		1 (100%)	

Table 2. *Cont.*

Study	Sports	Number of Patient Practicing Sport (%)	Number of Evaluated Patients	Rate of Return to Sport for Single Sport (%)	Overall Rate of Return to Sport (%)
Simovitch et al. [22]	Golf			50 (75%)	
	Swimming			19 (29%)	
	Water aerobics			16 (24%)	
	Deep sea fishing			14 (21%)	
	Firearm sports	67 (26%)	255	14 (21%)	64 (95%)
	Weight lifting			12 (18%)	
	Softball			7 (11%)	
	Tennis			7 (11%)	
	Table tennis			5 (7%)	
	Scuba diving			5 (7%)	
	Racquetball			3 (5%)	
	Surfing			1 (2%)	
	Water skiing			1 (2%)	
Garcia 2016 et al. [19]	Golf	6 (8.3%)		5 (83.3%)	
	Swimming	12 (16%)		9 (75%)	
	Baseball	1 (1.4%)		1 (100%)	
	Basketball	1 (1.4%)		1 (100%)	
	Nature sports	7 (9.7%)	72	7 (100%)	65 (90.27%)
	Fitness	15 (21%)		14 (93%)	
	Single tennis	5 (7%)		4 (80%)	
	Running	14 (19.4%)		13 (92.9%)	
	Cycling	5 (7%)		5 (100%)	
	Softball	2 (2.7%)		2 (100%)	
	Double tennis	4 (5.5%)		4 (100%)	

Table 2. *Cont.*

Study	Sports	Number of Patient Practicing Sport (%)	Number of Evaluated Patients	Rate of Return to Sport for Single Sport (%)	Overall Rate of Return to Sport (%)
Barnes et al. [23]	High intensity activities (hunting, golf, skiing …)	NR	78	18 (23.1%)	100%
	Moderate intensity activities (swimming, bowling …)			38 (48.7%)	
	Low intensity activities (riding bike, walking, dancing …)			22 (28.2%)	
Kirowicki et al. [26]	Golf	RTSA: 16 (22%) ATSA: 31 (27%)	RTSA: 71 ATSA 115	NR	RTSA 71/114 (62%); ATSA 115/162 (70%)
	Swimming	RTSA: 13 (18%) ATSA: 19 (16%)			
	Walking	RTSA: 16 (22%) ATSA: 18 (15%)			
	Gym exercises	RTSA: 8 (11%) ATSA: 24 (20%)			
	Racquet sport	RTSA: 4 (5%) ATSA: 13 (11%)			
	Group fitness	RTSA: 5 (7%) ATSA: 10 (8%)			
	Fishing and target shooting	RTSA: 5 (7%) ATSA: 4 (3%)			
	Adventure sport	RTSA: 1 (1%) ATSA: 9 (8%)			

NR: not reported.

3.5. Clinical Outcome Data

Outcome measures reported in the included studies are summarized in Table 3. The most frequently reported score was the American Shoulder and Elbow Surgeons (ASES) score, used in 6 (54%) of 11 studies [18–20,22,23,26], and the visual analog scale for pain (VAS) used in 4 (36%) studies [18–20,22] with an average of 76.23 (95% CI 0.81–0.90, $p < 0.01$) and 0.8 (95% CI 0.81–0.90, $p < 0.01$) points respectively (Figures 9 and 10). Constant score was used in two studies [21,22] and the evaluation of range of motion (ROM) was used in two studies [22,23].

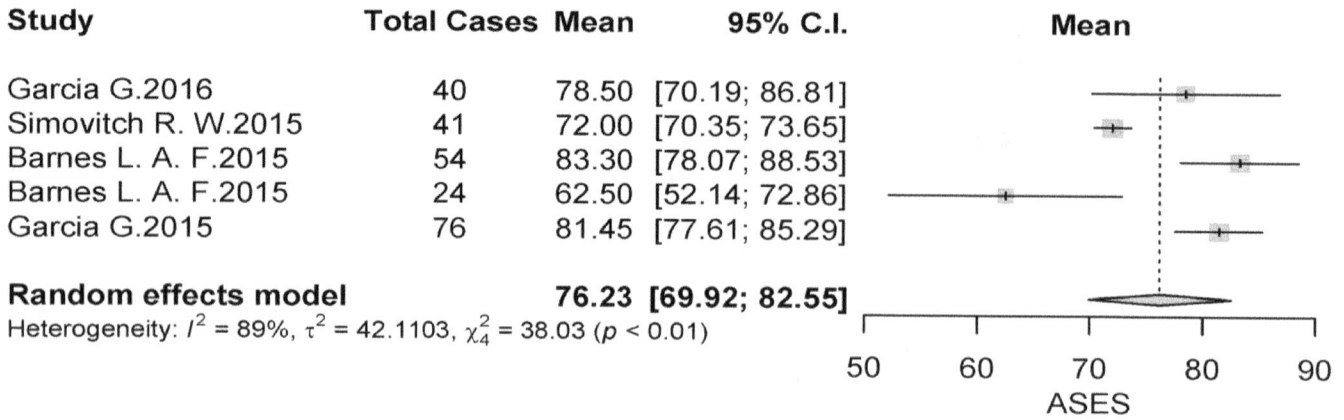

Study	Total Cases	Mean	95% C.I.	Mean
Garcia G.2016	40	78.50	[70.19; 86.81]	
Simovitch R. W.2015	41	72.00	[70.35; 73.65]	
Barnes L. A. F.2015	54	83.30	[78.07; 88.53]	
Barnes L. A. F.2015	24	62.50	[52.14; 72.86]	
Garcia G.2015	76	81.45	[77.61; 85.29]	
Random effects model		**76.23**	**[69.92; 82.55]**	

Heterogeneity: $I^2 = 89\%$, $\tau^2 = 42.1103$, $\chi^2_4 = 38.03$ ($p < 0.01$)

ASES axis: 50 60 70 80 90

Figure 9. Forest plot chart of ASES score.

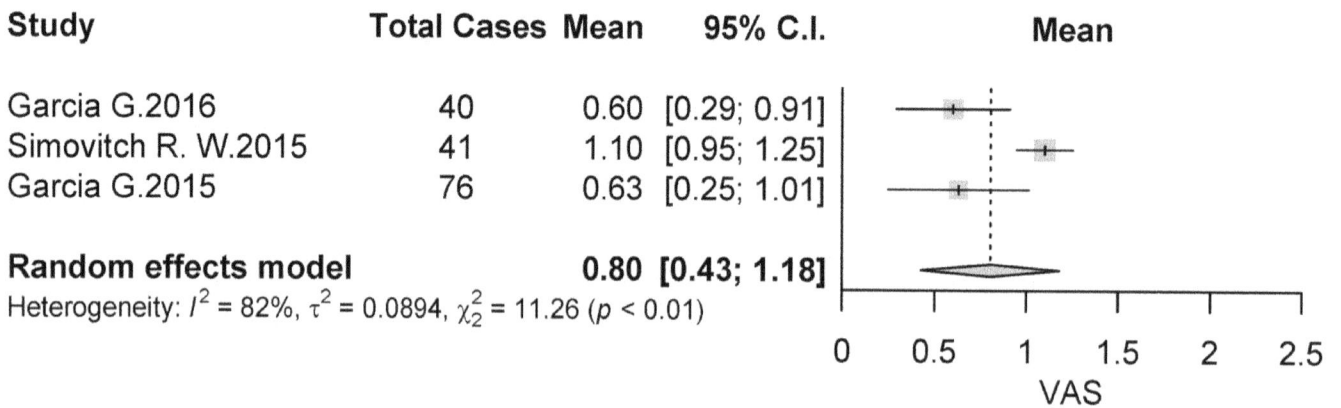

Study	Total Cases	Mean	95% C.I.	Mean
Garcia G.2016	40	0.60	[0.29; 0.91]	
Simovitch R. W.2015	41	1.10	[0.95; 1.25]	
Garcia G.2015	76	0.63	[0.25; 1.01]	
Random effects model		**0.80**	**[0.43; 1.18]**	

Heterogeneity: $I^2 = 82\%$, $\tau^2 = 0.0894$, $\chi^2_2 = 11.26$ ($p < 0.01$)

VAS axis: 0 0.5 1 1.5 2 2.5

Figure 10. Forest plot chart of VAS score.

Table 3. Clinical outcome data of the included studies.

Authors	Implant	Outcomes		Complication (Number)	Main Conclusion
		Preoperative	Postoperative		
Bulhoff et al. [17]	ATSA	NR	NR	NR	- Patients with active sports participation before TSA are successfully able to return to sports activities after surgery. - Patients who are not participating in sports just before surgery are unlikely to resume sports after surgery.
Bulhoff et al. [16]	RTSA	NR	NR	aseptic loosening of glenoid component (1), dislocation (2)	Patients with glenohumeral osteoarthritis and rotator cuff disease being active prior to RSA surgery are able to successfully return to their level of sports participation afterwards.
Liu et al. [18]	RTSA	ASES SCORE (overall mean change) +39 VAS (overall mean reduction) −5.64		None	Despite traditional sport restrictions placed on RTSA, patients undergoing RTSA can return to sports at rates higher than those undergoing HHA, with fewer postoperative complaints.
Kolling et al. [25]	RTSA	NR		NR	- Most patients carried out their main sports activity after surgery with a moderate level of intensity (83%) and between one to three times per week (69%). - 42% indicated that returning to sports was among their key demands after RSA.

Table 3. *Cont.*

Authors	Implant	Outcomes		Complication (Number)	Main Conclusion
		Preoperative	Postoperative		
Schumann et al. [21]	ATSA		**CONSTANT SCORE (mean ± SD)**	NR	The probability of being able to do sports postoperatively—if done preoperatively—is high. Long-term studies are needed to determine whether the greater loading on the joint will lead to more rapid wear and a higher rate of loosening with time.
		NR	GI: 70.8 ± 13.8; GII: 77.2 ± 10.6; GIII: 69.3 ± 9.7	-	
			SF-36 (mean ± SD)		
		NR	Physical component: GI 41.0 ± 11.2; GII: 46.2 ± 9.0; GIII: 42.2 ± 10.6; Mental component GI: 55.6 ± 9.3; GII 55.7 ± 6.4; GIII: 47.7 ± 12.9	-	
			DASH SCORE (mean ± SD)		
		NR	GI: 76.6 ± 19.3; GII: 83.4 ± 12.7; GIII: 69.6 ± 18.6		
			SPADI SCORE (mean ± SD)		
		NR	GI: 78.6 ± 20.5; GII: 83.7 ± 16.5; GIII: 68.7 ± 19.2		
Garcia et al. [19]	ATSA		**ASES SCORE (mean)**	NR	Rate of return to sports was significantly better after TSA, although further studies are needed to review glenoid loosening. HA patients had significantly more pain, worse satisfaction, and a decreased ability to return to sports.
		34.0	78.5	-	
			VAS (mean)	-	
		6.1	0.6		

Table 3. *Cont.*

Authors	Implant	Outcomes		Complication (Number)	Main Conclusion
		Preoperative	Postoperative		
Papaliodis et al. [24]	ATSA	VAS (mean average improvement) 4.3		NR	Patients who undergo TSA for primary glenohumeral arthritis can safely return to golfing activity with a significant decrease in their perceived pain level. Statistically significant findings included an increase in driving distance by 12.5 yd and an improvement in handicap by 1.4.
Simovitch et al. [22]	RTSA	CONSTANT SCORE (mean ± SD)		type II acromion stress fracture (1); postoperative infection (1), postoperative dislocation (1)	RTSA in senior athletes can be safely performed with good clinical results. No prominent mode of mechanical or clinical failure has been identified with short-term follow-up.
		25 ± 1.9	84 ± 1.7		
		ASES SCORE (mean ± SD)			
		31 ± 1.9	72 ± 4.5		
		ROM (mean ± SD)			
		Flexion: 78 ± 16; Abduction: 67 ± 14.6; External rotation: 26 ± 5.2	Flexion: 152 ± 12; Abduction: 148 ± 11.6; External rotation: 44 ± 5.7		
		VAS (mean ± SD)			
		7.2 ± 0.5	1.1 ± 0.5		
		SSV (mean ± SD)			
		27 ± 4.3	90 ± 4		

Table 3. *Cont.*

Authors	Implant	Outcomes		Complication (Number)	Main Conclusion
		Preoperative	**Postoperative**		
Barnes et al. [23]	RTSA	**ASES SCORE (mean)**		dislocation (3), aseptic loosening (1); dissociated glenosphere baseplates (1); deep infections (2); superficial infection (1)	RTSA results in good pain relief and motion, with a variety of postoperative overhead activities enjoyed by some patients who are not limited by comorbidities.
		NR	77.5		
		ROM (mean)			
		NR	active forward elevation: 140°, active external rotation: 48°, active internal rotation: S1		
		VAS (mean)			
		NR	2.3		
Kurowicki et al. [26]	RTSA ATSA	**ASES SCORE (mean)**		NR	- Both TSA and RSA allow for participation in work and sports, with TSA patients reporting better overall ability to participate. - For sports involving shoulder function, TSA patients more commonly report maximal ability to participate than RSA patients.
		NR	RTSA: 77.14 ATSA: 83.03		
Garcia et al. [20]	RTSA	**ASES SCORE (mean ± SD)**		None	- Patients undergoing RTSA had an 85% rate of return to 1 or more sporting activities at an average of 5.3 months after surgery. - Noncontact, high-demand activities (swimming, skiing, golf, and tennis) had lower return rates than lower demand activities. - Age greater than 70 years old was a significant predictor of decreased return to activities.
		34.3 ± 17.2	81.45 ± 17.1		
		VAS (mean ± SD)			
		6.57 ± 2.4	0.63 ± 1.7		

ATSA: anatomic shoulder arthroplasty; RTSA: reverse total shoulder arthroplasty; NR: not reported; ASES score: American Shoulder and Elbow Surgeons Score; VAS: visual analogue scale; SF-36: Short For;-36; DASH score: Disabilities of the Arm, Shoulder and Hand Score; SPADI score: Shoulder Pain and Disability Index Score; ROM: range of motion; SSV: subjective shoulder value; SD: standard deviation.

3.6. Rehabilitation Protocols

Only 5 out of 11 included papers reported the postoperative rehabilitation protocol [17,18,22,23,25]. Those authors advised a shoulder sling immobilization for the first four weeks, leaving free elbow and wrist movements. [17,18,22,23,25] In general, only passive ROM was allowed for the first 4 weeks, waiting for the sixth postoperative week to start active exercises. [17,18,22,23,25] Strengthening exercises were generally allowed from the twelfth postoperative week [18,22], even if Barnes et al. started them from the eighth [23]. On the contrary, Kolling et al. [25] permitted active mobilization and water therapy for shoulder strength and coordination from the second week after surgery. The surgical approach was evaluated in order to correlate subscapular repair to restrictions in the rehabilitative protocol. Among the five surgeons who performed the subscapularis tendon repair [16,17,21,23,25], only Kolling et al. [25] chose to limit external rotation movements to protect the reinserted tendon until the end of the second postoperative week. The postoperative rehabilitation protocols and the surgical approach are reported in Table 4.

Table 4. Rehabilitative protocols and surgical approach.

Authors	Rehabilitative Protocols	Surgical Approach
Bulhoff et al. [17]	1. Abduction pillow (20°) and internal rotation (20°) for the first 4 weeks. 2. Day 1 to 6th week: daily actively assisted exercise with a physiotherapist. 3. From 6th week: active and free range of motion.	Deltopectoral approach with subscapularis repair
Bulhoff et al. [16]	NR	Deltopectoral approach with subscapularis repair
Liu et al. [18]	1. Sling immobilization for the first 4 weeks. 2. From 2nd week: passive ROM at 2 weeks. 3. From 6th week: active ROM. 4. From 12th week: strengthening exercises and prior recreational activities and work were encouraged. Restriction: avoid contact sports	NR
Kolling et al. [25]	1. Sling immobilization during the night for the first 4 weeks. 2. From day 1 to 2nd week: passive motion with only limited external rotation movements to protect the reinserted subscapularis tendon. 3. From 2nd to 5th week: active mobilization and water therapy to gain shoulder strength and coordination. 4. After 12th week: resume any prior sports activities including non-contact sports.	Deltopectoral approach with subscapularis repair
Schumann et al. [21]	NR	Deltopectoral approach with subscapularis repair
Garcia et al. [19]	NR	Deltopectoral approach
Papaliodis et al. [24]	NR	NR

Table 4. *Cont.*

Authors	Rehabilitative Protocols	Surgical Approach
Simovitch et al. [22]	1. Abduction sling for the first 4 weeks. 2. From day 1 to 4th week: passive ROM and isometric exercises. 3. From 6th week: active ROM. 4. From 12th week: strengthening exercises. 5. From 16th week: return to sports.	Deltopectoral approach without subscapularis repair
Barnes et al. [23]	1. Sling immobilization for the first 4 weeks (only wrist and elbow motion allowed) 2. From 4th week: active shoulder ROM. 3. From 8th week: strengthening exercises.	Deltopectoral approach with subscapularis repair
Garcia et al. [20]	NR Restriction: avoid contact sports.	NR
Kirowicki et al. [26]	NR	NR

NR: not reported; ROM: range of motion.

4. Discussion

In the present review, we found that the overall rate of return to sport after ATSA and RTSA in elderly patients is 82%. Specifically, 90% of patients who underwent ATSA and 77% of patients who underwent RTSA were able to practice sports again. The fact that the pooled analysis demonstrated the highest rate of return to sports in ATSA is not unexpected. Several studies demonstrated greater range of motion, higher functional outcomes scores, and improved patient satisfaction when comparing ATSA and RTSA [27,28]. Among sports commonly performed after surgery, swimming has the highest rate (84%) followed by fitness (77%), golf (77%) and tennis (69%). Therefore, the most practiced sports after surgery are the non-contact ones, probably due to a defensive attitude of patients and surgeons. Golant et al. [29] have highlighted that, in the available literature, there is an extensive variation in surgeon recommendations on activity restrictions after TSA, and that information regarding return to sports activities after shoulder arthroplasty is also lacking. In particular, they find that surgeons recommend noncontact low-load sports at the expense of contact ones. Healy et al. [30] surveyed 35 members of the American Shoulder and Elbow Surgeons regarding their recommendations for sports participation after shoulder arthroplasty. They concluded that sports that may impart high loads on the glenohumeral joint, such as football, should be avoided, whereas low-impact sports, such as cross-country skiing and swimming, may be allowed.

Papaliodis et al. [24] demonstrated that return to sports is possible, reporting a significant decrease in shoulder pain during sports activity. In this study, all patients practiced golf. Thirty one of 35 patients could return to play golf after an average time of 8.4 months postoperatively (range, 2–24 months). Fifteen patients reported subjective improvement in their ability, 12 reported no change, and only 4 reported less ability. Schumann et al. [21] evaluated the return to sports activity after TSA in 55 patients. The most practiced sports were swimming (10 patients, 20.4%), golfing (8 patients, 16.3%), cycling (8 patients, 16.3%), and fitness (8 patients, 16.3%). Six patients did not resume sport activity after TSA. Of the considered patients, 33 of the 55 were able to resume sport within six months after surgery. Another 16 patients returned to practice sport within two years after TSA. In the study of Garcia et al. [20], 85.5% of patients resumed sports activity. Low contact sports and low demand sports had the highest rate of return to practice, (fitness: 81.5%, 22/27; swimming: 66.7%, 22/33; running 57.1%, 4/7; cycling 50.0%, 6/12; golf 50%, 10/20). Of the considered cohort, 47.6% resumed sport at a higher level than preoperative, while only 10.9% did not reach their preoperative activity level.

Moreover, the papers included in this systematic review confirmed a pain reduction after shoulder surgery. In the study of Liu et al. [18], the difference between preoperative and postoperative VAS was 5.64 points. In the study of Garcia et al. [20], the postoperative VAS score was 5.64 points lower than preoperative. Similar results were showed by Simovitch et al. [22], with a mean difference between preoperative and postoperative VAS of 6.1 points. Additionally, they showed that postoperative pain reduction was associated with an improvement of ROM and ASES scores [22]. Three studies reported the difference between preoperative and postoperative ASES and, in all of them, an improvement in postoperative values can be observed [18,20,22]. Barnes et al. [23] reported only the mean postoperative ASES which was 77.5, but even in this case, the improvement of ASES scores and VAS was associated with return to sport at the same or better preoperative level.

The present meta-analysis has shown that patients returned to sport activities at the same or a higher level in 75% of cases. This confirms that most patients undergoing shoulder arthroplasty (regardless of type) can safely return to at least one sport, with many returning to the same level of play, although a 100% guarantee should not be provided. Bulhoff et al. [17] assessed that, in their cohort, the postoperative activity levels and frequencies in sports practice were higher than before surgery. Moreover, patients were satisfied with their performances. Kolling et al. [25] selected 69 patients who clearly expressed their desire to resume sports activities after surgery and 60% of these patients were satisfied with their postoperative performance level and, within a year from surgery, 86% returned to practice sport at the same preoperative level or higher.

The postoperative rehabilitation protocol was reported in five studies [17,18,22,23,25]. Available protocols provided general information about time of immobilization and gradual recovery of shoulder motion and strength. Generally, the majority of surgeons followed similar indications: sling immobilization for at least four weeks, passive ROM for the first four weeks, active exercise from about the sixth postoperative week and strength training from the 12th postoperative week. On the contrary, Kolling et al. [25] permitted active mobilization and water therapy for shoulder strength and coordination in the second week after surgery. Unfortunately, the current literature lacks a detailed description of the rehabilitative steps and specific information about training for the athletic population. Moreover, to the best of our knowledge, no high-level evidence trials have been performed to test the efficacy of different post-operative rehabilitation protocols for patients who underwent TSA. However, some authors demonstrated that patients who received a physician-directed rehabilitation program had a significantly better range of motion as compared to patients only supervised by physiotherapists [12].

This systematic review has a few limitations including the number of studies and their heterogeneous methodological approach. Moreover, designs and implantation techniques may have varied significantly across the analyzed studies, thus reflecting the sparse available evidence on the subject and the absence of randomized controlled trials. Importantly, none of these studies mentions the abilities and experience of the surgeon. Since ATSA involves greater operative time and attention, surgical experience could be a determining factor in the decision to perform a reverse or anatomic total shoulder arthroplasty. In order to create a more homogenous cohort, future studies should account for these individual surgeon factors in the methodology. Moreover, all the included studies were affected by a high risk of bias and, in some of them, the follow-up period was quite short to detect important postoperative complications after return to sport, such as loosening or periprosthetic fractures. Patients and sports were heterogeneous as well as the postoperative rehabilitation protocol assessed. Great variability was observed in the postoperative treatment protocols following shoulder arthroplasty. Therefore, it is very difficult to identify common patterns, making it impossible to do a metanalysis of postoperative rehabilitation protocols. Moreover, we performed the metanalysis only on postoperative ASES and VAS scores since their preoperative data were not reported in the included studies, hindering the assessment of significant improvements of these postoperative outcomes. Finally, important postoperative clinical outcomes, such as postoperative ROM, were often not reported.

5. Conclusions

After ATSA and RTSA, elderly patients can satisfactorily resume their sports activities. The rate of return to sports following ATSA is slightly higher than RTSA, probably due to differences in the patient population, surgical indication, and biomechanical issues. Most patients are able to return to practice sport at the same or a higher preoperative level. The most practiced sports after surgery are low contact activities such as fitness, swimming, golf, and tennis. Unfortunately, there is a lack of research data on the advantages and disadvantages of existing rehabilitation protocols and no standard of practice could be deduced. Therefore, more prospective randomized studies are needed to establish which kind of postoperative protocol is best following ATSA and RTSA.

Author Contributions: Conceptualization, R.P. and V.D.; methodology, E.A. and M.C.; writing—original draft preparation, M.C., E.A. and C.D.A.; writing—review and editing, E.A., L.A.D.B., A.M.A., A.D.V. and R.B.; supervision, C.F. and A.M.; funding acquisition, R.P. All authors have read and agreed to the published version of the manuscript.

References

1. Deshmukh, A.V.; Koris, M.; Zurakowski, D.; Thornhill, T.S. Total shoulder arthroplasty: Long-term survivorship, functional outcome, and quality of life. *J. Shoulder Elbow Surg.* **2005**, *14*, 471–479. [CrossRef] [PubMed]

2. Westermann, R.W.; Pugely, A.J.; Martin, C.T.; Gao, Y.; Wolf, B.R.; Hettrich, C.M. Reverse Shoulder Arthroplasty in the United States: A Comparison of National Volume, Patient Demographics, Complications, and Surgical Indications. *Iowa Orthop. J.* **2015**, *35*, 1–7. [PubMed]

3. Chalmers, P.N.; Keener, J.D. Expanding roles for reverse shoulder arthroplasty. *Curr. Rev. Musculoskelet. Med.* **2016**, *9*, 40–48. [CrossRef] [PubMed]

4. Waldstein, W.; Kolbitsch, P.; Koller, U.; Boettner, F.; Windhager, R. Sport and physical activity following unicompartmental knee arthroplasty: A systematic review. *Knee Surg. Sports Traumatol. Arthrosc.* **2017**, *25*, 717–728. [CrossRef]

5. Mont, M.A.; LaPorte, D.M.; Mullick, T.; Silberstein, C.E.; Hungerford, D.S. Tennis after total hip arthroplasty. *Am. J. Sports Med.* **1999**, *27*, 60–64. [CrossRef]

6. Huch, K.; Müller, K.A.; Stürmer, T.; Brenner, H.; Puhl, W.; Günther, K.P. Sports activities 5 years after total knee or hip arthroplasty: The Ulm Osteoarthritis Study. *Ann. Rheum. Dis.* **2005**, *64*, 1715–1720. [CrossRef]

7. Magnussen, R.A.; Mallon, W.J.; Willems, W.J.; Moorman, C.T. Long-term activity restrictions after shoulder arthroplasty: An international survey of experienced shoulder surgeons. *J. Shoulder Elbow Surg.* **2011**, *20*, 281–289. [CrossRef]

8. Wolff, A.L.; Rosenzweig, L. Anatomical and biomechanical framework for shoulder arthroplasty rehabilitation. *J. Hand Ther.* **2017**, *30*, 167–174. [CrossRef]

9. Bade, M.J.; Struessel, T.; Dayton, M.; Foran, J.; Kim, R.H.; Miner, T.; Wolfe, P.; Kohrt, W.M.; Dennis, D.; Stevens-Lapsley, J.E. Early High-Intensity Versus Low-Intensity Rehabilitation After Total Knee Arthroplasty: A Randomized Controlled Trial. *Arthritis Care Res. (Hoboken)* **2017**, *69*, 1360–1368. [CrossRef]

10. Nassar, I.; Fahey, J.; Mitchell, D. Rapid recovery following hip and knee arthroplasty using local infiltration analgesia: Length of stay, rehabilitation protocol and cost savings. *ANZ J. Surg.* **2020**, *90*, 355–359. [CrossRef]

11. Hughes, M.; Neer, C.S. Glenohumeral joint replacement and postoperative rehabilitation. *Phys. Ther.* **1975**, *55*, 850–858. [CrossRef]

12. Mulieri, P.J.; Holcomb, J.O.; Dunning, P.; Pliner, M.; Bogle, R.K.; Pupello, D.; Frankle, M.A. Is a formal physical therapy program necessary after total shoulder arthroplasty for osteoarthritis? *J. Shoulder Elbow Surg.* **2010**, *19*, 570–579. [CrossRef]

13. Uschok, S.; Herrmann, S.; Pauly, S.; Perka, C.; Greiner, S. Reverse shoulder arthroplasty: The role of physical therapy on the clinical outcome in the mid-term to long-term follow-up. *Arch. Orthop. Trauma Surg.* **2018**, *138*, 1347–1352. [CrossRef]

14. Shamseer, L.; Moher, D.; Clarke, M.; Ghersi, D.; Liberati, A.; Petticrew, M.; Shekelle, P.; Stewart, L.A.; Group, P.-P. Preferred reporting items for systematic review and meta-analysis protocols (PRISMA-P) 2015: Elaboration and explanation. *BMJ* **2015**, *350*, g7647. [CrossRef]

15. Slim, K.; Nini, E.; Forestier, D.; Kwiatkowski, F.; Panis, Y.; Chipponi, J. Methodological index for non-randomized studies (minors): Development and validation of a new instrument. *ANZ J. Surg.* **2003**, *73*, 712–716. [CrossRef]

16. Bülhoff, M.; Sowa, B.; Bruckner, T.; Zeifang, F.; Raiss, P. Activity levels after reverse shoulder arthroplasty. *Arch. Orthop. Trauma Surg.* **2016**, *136*, 1189–1193. [CrossRef]

17. Bülhoff, M.; Sattler, P.; Bruckner, T.; Loew, M.; Zeifang, F.; Raiss, P. Do patients return to sports and work after total shoulder replacement surgery? *Am. J. Sports Med.* **2015**, *43*, 423–427. [CrossRef]

18. Liu, J.N.; Garcia, G.H.; Mahony, G.; Wu, H.H.; Dines, D.M.; Warren, R.F.; Gulotta, L.V. Sports after shoulder arthroplasty: A comparative analysis of hemiarthroplasty and reverse total shoulder replacement. *J. Shoulder Elbow Surg.* **2016**, *25*, 920–926. [CrossRef]

19. Garcia, G.H.; Liu, J.N.; Mahony, G.T.; Sinatro, A.; Wu, H.H.; Craig, E.V.; Warren, R.F.; Dines, D.M.; Gulotta, L.V. Hemiarthroplasty Versus Total Shoulder Arthroplasty for Shoulder Osteoarthritis: A Matched Comparison of Return to Sports. *Am. J. Sports Med.* **2016**, *44*, 1417–1422. [CrossRef]

20. Garcia, G.H.; Taylor, S.A.; DePalma, B.J.; Mahony, G.T.; Grawe, B.M.; Nguyen, J.; Dines, J.S.; Dines, D.M.; Warren, R.F.; Craig, E.V.; et al. Patient Activity Levels After Reverse Total Shoulder Arthroplasty: What Are Patients Doing? *Am. J. Sports Med.* **2015**, *43*, 2816–2821. [CrossRef]

21. Schumann, K.; Flury, M.P.; Schwyzer, H.K.; Simmen, B.R.; Drerup, S.; Goldhahn, J. Sports activity after anatomical total shoulder arthroplasty. *Am. J. Sports Med.* **2010**, *38*, 2097–2105. [CrossRef]

22. Simovitch, R.W.; Gerard, B.K.; Brees, J.A.; Fullick, R.; Kearse, J.C. Outcomes of reverse total shoulder arthroplasty in a senior athletic population. *J. Shoulder Elbow Surg.* **2015**, *24*, 1481–1485. [CrossRef]

23. Fink Barnes, L.A.; Grantham, W.J.; Meadows, M.C.; Bigliani, L.U.; Levine, W.N.; Ahmad, C.S. Sports activity after reverse total shoulder arthroplasty with minimum 2-year follow-up. *Am. J. Orthop. (Belle Mead NJ)* **2015**, *44*, 68–72.

24. Papaliodis, D.; Richardson, N.; Tartaglione, J.; Roberts, T.; Whipple, R.; Zanaros, G. Impact of Total Shoulder Arthroplasty on Golfing Activity. *Clin. J. Sport Med.* **2015**, *25*, 338–340. [CrossRef]

25. Kolling, C.; Borovac, M.; Audigé, L.; Mueller, A.M.; Schwyzer, H.K. Return to sports after reverse shoulder arthroplasty-the Swiss perspective. *Int. Orthop.* **2018**, *42*, 1129–1135. [CrossRef]

26. Kurowicki, J.; Rosas, S.; Law, T.Y.; Levy, J.C. Participation in Work and Sport Following Reverse and Total Shoulder Arthroplasty. *Am. J. Orthop. (Belle Mead NJ)* **2018**, *47*. [CrossRef]

27. Flurin, P.H.; Roche, C.P.; Wright, T.W.; Marczuk, Y.; Zuckerman, J.D. A Comparison and Correlation of Clinical Outcome Metrics in Anatomic and Reverse Total Shoulder Arthroplasty. *Bull. Hosp. Jt. Dis.* **2015**, *73* (Suppl. 1), S118–S123.

28. Eichinger, J.K.; Miller, L.R.; Hartshorn, T.; Li, X.; Warner, J.J.; Higgins, L.D. Evaluation of satisfaction and durability after hemiarthroplasty and total shoulder arthroplasty in a cohort of patients aged 50 years or younger: An analysis of discordance of patient satisfaction and implant survival. *J. Shoulder Elbow Surg.* **2016**, *25*, 772–780. [CrossRef]

29. Golant, A.; Christoforou, D.; Zuckerman, J.D.; Kwon, Y.W. Return to sports after shoulder arthroplasty: A survey of surgeons' preferences. *J. Shoulder Elbow Surg.* **2012**, *21*, 554–560. [CrossRef]

30. Healy, W.L.; Iorio, R.; Lemos, M.J. Athletic activity after joint replacement. *Am. J. Sports Med.* **2001**, *29*, 377–388. [CrossRef]

11

Biohumoral Indicators Influenced by Physical Activity in the Elderly

Chiara Fossati [1], **Guglielmo Torre** [2,*], **Paolo Borrione** [1], **Arrigo Giombini** [1], **Federica Fagnani** [1], **Matteo Turchetta** [3], **Erika Albo** [2], **Maurizio Casasco** [4], **Attilio Parisi** [1] and **Fabio Pigozzi** [1]

[1] Department of Movement, Human and Health Sciences, University of Rome "Foro Italico", 00135 Rome, Italy; chiara.fossati@uniroma4.it (C.F.); paolo.borrione@uniroma4.it (P.B.); arrigo.giombini@uniroma4.it (A.G.); federica.fagnani@uniroma4.it (F.F.); attilio.parisi@uniroma4.it (A.P.); fabio.pigozzi@uniroma4.it (F.P.)

[2] Department of Orthopaedic and Trauma Surgery, Campus Bio-Medico University of Rome, 00128 Roma, Italy; e.albo@unicampus.it

[3] Department of Orthopaedics, Policlinico Casilino, 00169 Rome, Italy; matteoturchetta1@gmail.com

[4] Italian Federation of Sports Medicine, 00196 Rome, Italy; presidente@fmsi.it

* Correspondence: g.torre@unicampus.it

Abstract: In the scientific landscape, there is a growing interest in defining the role of several biomolecules and humoral indicators of the aging process and in the modifications of these biomarkers induced by physical activity and exercise. The main aim of the present narrative review is to collect the available evidence on the biohumoral indicators that could be modified by physical activity (PA) in the elderly. Online databases including Pubmed, Web of science (Medline), and Scopus were searched for relevant articles published in the last five years in English. Keywords and combination of these used for the search were the following: "biological", "indicators", "markers", "physical", "activity", and "elderly". Thirty-four papers were analyzed for inclusion. Twenty-nine studies were included and divided into four categories: cardiovascular (CV) biomarkers, metabolic biomarkers, inflammatory markers-oxidative stress molecules, and other markers. There are many distinct biomarkers influenced by PA in the elderly, with promising results concerning the metabolic and CV indexes, as a growing number of studies demonstrate the role of PA on improving parameters related to heart function and CV risk like atherogenic lipid profile. Furthermore, it is also a verified hypothesis that PA is able to modify the inflammatory status of the subject by decreasing the levels of pro-inflammatory cytokines, including interleukin-1 (IL-1), interleukin-6 (IL-6), and tumor necrosis factor-alpha (TNF-α). PA seems also to be able to have a direct effect on the immune system. There is a strong evidence of a positive effect of PA on the health of elderly people that could be evidenced and "quantified" by the modifications of the levels of several biohumoral indicators.

Keywords: physical activity; elderly; biomarkers; noncommunicable diseases; hypertension; diabetes

1. Introduction

Successful aging is one of the main health-related concerns of nowadays, as the public burden related to aging becomes even more consistent, especially in terms of assistance and expense. Physical activity (PA) plays a key role in aging, as many studies have evinced its beneficial effects in primary and secondary prevention of noncommunicable diseases (NCDs) and its influence in the aging process of tissues. Furthermore, PA has a relevant role in mental wellness, in decreasing dementia and stress reactions [1], as well as in increasing the life expectancy. The World Health Organization (WHO) recommends a minimum of 150 min of moderate exercise or 75 min of vigorous training per week for adults, including older adults. Physical inactivity is considered the fourth major risk factor for global mortality [1], leading to approximately 3 million deaths per year [2]. According to actual data from Europe, there is a lack of active lifestyles in daily life, as older adults spend an average of 9.4 h per day in sedentary activities [3] and only 7% practice regular exercise [1]. Age is indeed the most relevant risk factor for inactivity [4], since for older people, it is significantly more challenging to get engaged in exercise when compared to younger subjects. Conceivably, a comprehensible vicious circle develops, since the presence of systemic diseases prevents the subject from being engaged in exercise and the lack of activity yields a worsening of such systemic pathologic conditions. A major role of physical inactivity has been reported in the onset and worsening of cardiovascular (CV) disease, type 2 diabetes mellitus (T2DM), atherosclerosis, neurodegeneration, and cancer. The combination of these diseases as well as the presence of osteoporosis and sarcopenia configures a frailty syndrome, considered the main cause of disability in the elderly [5].

One of the main challenges of modern medicine and public health is efficient monitoring of health conditions of the elderly to better understand the aging process and to prevent the development of such a vicious mechanism. In the scientific landscape, there is a growing interest in defining the role of several biomolecules and humoral indicators [6] of the aging process and in the modifications of these biomarkers induced by physical activity and exercise [7]. However, the role of PA on these modifications is far from being completely elucidated.

The main objective of the present narrative review is to collect the available evidence above the biohumoral indicators that could be modified by PA in the elderly in order to understand by the use of quantitative indicators its role in protecting the health and functional wellbeing of this age group.

2. Methods

2.1. Criteria for Considering Studies for This Review

Types of studies considered for inclusion in the present review were randomized controlled trials (RCT), prospective cohort studies (PCS), case-control studies (CCS), and letters to the editor. Studies considered should concern biohumoral indicators, biomolecules, and markers that are influenced by PA in elderly.

2.2. Search Methods for Identification of Studies

Online databases including Pubmed, Web of science (Medline), and Scopus were searched for relevant articles published in the last five years in English. Keywords and combination of these used for the search were the following: "biological", "indicators", "markers", "physical", "activity", and "elderly". The studies retrieved were firstly screened by title, and then, the whole abstract was examined for the relevant ones.

After a first selection and exclusion of nonrelevant papers and papers which did not focus on elderly (mean age < 60 years old), the full-text of the potentially eligible articles was retrieved and read for possible inclusion. To enrich the electronic search with further studies, the bibliography of the relevant articles was manually searched to identify potentially eligible papers missed at the electronic search. Thirty-four papers were analyzed for inclusion, 3 of these were then excluded (2 did not concern clinical research, and 1 investigated functional status and not PA). Two more were excluded because they were systematic reviews (Figure 1). Studies included were divided into four categories depending on the type of biohumoral indicators that were investigated: CV biomarkers, metabolic biomarkers, inflammatory markers-oxidative stress molecules, and other markers. The following categories of population were considered by the studies included in the review: community dwelling "healthy" elderly, elderly with pathology/activity limitation, frail elderly, hypertensive patients, diabetic patients, metabolic syndrome patients, and breast cancer patients. After extraction of data concerning the paper, a summary of the results was reported in the text.

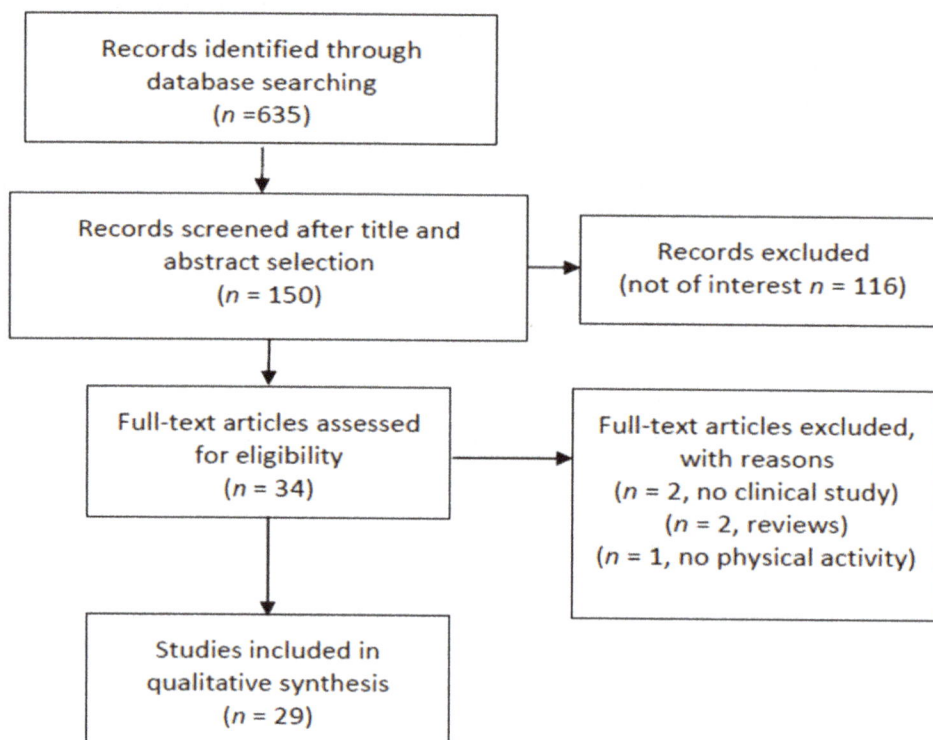

Figure 1. Flow chart of the inclusion process.

3. Results

3.1. Effect of PA on Inflammatory Markers and Oxidative Stress Mediators

It is well known that inflamm-aging, which is an age-related chronic progressive increase in the pro-inflammatory status, plays an important role in the process of aging and age-related conditions like cognitive decline and chronic comorbidities [8,9]. Several research studies evidenced that healthy aging could be related both to a lower pro-inflammatory status and to an efficient anti-inflammatory response. The imbalance between these two pathways can be a risk factor for frailty and chronic age-related pathologies leading to poor quality of life [10]. Oxidative stress occurs from the imbalance between the production of reactive oxygen and nitrogen species (RONS) and the antioxidant defences. It has been hypothesized that oxidative stress could have a role in the aging process as the age-related modifications could be caused by the accumulation of RONS-induced damages that lead to a progressive loss of function in tissues and organs [11]. Several research studies have investigated the influence of PA on inflammatory and oxidative stress biohumoral markers in the elderly. It has been demonstrated that an active lifestyle can influence the age-related inflammatory profile [12], reducing the secretion of pro-inflammatory factors and increasing the release of anti-inflammatory cytokines. Nevertheless, the effect of different type and intensity of exercise on these pathways has not been fully clarified yet. Monteiro-Junior et al. performed a systematic review and meta-analysis on studies investigating the effect of chronic exercise on interleukin-6 (IL-6), tumor necrosis factor-alpha (TNF-α), and C-reactive Protein (CRP) in a population of ≥60 elderly persons (8 articles were analyzed after screening and application of inclusion/exclusion criteria) [13]. IL-6 and CRP but not TNF-α significantly decreased after the exercise intervention (overall effect $p < 0.05$). A systematic review by Cronin et al. investigated the effect of aerobic and resistance exercise on inflammatory markers (CRP, IL-6, interleukin-8 (IL-8), interleukin-1 beta (IL-1β), and TNF-α) in healthy, physically inactive subjects (11 articles included). Results from studies investigating an elderly population (3 studies of the 11) showed the greatest reduction of inflammatory markers (CRP and IL-6), while results from studies including younger subjects were inconsistent. These different results in the different age groups are probably due to higher basal level of these markers in the elderly and to the resulting higher potential for them to be lowered by PA in this population [14]. Another cross-sectional study investigated the association between inflammatory markers (IL-6 and soluble receptor for TNF-α (sTNFR1)) and muscle/functional performances (assessed by 10 m gait speed) in 221 community-dwelling elderly women aged of $\geq$65 years. Results did not show any negative correlation between levels of IL-6 and sTNFR1 and muscle or physical performance, probably because the levels of these mediators were not high enough to influence muscles and functionality of the sample [15]. A cross-sectional (1139 subjects included) and longitudinal study (490 subjects with two measures of PA one year apart were included) on elderly men [16] investigated the influence of different levels of PA and sedentary behaviour (SB) on markers of inflammation (IL-6, CRP, and tissue plasminogen activator (tPA), von Willebrand factor (vWF), D-Dimer (ng/mL), and insulin-like growth factor-1 (IGF-1). PA and SB were measured using Actigraph GT3X accelerometers. Results showed that the individuals who spent more time in Moderate to Vigorous PA (MVPA) had lower levels of IL-6, CRP, tPA, vWF, and D-dimer and higher levels of IGF-1 ($p \leq 0.006$) in contrast with men with higher levels of SB that resulted in having higher levels of IL-6, CRP, tPA, and D-dimer and lower levels of IGF-1 ($p \leq 0.03$). Moreover, each additional 10 min of MVPA showed to have a lowering effect on IL-6, CRP, tPA, vWF, and D-dimer (3.2%, 5,6%, 2.2%,1.2%, and 1.8% respectively) that, for CRP, vWF, and D-dimer, was independent from levels of SB. A cross-sectional study performed by Do-Yeon et al. [17] investigated the association of quality of diet and physical performance assessed by the Short Physical Performance Battery (SPPB) with IL-6 and TNF-α in 78 frail, elderly South Korean individuals aged $\geq$ 65 years. The results evidenced that high physical performances (as assessed by SPPB) were associated with lower levels of TNF-α ($p = 0.001$).

Plasma levels of IL-6 and TNF-α were also measured in a population of elderly subjects with hypertension undergoing aerobic training or aerobic and resistance training for 10 weeks. In the group of subjects that underwent both aerobic and resistance training, TNF-α levels were lower ($p = 0.01$), while IL-6 was reduced in subjects undergoing aerobic training compared to untrained controls ($p = 0.04$) [18]. Moreover, direct measurement of the levels of oxidative products has been carried out in some studies. Alghadir et al. showed that, in a population of elderly undergoing a 24-week program of PA, there was a significant decrease in oxidative stress markers, including high sensitivity C-reactive protein (hsCRP), malondialdehyde (MDA), and 8-hydroxyguanine (8-OHdG) when compared to subjects who did not exercise [19]. Similarly, a 12-week program of Nordic walking in elderly women showed a decrease in levels of MDA oxidation products ($p = 0.01$) [20]. In another study, a thorough evaluation of the oxidative status of the included subject (61 women and 34 men aged $\geq$ 60 years) was carried out through determination of plasma total antioxidant status (TAS), plasma antioxidant enzyme activities, i.e., glutathione peroxidase (GPx), catalase (CAT), superoxide dismutase (SOD), and membrane lipid peroxidation (TBARS). Accelerometers were used to evaluate PA. Among the female sample, TAS was significantly lower and CAT activity was significantly higher in the group that met the criteria of recommended levels of PA for healthy adults (daily step goal of 10,000 steps) than in the group that did not meet these criteria. Correlation analysis showed an inverse association between PA and TAS, while moderate to vigorous physical activity (MVPA) was related to an increase in GPx antioxidant activity in the elderly women sample. In elderly male subjects, a significant correlation was found between CAT activity and the level of PA related to the lifestyle [21]. On the same research line, in a large study involving 1449 subjects, SOD activity and plasma levels of malondialdehyde (MDA) and 4-hydroxynonenal (4-HNE) were determined. Results from a subpopulation of elderly subjects with hypertension showed that different types of PA induced an improvement in antioxidant activity and a reduction in MDA levels; however, these results were not always significant for all the types of PA advocated [22]. Other direct markers of inflammation are those related to the activation of the immune system, including the toll-like receptor (TLR) on white blood cells. This marker has been investigated in a clinical trial, evaluating the effect of an 8-week program of resistance training in elderly subjects. Results showed that, in those patients that completed the program, the expression of TLR-2 and TLR-4 was reduced ($p < 0.04$ and $p < 0.03$, respectively). Furthermore, C-reactive protein levels also decrease in the training group [23]. Similarly, another trial by the same research group demonstrated that whole-body vibration training had a significant effect in the reduction of TLR-2 and TLR-4 in a population of elderly subjects [23]. Furthermore, a cross-sectional study which evaluated TLR activity and cytokines expression reported results stratified by Metabolic Equivalent of Tasks (MET), showing that elderly subjects with higher MET levels and exercise levels had decreased blood levels of IL-6 ($p = 0.001$) but not of TNF-α ($p = 0.148$) and myeloperoxidase ($p = 0.799$). TLR-2 levels significantly decreased both in males and females, according to MET levels, while TLR-4 did not show any significant decrease [24]. Results of the included studies were reported in Table 1.

Table 1. Inflammatory markers and oxidative stress mediators.

Study	Physical Activity	Participants	Biomarkers	Main Findings
Alghadir et al. 2016 [19]	Moderate aerobic for 24 weeks	100 (age 65–95 y)	MDA, 8-OHdG, TAC, and hs-CRP	Physically active persons showed a higher cognitive performance along with reduction in the levels of MDA, 8-OHdG, and hs-CRP and increase in TAC activity compared with sedentary participants.
Felicio et al. 2014 [15]	Muscle performance and handgrip were measured using dynamometer	221 women (mean age 71 y)	IL-6, SNTFR	IL-6 (0.87 pg/mL) correlated with the power of the knee extensors ($r = 0.14$; $p = 0.03$) and the power of the knee flexors ($r = 0.16$; $p = 0.01$). IL-6, level of physical activity, and depressive status explained 5.5% ($R^2 = 0.055$, $p < 0.01$) of average power of knee extensors variability.
Ferrer et al. 2018 [24]	Metabolic equivalent of task measurement; Minnesota leisure-time physical activity level	116 (age 55–80 y)	IL-6 and TLR protein array	Exercise induced a decrease in the IL-6 circulating levels and the TLR2 protein levels in PBMCs. Anti-inflammatory IL-10 was increased in active subjects.
Fraile-Bermudez et al. 2015 [21]	Level of physical activity measured through accelerometers	61 women and 34 men (mean age 70 y)	GPx, SOD, CAT, and TBARS	In active women, lower levels of TAS were found. Moderate to vigorous physical activity was negatively correlated with TAS but was correlated with increase in the GPx activity. The counts per minute were positively correlated with CAT activity.
Kim et al. 2017 [17]	Grip strength and SPPB	78 (mean age 78.3 y)	IL-6 and TNF-α	Higher SPPB score was associated with lower levels of TNF-α.
Kortas et al. 2017 [20]	Nordic walking for 12 weeks	35 women (mean age 68 y)	MDA and AOP	Statistically significant decreasing of MDA level and concentration of AOP
Lima et al. 2015 [18]	Aerobic training vs. arobic + resistance training for 10 weeks	44 (age 60–75 y)	IL-6 and TNF-α	IL-6 was reduced in aerobic training group compared to controls ($p = 0.04$), and TNF-α levels were lower in aerobic + resistance group compared to controls ($p = 0.01$).
Mendoza-Nunez et al. 2018 [25]	Tai-Chi	110 affected by MetS	TAS, TNF-α, IL-6, IL-8, and IL-10	Activity group showed a statistically significant increase in TAS and a decrease in the oxidative stress score ($p < 0.05$).
Parsons et al. 2017 [16]	Level of physical activity measured through GT3X accelerometers	1139 (mean age 79 y)	IL-6, CRP, tPA, vWF, and D-Dimer	Higher physical activity was associated with lower levels of IL-6, CRP, tPA, vWF, and D-Dimer. Furthermore, each additional 10 min of moderate to vigorous activity was associated with a 3.2% lower IL-6, 5.6% lower CRP, 2.2% lower tPA, 1.2% lower vWF, and 1.8% lower D-dimer.

Table 1. *Cont.*

Study	Physical Activity	Participants	Biomarkers	Main Findings
Rodriguez-Miguelez et al. 2014 [23]	Resistance exercise training	26 (mean age 69.5 y)	IL-10, TNF-α, and CRP	TNF-α remained unchanged in both trained subjects and controls. IL-10 was upregulated in trained subjects. CRP values decreased in trained subjects only.
Yu et al. 2018 [22]	Walking, square dancing, Taiji, and yoga	1449 (age 45–79 y), with or without hypertension	SOD, MDA, and 4-HNE	In individuals with hypertension, MDA levels decreased (if walking/square dancing), SOD activity increased (if walking/square dancing), and 4-HNE levels decreased (if Taiji/yoga). In individuals without cardiovascular disease, MDA levels decreased (if any activity), SOD activity increased (if walking/square dancing), and 4-HNE levels decreased (if Taiji/yoga)

Where not specified, the patients where healthy community-dwelling elderly subjects. MDA = malondialdehyde, 8-OHdG = 8-hydroxyguanine, TAS = Total Antioxidant Status, TAC = Total Antioxidant Capacity, and hs-CRP = high-sensitivity C-reactive Protein, MetS = Metabolic Syndrome, tPA = tissue plasminogen activator, vWF = von Willebrand factor, SNTFR = soluble receptor for tumor necrosis factor alpha, AOP = advanced oxidation products, SPPB = Short Physical Performance Battery, GPx = glutathione peroxidase, CAT = catalase and SOD = superoxide dismutase, TBARS = membrane lipid peroxidation, PBMC = peripheral mononuclear blood. Cells, 4-HNE = hydroxynonenal, y = years, TLR = toll like receptor, IL = interleukin-1, TNF-α = tumor necrosis factor-alpha, CRP = C-reactive Protein.

3.2. Effect of PA on Cardiac Biomarkers

A sedentary lifestyle and the lack of a scheduled activity during daily life are well-established risk factors for cardiovascular disease (CVD) because of negative effects on cardiac and endothelial function, including a pro-atherogenic action [26,27]. The classical and nonclassical risk factors for CV disease were investigated in a recent paper, where the single factors were measured at different time-points of a specific PA program in a sample of elderly women (aged 65.0 ± 7.3 years). Body mass index (BMI), waist and hip circumferences, resting systolic and diastolic blood pressure (BP), and resting heart rate were significantly reduced after 2 weeks of a program based on general fitness, yoga, body balance, and self-guided PA. Exercise capacity, low-density lipoprotein (LDL) and high-density lipoprotein (HDL-C), cholesterol, and other atherogenic lipid indices (ALI) also improved after 2 weeks. At three months of the PA program, the values of these markers improved even more, with a significant reduction of calculated CVD risk at ten years [1]. PA also stimulates endothelium to synthesize and release the tissue-plasminogen activator (tPA), and some evidence suggested that also E-selectin may be influenced by PA [26]. A plethora of factors are actually influenced by PA, including C-reactive protein (CRP), interleukin-6 (IL-6), tPA, E-selectin, and adipokines, and several studies attempted to address the influence of PA on the cardiovascular system. A recent paper by Elhakeem et al. evaluated heart rate and data collected by movement sensors to derive overall PA energy expenditure (KJ/kg per day) and time spent in sedentary behaviours (<1.5 metabolic equivalent of tasks), in light PA (1.5–3 metabolic equivalent of tasks), and in moderate-to-vigorous intensity PA (>3 metabolic equivalent of tasks). Results of the linear regressions analysis showed a significant association between time spent in PA (both in light and moderate to vigorous) and blood levels of CRP, IL-6, leptin, and adiponectin, especially in women [26]. Furthermore, the same study reported a positive association between cardiorespiratory fitness and favourable biomarkers levels. Among other biomarkers, a recent cross-sectional study on 1130 men evaluated the influence of PA on the behaviour of N-terminal pro-brain natriuretic peptide (NT-proBNP) and high sensitivity Troponin T (hsTnT), which are both markers of cardiac injury. The results showed that the total amount of PA in patients aged 70–91 years was nonlinearly associated to lower NT-proBNP and hsTnT. Higher levels of PA were associated with lower levels of NT-proBNP but significantly only below a certain threshold of activity per day (measured by accelerometer count, step count, and minutes of moderate/vigorous activity). Similarly,

PA level was also associated with lower levels of hsTnT, with significant correlations only below threshold levels of counts, steps, moderate/vigorous activity, and light activity [16]. On the same research line, Van der Linden et al. hypothesized that the frail elderly population is characterized by high levels of basal cardiac Troponin T (cTnT) and may benefit from the potential effects of an exercise intervention. The greatest part of the population evaluated had cTnT levels above the 99th percentile. However, results showed no evident effect of a 24-week resistance-training program on the cTnT levels [28]. Results of the included studies were reported in Table 2.

Table 2. Cardiovascular risk biomarkers.

Study	Type of Exercise	Participants	Biomarkers	Main Findings
Elhakeem et al. 2018 [26]	Light and moderate-to-vigorous activity, monitored with sensors worn for 5 consecutive days	795 men and 827 women (age 60 to 64 y)	E-selectine, leptin, and adiponectine	Greater time in light PA and moderate-to-vigorous intensity PA and less sedentary time were associated with more favorable biomarker levels.
Koh et al. 2018 [29]	Aerobic capacity (VO$_2$), physical activity frequency, intensity, and duration	141 (mean age 70.6 y)	Ecographic and cardiac magnetic resonance imaging parameters	Compared to participants with high VO$_2$, participants with low VO$_2$ had lower ratio of peak velocity flow in early diastole to peak velocity flow in late diastole by atrial contraction of >0.8 ($p = 0.001$) and lower left atrial conduit strain ($p = 0.045$)
Parsons et al. 2018 [16]	Level of physical activity measured through GT3X accelerometers	1130 men (age 70 to 91 y)	NT-proBNP and hsTnT	For each additional 10 min of moderate/vigorous activity, NT-proBNP was lower by 35.7% and hsTnT was lower by 8.4%, in men who undertook <25 or 50 min of moderate/vigorous activity per day, respectively.
Van der Linden et al. 2014 [28]	24-week supervised resistance-type exercise training program vs. normal activity monitoring	52 pre-frail elderly (age ≥ 65 y)	cTnT	The majority of participants had cTnT levels above the 99th percentile. These data confirm the hypothesis that chronically elevated cTnT concentrations are highly prevalent among (pre)frail elderly subjects.
Zmijewski et al. 2015 [27]	Organized, group-based physical activity	35 women (mean age 65 y)	BP, resting HR, EC, HDL, and LDL	Two-week effects included significant decreases in BMI, waist and hip circumferences, resting BP, and resting HR; improved EC; and improved LDL, HDL, and TC, with a reduction in 10-year estimated risk of death from CVD. Three-month effects included a further decrease in systolic BP, improvements in EC and HDL, and maintenance of lower levels of CVD risk.

Where not specified, the patients where healthy community-dwelling elderly subjects. PA = physical activity, TC = Total Cholesterol, TAG = triacylglycerols, HDL = High-Density Lipoproteins, LDL = Low-Density Lipoproteins, BP = blood pressure, HR = heart rate, EC= exercise capacity, BMI = Body Mass Index, CVD = Cardiovascular Disease, NT-proBNP = N-terminal pro-brain natriuretic peptide, hsTnT = high sensitivity Troponin T, cTnT = cardiac Troponin T.

3.3. Effect of PA on Metabolic Parameters

There is a consistent and rising evidence that metabolic pathways and endocrine system as well as immune system and defense mechanisms are definitely affected by the aging process. Specifically, in the elderly, the carbohydrates metabolism is impaired and utilization of blood glucose is decreased [30]; furthermore, in this population, lipid profile results were imbalanced by the altered fat utilization and the lack of PA [31]. Vitamin D levels, the main factor influencing bone health, also result in impairment for a plethora of alterations in kidney and other endocrine organs [32]. There is a growing interest and development of new data analysis methods for the assessment of metabolic status and metabolic changes that occur in the individual during and after activities [33]. It is a common hypothesis that the prevention of metabolic noncommunicable diseases passes through the opportunity to understand which kind of activities may be useful in improving the metabolome of the elderly. In a recent study based on aged Korean woman, the effect of combined aerobic and anaerobic exercise on glucose metabolism was investigated by assessing insulin resistance, Growth Hormone (GH), Insulin-like growth factor-1 (IGF-1), Deidrossiepiandrostenedione (DHEA-S), and estrogen values. The authors found that blood glucose levels decreased significantly when compared to non-exercise controls while GH and DHEA-S increased. Interaction effects were found for IGF-1, GH, and DHEA-S. From these results, it seems that, in older women, the combination of aerobic and anaerobic exercise improves insulin resistance, avoiding the decline of glucose metabolism function [30]. Combined exercise was also investigated in another study; specifically, the effect of resistance training and multicomponent exercise was compared. Main findings included the evaluation of aerobic functionality, lipid profile, and inflammatory markers. The results showed that only epidermal growth factor (EGF) levels and adiponectin (ADN) levels were different between groups, with an increase of the EGF in the group of elderly undergoing multimodal fitness program and a significant ADN reduction in the resistance training group [31]. In a study carried out on 85 healthy older subjects, the levels of vitamin D, creatinine kinase, lactic acid dehydrogenase, troponin I, total antioxidant capacity, body composition, and PA were evaluated to find possible correlations among these parameters. Main findings showed that, in physically active subjects, there was a significant increase in the vitamin D serum levels, calcium, and total antioxidant capacity, with an associated reduction in the levels of muscle fatigue biomarkers: creatine kinase, lactic acid dehydrogenase, troponin I, and hydroxyproline. Based on these results, improved biohumoral markers of bone and muscle health correlated with the improvement in muscle relief and performance of physically active participants [32]. Similarly, a study investigating the beneficial effects of Tai-Chi in older adults showed a statistically significant difference in glycosylated haemoglobin levels compared to untrained controls as well as a significant increase in total antioxidant status [25]. Another study evaluating the association between peak oxygen uptake (a marker of aerobic capacity) and metabolic/cardiovascular parameters showed that subjects with lower VO_2 had a higher risk to present altered cardiovascular parameters and had higher levels of accumulation of wide-spectrum acyl-carnitines, alanine, and glutamine [29]. The role of microRNA in diabetes mellitus type 2 (T2DM) is growing in interest in the scientific literature. Reduced levels of the microRNAs miR-146a and miR-155 contribute to a pro-inflammatory state associated with T2DM. The effect of strength and cardiovascular training on T2DM patients has been investigated compared to a group of nondiabetic subjects, showing a significant increase of miR-146a and a decrease of blood glucose levels, which were more pronounced in diabetic patients after strength training [34]. In a Swedish study aimed at evaluating the wellbeing of the elderly, the Psychological General Wellbeing (PGWB) index has been put into correlation with several metabolic biomarkers, including the levels of several types of lipoproteins, BMI, and blood pressure. The only significant results found was a positive association between the high-density lipoprotein and the level of general health, according to the PGWB [35]. Caminiti et al. investigated hormonal responses (levels of total and free testosterone, IGF-1, GH, and Sex-Hormone binding protein (SHBG)) after two different types of aerobic PA (interval training (IT) and continuous training (CT)) in chronic heart failure (CHF) elderly patients. Results showed a greater increase in total and free testosterone levels and in IGF-1 in the IT group compared to the CT group. On the contrary, levels of testosterone and IGF-1 remained unchanged after CT. GH significantly increased and SHBG decreased in both groups without between-groups differences. The level of hormonal response was related neither to an improvement of exercise capacity nor to the training load, but it seemed to be related to exercise intensity [36]. Results of the included studies were reported in Table 3.

Table 3. Metabolic biomarkers.

Study	Type of Exercise	Participants	Biomarkers	Main Findings
Al-Eisa et al. 2016 [32]	Physical activity assessed through estimated energy expenditure scores	85 (age 64 to 96 y)	TAG, TC, LDL, HDL, 25(OH)D, TAC, CK, LDH, Troponin I, and hydroxyproline	Significant reduction of TC, TAG, LDL, and HDL occurred in subjects with moderately active and active subjects. Significant increase in 25(OH)D and TAC and a reduction in the levels of muscle fatigue biomarkers occurred in physically active subjects.
Biddle et al. 2018 [33]	Physical behaviors (time spent per day): stepping, sleeping, sitting, and standing	435 (mean age 66.7 y)	Fasting and 2 h glucose and insulin levels, and HbA1c	Reallocating 30 min from sleep, sitting, or standing to stepping was associated with 5–6 fold lower 2-h glucose, 15–17 fold lower 2-h insulin, and higher insulin sensitivity.
Ha and Son 2018 [30]	Aerobic + anaerobic exercise for 12 weeks vs. controls	20 Korean women	Insulin resistance, GH, IGF-1, DHEA-S, and estrogen	GH level increased significantly in the exercise group. The DHEA-S level significantly increased in the exercise group. The estrogen level increased significantly in the exercise group.
Hurtig-Wennlof et al. 2014 [35]	International Physical Activity Questionnaire modified for the elderly.	389 community-dwelling elderly (mean age 74 y)	LDL, HDL, Apolipoprotein A1, and B. PGWB	PGWB correlated significantly with all parameters, positively with LDL, HDL ApoA1 (respective Spearman's rho 0.03, 0.05, and 0.013), and negatively with ApoB (rho −0.031).
Kortas et al. 2017 [20]	Nordic walking for 12 weeks	35 women (mean age 68 y)	TC, TAG, HDL, LDL, and ferritin	The training induced a rise of HDL cholesterol ($p < 0.05$), whereas other lipid parameters remained unchanged. Decrease of blood ferritin ($p < 0.05$)
Leite et al. 2015 [31]	Resistance training vs. multicomponent exercise for 12 weeks	24 women and 15 men (age 65 to 75 y)	LDL, HDL, glucose, TAG, NEFA, adiponectine, ferritin, and EGF	Among the evaluated biomarkers, only high molecular weight adiponectin decreased significantly within the RT group ($p = 0.03$) after the exercise protocol. Between-group differences included only ferritin ($p = 0.02$) and EGF ($p = 0.01$).
Mendoza-Nunez et al. 2018 [25]	Tai-Chi	110 affected by MetS	HbA1c	Decrease in HbA1c concentration was observed in the TC group compared with the control group ($p < 0.05$).
Santos Morais et al. 2017 [34]	Strength training and guided walk (monitored through Polar Team software)	23 (mean age 68.2 y), of whom 13 were diabetics	miR-126, miR-146a, and miR-155 in	Diabetic patients had higher reduction in blood glucose than nondiabetics, which was paralleled by a positive change of the circulating levels of miR-146a but not of the other miRs.

Where not specified, the patients where healthy community-dwelling elderly subjects. MetS = Metabolic Syndrome, TC = Total Cholesterol, TAG = triacylglycerols, HDL = High-Density Lipoproteins, LDL = Low-Density Lipoproteins, HbA1c = glycosylated haemoglobin, GH = growth hormone, IGF-1 = Insulin-like Growth Factor 1, DHEA-S = deidroepiandrosterone sulphate, NEFA = Non Esterified Fatty Acid, EGF = Epidermal Growth Factor, 25(OH)D = 25-hydroxy vitamin D, TAC = Total Antioxidant Capacity, CK = Creatinine Kinase, LDH = Lactic acid DeHidrogenase, VO$_2$ = peak Oxigen Uptake, PGWB = Psychological Geneal Wellbeing, miR = micro RNA.

3.4. Effect of PA on Other Biohumoral Markers

A plethora of other biomarkers has been investigated to understand and highlight the effect of PA on their levels. In a cohort of postmenopausal women with breast cancer, the levels of progesterone, estrogens, and their precursors were measured on tissue samples and correlated to BMI and PA status. An interesting result is that estradiol, estrone, and testosterone levels were significantly associated with BMI in women with Estrogen Receptor positive (ER+) breast cancer. Furthermore, an inverse association was found between time spent in PA and serum estradiol levels among ER+ subjects, although this difference was not significant on tissue samples [37]. Another relevant biomarker that has been recently proposed as a predictor of changes in physical function is the C-terminal Agrin Fragment

(CAF), a product of the catabolism of neuromuscular junction molecule Agrin. A cohort of 333 older subjects has been followed for 1 year to evaluate the effect of a 12-month program of health education only or a 12-month program of walking, strengthening, flexibility, and balance exercises. However, the large trial failed to demonstrate a significant association between CAF levels and the 12-month activity program [38]. Two large studies investigated the role of PA on kidney function. A study on 1041 older subjects investigated the association between muscular strength and kidney disfunction, by measuring cystatin C levels and maximal muscle strength. The odds ratio of having elevated cystatin C was higher in those subjects with lower muscle strength. Similarly, those subjects with lower muscle strength had also lower estimated glomerular filtration rate from cystatin C (eGFRcysC) [39]. The second study evaluated a cohort of 1352 men, in which the higher levels of PA and lower levels of sedentary behaviours reduced the odds ratio for decreased eGFR [16]. Moreover, a recent paper investigated the possible role of PA on renal proximal tubule stress levels through the evaluation of urinary levels of liver-type fatty acid-binding protein (L-FABP). The intent of the study was two-fold: in a cross-sectional evaluation, urinary L-FABP levels were significantly lower in those subjects with higher PA levels than in those with lower PA levels; in the interventional study, those subjects that underwent 12 weeks of aerobic training had significantly decreased levels of urinary L-FABP [40].

4. Discussion

There is growing evidence on the effects of PA in the elderly, and the clinical tools for the assessment of these effects are the focus of several recent research studies. According to the results of the present review, there are many distinct biomarkers influenced by PA in the elderly, although none of them have sufficient evidence for clinical use as the majority of these biomolecules have been investigated in one or very few studies. However, promising results are available, especially concerning the metabolic and cardiovascular indexes, as a growing number of studies demonstrate the role of PA on improving parameters related to heart function and CV risk like atherogenic lipid profile [41]. Prospective observational studies confirm that high–moderate levels of leisure time PA are able to decrease the risk of CV disease in both sexes with an effect size that ranges between 20–30% and 10–20% respectively, showing a dose–effect relationship [41]. Research studies have evidenced that the association between higher levels of PA and lower CV disease rates can be explained in large part by the reduction of known risk factors, with inflammatory/hemostatic biomarkers making the largest contribution to lowered risk, followed by a positive effect on blood pressure, lipids, and body mass index [42]. Furthermore, it is also a verified hypothesis that PA is able to modify the inflammatory status of elderly subjects by decreasing the levels of pro-inflammatory cytokines, including IL-1, IL-6, and TNF-α [13,14]. Several studies have investigated the effect of exercise on inflammatory factors; it has been evidenced that acute bouts of exercise result in a transient, mostly pro-inflammatory effect, which is proportional to the amount of exercise and to the entity of muscle injury [43,44]. On the other hand, regular PA has been associated with a chronic anti-inflammatory effect. The mechanisms underlying this action are not well defined and include reduction of body weight [45], reduction of basal levels of pro-inflammatory cytokines and pro-atherogenic adipokines, enhancement of the expression of antioxidant and anti-inflammatory mediators in the vascular wall, and insulin-sensitizing pathways [46,47]. Moreover, regular exercise has been demonstrated to be able to attenuate the age-associated increase in oxidative stress and nuclear factor-κB activation in animals [48] and to reduce toll-like receptor signaling [23], which may explain its chronic anti-inflammatory effect.

As for the influence of PA on oxidative stress and antioxidant systems, a recent review by Nocella et al. [7] highlighted that high-intensity physical exercise can cause redox imbalance, leading to several types of injuries and muscle damage, while the studies reported in this review show an improvement in antioxidant activity and reduction of oxidative stress in elderly performing regular PA. Similar to our results, some studies demonstrated that exercise and regular PA have a positive impact on oxidative stress and inflammation during aging [49,50]. The balance between Reactive oxygen species (ROS) production and antioxidant systems is a very important, as ROS plays a dual role: at low or moderate levels, they have a beneficial action on cellular responses, while at high concentrations, they cause inflammation and oxidative damage to cells and tissues [51,52]. This is crucial for the aging process, as inflammatory processes and oxidative stress are biochemical alterations related to the etiology and complications of several age-related diseases such as T2DM, Alzheimer's disease, CV disease, and cancer. It has been evidenced that regular practice of PA has a positive effect on the aging process, with an action on biochemical changes related to aging and on the risk of chronic diseases. This action has the consequence of enhancing quality of life in aging individuals and of increasing longevity [53,54]. It has also been evidenced that PA could modify blood glucose levels and glycosylated haemoglobin levels in nondiabetic elderly subjects [42]. One study has also demonstrated a significant increase in miR-146a (reduced concentrations of miR-146a contribute to a pro-inflammatory state associated with T2DM) with a decrease in serum blood glucose levels, which was more evident in the group of diabetic patients compared to healthy individuals after strength training [34]. In agreement with our results, literature shows that PA (both endurance and strength training) has an important role in the prevention and control of T2DM, producing acute and chronic physiological effects [55,56]. It has been demonstrated that insulin action in muscle and liver can be modified by acute bouts of exercise and by regular PA. Regular training increases muscle capillary density and insulin signaling proteins [57]. Moreover, it has been evidenced that both aerobic and resistance training promote adaptations in skeletal muscle, adipose tissue, and liver associated with enhanced insulin action, regardless of weight loss [58].

Some studies reported in this review showed that PA was able to raise testosterone, GH, and vitamin D levels in elderly populations [32]. Our results comply with the results of some cross-sectional studies performed on middle-aged and older men which indicate that circulating testosterone concentrations may be higher in men who regularly exercise [59,60], and this is very important in the elderly in order to counteract the physiological age-associated decline of serum testosterone. It should be noted that low levels of testosterone in men have been associated with decreased sexual function, loss of muscle mass and strength, osteoporosis, declining cognitive function, and poorer quality of life [61]. As for the effects of PA on GH levels, neuroendocrine mechanisms underlying exercise-facilitated GH secretion are complex; they probably include somatostatin withdrawal, GH-releasing hormone (GHRH) release, and possibly co-secretagogue actions. The effect of PA on vitamin D levels could be related to the evidence that shows that long-term regular exercise programs are able to increase bone mineral density (BMD) in the elderly and to consequently reduce the risk of osteoporotic fractures [62], which are the most fearsome events in an aged person that frequently lead to disability, hospitalization, and death.

There is also some evidence from literature about the role of PA on other interesting markers like CAF and urinary L-FABP [40], but further studies should be designed to confirm and fully explain these results.

Concerning the kind of exercise that could have a positive effect on health indicators in the elderly, there is not strong evidence, as the majority of the studies in literature have focused on global levels of PA. Only a few of them investigated the effect of aerobic, resistance or combined training, or specific kind of activities (Tai-chi, Nordic walking, and whole-body vibrations) on biohumoral indicators. Well-designed clinical trials on the effect of a different kind of PA on health indicators are therefore needed to better understand the role of each kind of exercise on specific physiopathological pathways.

Moreover, most of the reported studies investigate a population of "healthy" community-dwelling elderly and only a few of them include people with chronic pathologies (Tables 1–3). This scarce evidence on elderly with chronic comorbidities limits the transposition of the results to clinical settings in which the majority of the individuals have multimorbidity [63].

5. Conclusions

The studies that are reported in this review give strong evidence of an effect of PA on the health of elderly people that is not generic and confused but could be evidenced and "quantified" by the modifications of the levels of biohumoral indicators. This represents an additional support to the concept of the role of PA in primary and secondary prevention of noncommunicable diseases. Therefore, the practice of PA and the reduction of sedentary behaviors should be encouraged in all ages, overcoming psychological barriers and false beliefs of the elderly. The evidence coming from further clinical research and new biotechnologies could help in having the opportunity to "tailor" the right type of exercise for the particular clinical and genetic features of each individual in order to build up an individualized preventive strategy.

Author Contributions: Conceptualization, C.F. and F.P.; methodology, G.T. and A.G.; writing—original draft preparation, G.T., P.B., and F.F.; writing—review and editing, M.T. and E.A.; supervision, M.C. and A.P. All authors have read and agreed to the published version of the manuscript.

References

1. Physical Activity Factsheets for the 28 European Union Member States of the Who European Region. Overview (2018). Available online: http://www.euro.who.int/en/health-topics/disease-prevention/physical-activity/publications/2018/factsheets-on-health-enhancing-physical-activity-in-the-28-eu-member-states-of-the-who-european-region (accessed on 22 February 2019).
2. Lim, S.S.; Vos, T.; Flaxman, A.D.; Danaei, G.; Shibuya, K.; Adair-Rohani, H.; Amann, M.; Anderson, H.R.; Andrews, K.G.; Aryee, M.; et al. A comparative risk assessment of burden of disease and injury attributable to 67 risk factors and risk factor clusters in 21 regions, 1990–2010: A systematic analysis for the Global Burden of Disease Study 2010. *Lancet Lond. Engl.* **2012**, *380*, 2224–2260. [CrossRef]
3. Harvey, J.A.; Chastin, S.F.M.; Skelton, D.A. How Sedentary are Older People? A Systematic Review of the Amount of Sedentary Behavior. *J. Aging Phys. Act.* **2015**, *23*, 471–487. [CrossRef]
4. Gomes, M.; Figueiredo, D.; Teixeira, L.; Poveda, V.; Paúl, C.; Santos-Silva, A.; Costa, E. Physical inactivity among older adults across Europe based on the SHARE database. *Age Ageing* **2017**, *46*, 71–77. [CrossRef]
5. Collino, S.; Martin, F.-P.; Karagounis, L.G.; Horcajada, M.N.; Moco, S.; Franceschi, C.; Kussmann, M.; Offord, E. Musculoskeletal system in the old age and the demand for healthy ageing biomarkers. *Mech. Ageing Dev.* **2013**, *134*, 541–547. [CrossRef] [PubMed]
6. Papalia, R.; Vadalà, G.; Torre, G.; Perna, M.; Saccone, L.; Cannata, F.; Denaro, V. The cytokinome in osteoarthritis, a new paradigm in diagnosis and prognosis of cartilage disease. *J. Biol. Regul. Homeost. Agents* **2016**, *30*, 77–83. [PubMed]
7. Nocella, C.; Cammisotto, V.; Pigozzi, F.; Borrione, P.; Fossati, C.; D'Amico, A.; Cangemi, R.; Peruzzi, M.; Gobbi, G.; Ettorre, E.; et al. Impairment between Oxidant and Antioxidant Systems: Short- and Long-term Implications for Athletes' Health. *Nutrients* **2019**, *11*, 1353. [CrossRef] [PubMed]
8. Franceschi, C.; Bonafè, M.; Valensin, S.; Olivieri, F.; De Luca, M.; Ottaviani, E.; De Benedictis, G. Inflamm-aging. An evolutionary perspective on immunosenescence. *Ann. N. Y. Acad. Sci.* **2000**, *908*, 244–254. [CrossRef]
9. Sartori, A.C.; Vance, D.E.; Slater, L.Z.; Crowe, M. The impact of inflammation on cognitive function in older adults: Implications for healthcare practice and research. *J. Neurosci. Nurs. J. Am. Assoc. Neurosci. Nurses* **2012**, *44*, 206–217. [CrossRef]
10. Franceschi, C.; Capri, M.; Monti, D.; Giunta, S.; Olivieri, F.; Sevini, F.; Panourgia, M.P.; Invidia, L.; Celani, L.; Scurti, M.; et al. Inflammaging and anti-inflammaging: A systemic perspective on aging and longevity emerged from studies in humans. *Mech. Ageing Dev.* **2007**, *128*, 92–105. [CrossRef]
11. Liguori, I.; Russo, G.; Curcio, F.; Bulli, G.; Aran, L.; Della-Morte, D.; Gargiulo, G.; Testa, G.; Cacciatore, F.; Bonaduce, D.; et al. Oxidative stress, aging, and diseases. *Clin. Interv. Aging* **2018**, *13*, 757–772. [CrossRef]
12. Walsh, N.P.; Gleeson, M.; Pyne, D.B.; Nieman, D.C.; Dhabhar, F.S.; Shephard, R.J.; Oliver, S.J.; Bermon, S.; Kajeniene, A. Position statement. Part two: Maintaining immune health. *Exerc. Immunol. Rev.* **2011**, *17*, 64–103. [PubMed]
13. Monteiro-Junior, R.S.; de Tarso Maciel-Pinheiro, P.; da Matta Mello Portugal, E.; da Silva Figueiredo, L.F.; Terra, R.; Carneiro, L.S.F.; Rodrigues, V.D.; Nascimento, O.J.M.; Deslandes, A.C.; Laks, J. Effect of Exercise on Inflammatory Profile of Older Persons: Systematic Review and Meta-Analyses. *J. Phys. Act. Health* **2018**, *15*, 64–71. [CrossRef] [PubMed]

14. Cronin, O.; Keohane, D.M.; Molloy, M.G.; Shanahan, F. The effect of exercise interventions on inflammatory biomarkers in healthy, physically inactive subjects: A systematic review. *QJM Int. J. Med.* **2017**, *110*, 629–637. [CrossRef]

15. Felicio, D.C.; Pereira, D.S.; Assumpção, A.M.; Jesus-Moraleida, F.R.; Queiroz, B.Z.; Silva, J.P.; Rosa, N.M.; Dias, J.M.; Pereira, L.S. Inflammatory mediators, muscle and functional performance of community-dwelling elderly women. *Arch. Gerontol. Geriatr.* **2014**, *59*, 549–553. [CrossRef] [PubMed]

16. Parsons, T.J.; Sartini, C.; Ash, S.; Lennon, L.T.; Wannamethee, S.G.; Lee, I.-M.; Whincup, P.H.; Jefferis, B.J. Objectively measured physical activity and kidney function in older men; a cross-sectional population-based study. *Age Ageing* **2017**, *46*, 1010–1014. [CrossRef] [PubMed]

17. Kim, D.-Y.; Kim, C.-O.; Lim, H. Quality of diet and level of physical performance related to inflammatory markers in community-dwelling frail, elderly people. *Nutrition* **2017**, *38*, 48–53. [CrossRef] [PubMed]

18. Lima, L.G.; Bonardi, J.M.T.; Campos, G.O.; Bertani, R.F.; Scher, L.M.L.; Louzada-Junior, P.; Moriguti, J.C.; Ferriolli, E.; Lima, N.K.C. Effect of aerobic training and aerobic and resistance training on the inflammatory status of hypertensive older adults. *Aging Clin. Exp. Res.* **2015**, *27*, 483–489. [CrossRef]

19. Alghadir, A.H.; Gabr, S.A.; Al-Eisa, E.S. Effects of Moderate Aerobic Exercise on Cognitive Abilities and Redox State Biomarkers in Older Adults. *Oxid. Med. Cell. Longev.* **2016**, *2016*, 1–8. [CrossRef]

20. Kortas, J.; Kuchta, A.; Prusik, K.; Prusik, K.; Ziemann, E.; Labudda, S.; Ćwiklińska, A.; Wieczorek, E.; Jankowski, M.; Antosiewicz, J. Nordic walking training attenuation of oxidative stress in association with a drop in body iron stores in elderly women. *Biogerontology* **2017**, *18*, 517–524. [CrossRef]

21. Fraile-Bermúdez, A.B.; Kortajarena, M.; Zarrazquin, I.; Maquibar, A.; Yanguas, J.J.; Sánchez-Fernández, C.E.; Gil, J.; Irazusta, A.; Ruiz-Litago, F. Relationship between physical activity and markers of oxidative stress in independent community-living elderly individuals. *Exp. Gerontol.* **2015**, *70*, 26–31. [CrossRef]

22. Yu, Y.; Gao, Q.; Xia, W.; Zhang, L.; Hu, Z.; Wu, X.; Jia, X. Association between Physical Exercise and Biomarkers of Oxidative Stress among Middle-Aged and Elderly Community Residents with Essential Hypertension in China. *BioMed Res. Int.* **2018**, *2018*, 1–11. [CrossRef] [PubMed]

23. Rodriguez-Miguelez, P.; Fernandez-Gonzalo, R.; Almar, M.; Mejías, Y.; Rivas, A.; de Paz, J.A.; Cuevas, M.J.; González-Gallego, J. Role of Toll-like receptor 2 and 4 signaling pathways on the inflammatory response to resistance training in elderly subjects. *AGE* **2014**, *36*, 9734. [CrossRef]

24. Ferrer, M.; Capó, X.; Martorell, M.; Busquets-Cortés, C.; Bouzas, C.; Carreres, S.; Mateos, D.; Sureda, A.; Tur, J.; Pons, A. Regular Practice of Moderate Physical Activity by Older Adults Ameliorates Their Anti-Inflammatory Status. *Nutrients* **2018**, *10*, 1780. [CrossRef] [PubMed]

25. Mendoza-Núñez, V.M.; Arista-Ugalde, T.L.; Rosado-Pérez, J.; Ruiz-Ramos, M.; Santiago-Osorio, E. Hypoglycemic and antioxidant effect of Tai chi exercise training in older adults with metabolic syndrome. *Clin. Interv. Aging* **2018**, *13*, 523–531. [CrossRef] [PubMed]

26. Elhakeem, A.; Cooper, R.; Whincup, P.; Brage, S.; Kuh, D.; Hardy, R. Physical Activity, Sedentary Time, and Cardiovascular Disease Biomarkers at Age 60 to 64 Years. *J. Am. Heart Assoc.* **2018**, *7*, e004284. [CrossRef] [PubMed]

27. Zmijewski, P.; Mazurek, K.; Kozdron, E.; Szczypiorski, P.; Frysztak, A. Effects of Organized Physical Activity on Selected Health Indices among Women Older than 55 Years. *Sci. World J.* **2015**, *2015*, 1–8. [CrossRef]

28. Van der Linden, N.; Tieland, M.; Klinkenberg, L.J.J.; Verdijk, L.B.; de Groot, L.C.P.G.M.; van Loon, L.J.C.; van Dieijen-Visser, M.P.; Meex, S.J.R. The effect of a six-month resistance-type exercise training program on the course of high sensitive cardiac troponin T levels in (pre)frail elderly. *Int. J. Cardiol.* **2014**, *175*, 374–375. [CrossRef] [PubMed]

29. Koh, A.S.; Gao, F.; Tan, R.S.; Zhong, L.; Leng, S.; Zhao, X.; Fridianto, K.T.; Ching, J.; Lee, S.Y.; Keng, B.M.H.; et al. Metabolomic correlates of aerobic capacity among elderly adults. *Clin. Cardiol.* **2018**, *41*, 1300–1307. [CrossRef]

30. Ha, M.-S.; Son, W.-M. Combined exercise is a modality for improving insulin resistance and aging-related hormone biomarkers in elderly Korean women. *Exp. Gerontol.* **2018**, *114*, 13–18. [CrossRef]

31. Leite, J.C.; Forte, R.; de Vito, G.; Boreham, C.A.G.; Gibney, M.J.; Brennan, L.; Gibney, E.R. Comparison of the effect of multicomponent and resistance training programs on metabolic health parameters in the elderly. *Arch. Gerontol. Geriatr.* **2015**, *60*, 412–417. [CrossRef]

32. Al-Eisa, E.S.; Alghadir, A.H.; Gabr, S.A. Correlation between vitamin D levels and muscle fatigue risk factors based on physical activity in healthy older adults. *Clin. Interv. Aging* **2016**, *11*, 513–522. [PubMed]

33. Biddle, G.; Edwardson, C.; Henson, J.; Davies, M.; Khunti, K.; Rowlands, A.; Yates, T. Associations of Physical Behaviours and Behavioural Reallocations with Markers of Metabolic Health: A Compositional Data Analysis. *Int. J. Environ. Res. Public. Health* **2018**, *15*, 2280. [CrossRef] [PubMed]

34. Santos Morais Junior, G.; Carolino Souza, V.; Machado-Silva, W.; Dallanora Henriques, A.; Melo Alves, A.; Barbosa Morais, D.; Nóbrega, O.; Brito, C.J.; Jerônimo dos Santos Silva, R. Acute strength training promotes responses in whole blood circulating levels of miR-146a among older adults with type 2 diabetes mellitus. *Clin. Interv. Aging* **2017**, *12*, 1443–1450. [CrossRef] [PubMed]

35. Hurtig-Wennlof, A.; Olsson, L.A.; Nilsson, T.K. Subjective well-being in Swedish active seniors and its relationship with physical activity and commonly available biomarkers. *Clin. Interv. Aging* **2014**, *9*, 1233–1239. [CrossRef]

36. Caminiti, G.; Iellamo, F.; Manzi, V.; Fossati, C.; Cioffi, V.; Punzo, N.; Murugesan, J.; Volterrani, M.; Rosano, G. Anabolic hormonal response to different exercise training intensities in men with chronic heart failure. *Int. J. Cardiol.* **2014**, *176*, 1433–1434. [CrossRef] [PubMed]

37. Kakugawa, Y.; Tada, H.; Kawai, M.; Suzuki, T.; Nishino, Y.; Kanemura, S.; Ishida, T.; Ohuchi, N.; Minami, Y. Associations of obesity and physical activity with serum and intratumoral sex steroid hormone levels among postmenopausal women with breast cancer: Analysis of paired serum and tumor tissue samples. *Breast Cancer Res. Treat.* **2017**, *162*, 115–125. [CrossRef]

38. Bondoc, I.; Cochrane, S.K.; Church, T.S.; Dahinden, P.; Hettwer, S.; Hsu, F.-C.; Stafford, R.S.; Pahor, M.; Buford, T.W.; Life Study Investigators. Effects of a One-Year Physical Activity Program on Serum C-Terminal Agrin Fragment (CAF) Concentrations among Mobility-Limited Older Adults. *J. Nutr. Health Aging* **2015**, *19*, 922–927. [CrossRef]

39. Volaklis, K.; Thorand, B.; Peters, A.; Halle, M.; Margot, H.; Amann, U.; Ladwig, K.; Schulz, H.; Koenig, W.; Meisinger, C. Muscular Strength is Independently Associated with Cystatin C: The KORA-Age Study. *Int. J. Sports Med.* **2018**, *39*, 225–231. [CrossRef]

40. Kosaki, K.; Kamijo-Ikemori, A.; Sugaya, T.; Tanahashi, K.; Sawano, Y.; Akazawa, N.; Ra, S.-G.; Kimura, K.; Shibagaki, Y.; Maeda, S. Effect of habitual exercise on urinary liver-type fatty acid-binding protein levels in middle-aged and older adults. *Scand. J. Med. Sci. Sports* **2018**, *28*, 152–160. [CrossRef]

41. Li, J.; Siegrist, J. Physical activity and risk of cardiovascular disease–a meta-analysis of prospective cohort studies. *Int. J. Environ. Res. Public. Health* **2012**, *9*, 391–407. [CrossRef]

42. Mora, S.; Cook, N.; Buring, J.E.; Ridker, P.M.; Lee, I.-M. Physical activity and reduced risk of cardiovascular events: Potential mediating mechanisms. *Circulation* **2007**, *116*, 2110–2118. [CrossRef] [PubMed]

43. Brown, W.M.C.; Davison, G.W.; McClean, C.M.; Murphy, M.H. A Systematic Review of the Acute Effects of Exercise on Immune and Inflammatory Indices in Untrained Adults. *Sports Med.—Open* **2015**, *1*, 35. [CrossRef] [PubMed]

44. Kasapis, C.; Thompson, P.D. The effects of physical activity on serum C-reactive protein and inflammatory markers: A systematic review. *J. Am. Coll. Cardiol.* **2005**, *45*, 1563–1569. [CrossRef] [PubMed]

45. Hamer, M. The relative influences of fitness and fatness on inflammatory factors. *Prev. Med.* **2007**, *44*, 3–11. [CrossRef]

46. Wilund, K.R. Is the anti-inflammatory effect of regular exercise responsible for reduced cardiovascular disease? *Clin. Sci. Lond. Engl. 1979* **2007**, *112*, 543–555. [CrossRef]

47. Hambrecht, R.; Wolf, A.; Gielen, S.; Linke, A.; Hofer, J.; Erbs, S.; Schoene, N.; Schuler, G. Effect of exercise on coronary endothelial function in patients with coronary artery disease. *N. Engl. J. Med.* **2000**, *342*, 454–460. [CrossRef]

48. Radák, Z.; Chung, H.Y.; Naito, H.; Takahashi, R.; Jung, K.J.; Kim, H.-J.; Goto, S. Age-associated increase in oxidative stress and nuclear factor kappaB activation are attenuated in rat liver by regular exercise. *FASEB J. Off. Publ. Fed. Am. Soc. Exp. Biol.* **2004**, *18*, 749–750.

49. Bassey, E.J. The benefits of exercise for the health of older people. *Rev. Clin. Gerontol.* **2000**, *10*, 17–31. [CrossRef]

50. Sallam, N.; Laher, I. Exercise Modulates Oxidative Stress and Inflammation in Aging and Cardiovascular Diseases. *Oxid. Med. Cell. Longev.* **2016**, *2016*, 7239639. [CrossRef]

51. Zhang, J.; Wang, X.; Vikash, V.; Ye, Q.; Wu, D.; Liu, Y.; Dong, W. ROS and ROS-Mediated Cellular Signaling. *Oxid. Med. Cell. Longev.* **2016**, *2016*, 4350965. [CrossRef]

52. Pham-Huy, L.A.; He, H.; Pham-Huy, C. Free radicals, antioxidants in disease and health. *Int. J. Biomed. Sci.* **2008**, *4*, 89–96. [PubMed]

53. Singh, M.A.F. Exercise and aging. *Clin. Geriatr. Med.* **2004**, *20*, 201–221. [CrossRef] [PubMed]

54. Gopinath, B.; Kifley, A.; Flood, V.M.; Mitchell, P. Physical Activity as a Determinant of Successful Aging over Ten Years. *Sci. Rep.* **2018**, *8*, 10522. [CrossRef] [PubMed]

55. Bassi, D.; Mendes, R.G.; Arakelian, V.M.; Caruso, F.C.R.; Cabiddu, R.; Júnior, J.C.B.; Arena, R.; Borghi-Silva, A. Potential Effects on Cardiorespiratory and Metabolic Status After a Concurrent Strength and Endurance Training Program in Diabetes Patients—A Randomized Controlled Trial. *Sports Med.—Open* **2015**, *2*, 31. [CrossRef] [PubMed]

56. McGarrah, R.W.; Slentz, C.A.; Kraus, W.E. The Effect of Vigorous- Versus Moderate-Intensity Aerobic Exercise on Insulin Action. *Curr. Cardiol. Rep.* **2016**, *18*, 117. [CrossRef]

57. Roberts, C.K.; Hevener, A.L.; Barnard, R.J. Metabolic syndrome and insulin resistance: Underlying causes and modification by exercise training. *Compr. Physiol.* **2013**, *3*, 1–58.

58. Bacchi, E.; Negri, C.; Targher, G.; Faccioli, N.; Lanza, M.; Zoppini, G.; Zanolin, E.; Schena, F.; Bonora, E.; Moghetti, P. Both resistance training and aerobic training reduce hepatic fat content in type 2 diabetic subjects with nonalcoholic fatty liver disease (the RAED2 Randomized Trial). *Hepatology* **2013**, *58*, 1287–1295. [CrossRef]

59. Ari, Z.; Kutlu, N.; Uyanik, B.S.; Taneli, F.; Buyukyazi, G.; Tavli, T. Serum testosterone, growth hormone, and insulin-like growth factor-1 levels, mental reaction time, and maximal aerobic exercise in sedentary and long-term physically trained elderly males. *Int. J. Neurosci.* **2004**, *114*, 623–637. [CrossRef]

60. Muller, M.; den Tonkelaar, I.; Thijssen, J.H.H.; Grobbee, D.E.; van der Schouw, Y.T. Endogenous sex hormones in men aged 40–80 years. *Eur. J. Endocrinol.* **2003**, *149*, 583–589. [CrossRef]

61. Kaufman, J.M.; Vermeulen, A. The decline of androgen levels in elderly men and its clinical and therapeutic implications. *Endocr. Rev.* **2005**, *26*, 833–876. [CrossRef]

62. Senderovich, H.; Tang, H.; Belmont, S. The Role of Exercises in Osteoporotic Fracture Prevention and Current Care Gaps. Where Are We Now? Recent Updates. *Rambam Maimonides Med. J.* **2017**, *8*. [CrossRef] [PubMed]

63. Parisi, A.; Massaa, G.; Rizzo, M.; Nataloni, C.; Pigozzi, F. Lo sportivo diabetico: Prescrizioni nutrizionali ed indicazione all'attività sportiva. *Med. Dello Sport* **2004**, *57*, 149–155.

12

Return to Sport Activity in the Elderly Patients after Unicompartmental Knee Arthroplasty

Rocco Papalia [1], Biagio Zampogna [1,*], Guglielmo Torre [1], Lorenzo Alirio Diaz Balzani [1], Sebastiano Vasta [1], Giuseppe Papalia [1], Antonio De Vincentis [2] and Vincenzo Denaro [1]

[1] Deaprtment of Orthopaedic and Trauma Surgery, Campus Bio-Medico University of Rome, Via A. Del Portillo, 21, 00128 Rome, Italy; r.papalia@unicampus.it (R.P.); g.torre@unicampus.it (G.T.); l.diaz@unicampus.it (L.A.D.B.); s.vasta@unicampus.it (S.V.); g.papalia@unicampus.it (G.P.); denaro@unicampus.it (V.D.)

[2] Department of Internal Medicine and Gerontology, Campus Bio-Medico University of Rome, Via A. Del Portillo, 21, 00128 Rome, Italy; a.devincentis@unicampus.it

* Correspondence: b.zampogna@unicampus.it

Abstract: In patients with knee osteoarthritis, when only medial or lateral compartment of the knee is involved, unicompartimental knee arthroplasty (UKA) is a reliable option for addressing the symptoms and restore function. The main aim of the present review is to systematically collect the available evidence concerning the return to sport activity in the elderly patients after UKA. An electronic search was carried out on the following databases; Pubmed-Medline, Cochrane central, and Scopus, searching for randomized controlled trials, prospective cohort studies, retrospective case-control studies, and case series. Data concerning the evaluation of the return to sport (RTS) and of functional outcomes in the elderly patients after UKA surgery. MINORS score was used to assess the risk of methodological biases. Odds ratios and raw proportions were used to report the pooled effect of UKA on the return to sport in comparative and non-comparative studies, respectively. Same level RTS in elderly patients was of 86% (pooled return proportion 0.86, 95%CI 0.78, 0.94), showing also better relative RTS and time to RTS of patients undergoing UKA, in comparison to those undergoing TKA. Sport-specific RTS showed that higher return rates were observed for low-impact sports, whereas high-impact sports prevented a full return to activities. UKA is a valid and reliable option for elderly patients to satisfactorily resume their sport practice, especially for low impact activities. The rate of return to sports following UKA is higher than TKA.

Keywords: knee osteoarthritis; unicompartimental knee arthroplasty; sport; activity; elderly

1. Introduction

In the present social scenario, the needs of elderly people are changing. It is not infrequent that patients want to stay active and be able to perform physical exercises and sport activities even in an advanced age [1,2]. However, these requests are often undermined by chronic painful conditions, such as osteoarthritis (OA), that do not allow the patient perform all desired activities [3]. In particular, knee OA is a common, debilitating condition that is increasingly widespread accordingly with the aging of the general population [1,2,4–6]. It is widely accepted that the definitive treatment for the end stage knee OA is the joint arthroplasty [7]. When only medial or lateral compartment of the knee is involved, unicompartimental knee arthroplasty (UKA) is a reliable option that is raising in popularity [8,9]. Indications to UKA have been widely discussed, but it is well known that this implant provides some advantages: lower invasiveness, shorter rehabilitation time, restoration of a wider range of motion, and physiological proprioception of the knee due to cruciate ligaments retention [10]. Several studies in literature reported the benefits of patients who underwent UKA in terms of pain relief and quality of life, with a good to excellent return to activities [11]. The opportunity to move and walk without pain, with also a good recovery of the motion, allows individuals to perform physical activity and sport, which is particularly important to prevent systemic diseases associated to sedentary life such as obesity, diabetes, cardiovascular accidents, and cancer [12–14]. One of the principal expectation for active patients before undergoing UKA surgery, is about their chances to perform physical activity and sport after surgery. Moreover, active patient is mostly interested in type and level of sport activity [15,16]. The current scientific literature answers those questions mainly with recommendations based on expert opinions and surgical society guidelines [17,18], but still lacks high level evidence-based guidelines, especially regarding the elderly population. The main aim of the present manuscript is therefore to systematically collect the available evidence concerning the return to sport activity in the elderly patients after UKA, with a special concern to the type of activity. A secondary endpoint of this investigation is to assess the functional outcomes in the same population.

2. Methods

A systematic review and meta-analysis was carried out using the Preferred Reporting Items for Systematic Reviews and Meta-analysis (PRISMA) guidelines [19]. The review was planned and conducted following the PRISMA checklist. According to PICO, the following elements have been used to frame the study question.

Population: Elderly patients.
Intervention: Unicompartmental Knee Arthroplasty (UKA).
Comparison: Total Knee Arthroplasty (TKA) or no comparison.
Outcomes: Return to sport activity and functional outcomes.

2.1. Criteria for Considering Studies for This Review

The studies considered for inclusion were randomized controlled trials (CRT), prospective cohort studies (PCS), retrospective case–control studies (RCS), and case series (CS). The main topic of the papers had to be the evaluation of the return to sport activity and of functional outcomes in the elderly patients after UKA surgery. Case Reports, Reviews, and Meta-analyses were not eligible for inclusion. Moreover, in vitro studies and cadaver studies were excluded from the review analysis. Given the specific focus on a selected population, only studies reporting outcomes of patients aged 65 or older were considered for inclusion (average population age > 65).

2.2. Primary Outcome Measures

The absolute numbers and proportions of patients returned to same level sport activities (RTS) was considered as the primary outcome measure and assessed throughout the included studies. Sport-specific return was extracted from the studies, to stratify results according to the type of activities.

2.3. Secondary Outcome Measures

The secondary endpoint was achieved by evaluating the following measures; Oxford Knee Score (OKS), Knee injury and Osteoarthritis Outcome Score (KOOS), Knee Society Score (KSS) and American Knee Society Score (AKSS), University of California Los Angeles (UCLA), Tegner and Lysholm scales, and the Western Ontario McMaster universities osteoarthritis index (WOMAC). These measures were evaluated across the included studies.

2.4. Search Strategy for Study Identification

The online search was carried out on the following databases; Pubmed-Medline, Cochrane central, and Scopus. The following search string was used; (Arthroplasty, Replacement [MeSH Terms])

AND joint, knee [MeSH Terms]) AND sports [MeSH Terms] and (arthroplasties, knee replacement [MeSH Terms]) AND sports [MeSH Terms]. The bibliography of the included studies and of recent review articles was screened for further relevant articles, potentially missed at the electronic search. After duplicates removal, all the retrieved studies were firstly screened by title to find studies dealing with UKA. Two independent reviewers (B.Z. and G.T.) evaluated the abstract of each of the papers considered for inclusion. Discordant opinions concerning study inclusion were discussed with a third experienced reviewer (R.P.). If abstract was not sufficient to define inclusion of a paper, the full-text was retrieved and evaluated. Articles included for review process were retrieved in full-text and read. The search process was summarized in Figure 1.

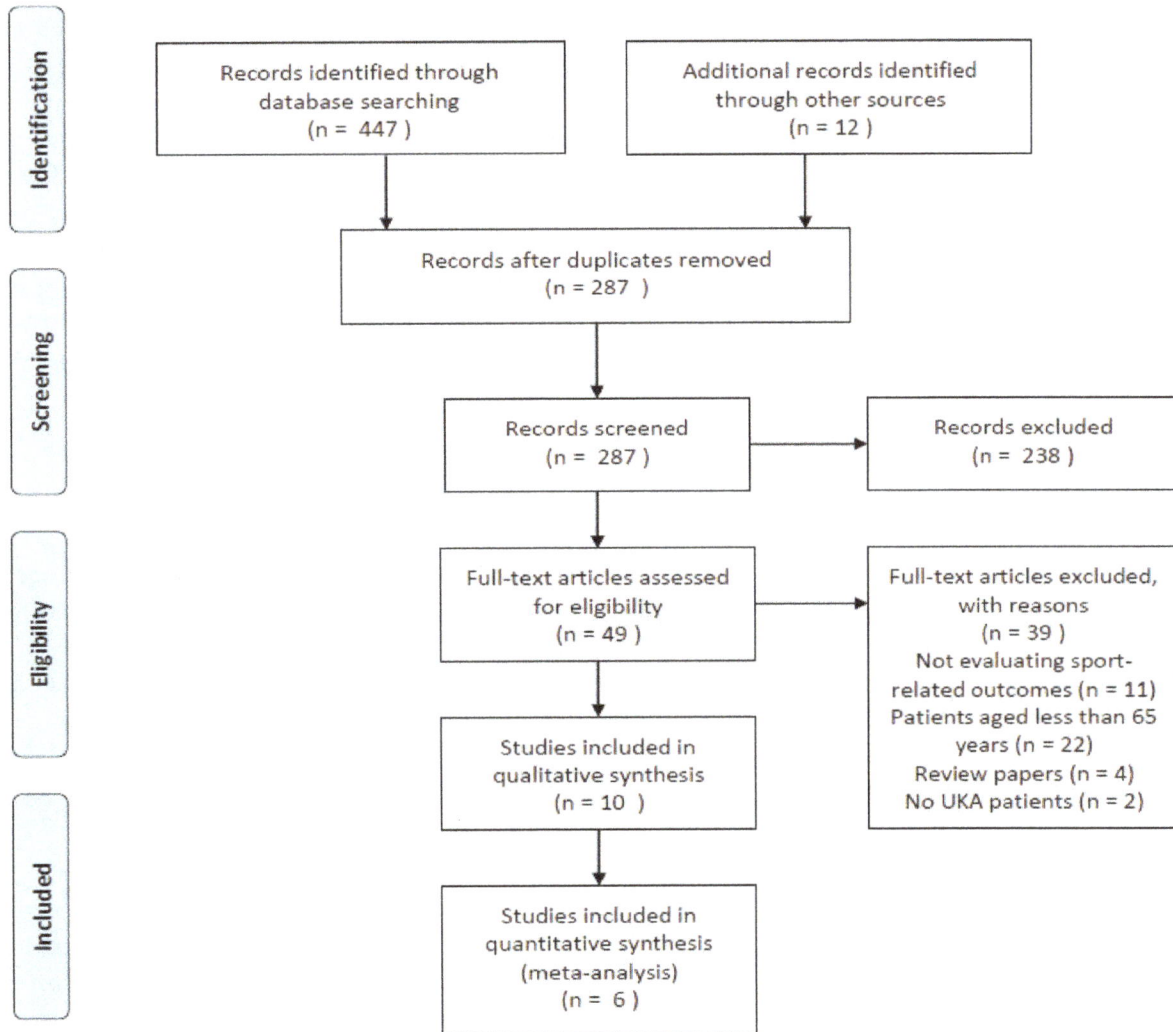

Figure 1. Study selection flowchart (UKA: Unicompartimental Knee Arthroplasty).

2.5. Data Collection and Analysis

Data were extracted independently by two reviewers (B.Z. and L.A.D.B.) and tabulated according to primary and secondary outcomes of this review. Discordant opinions in data extraction were solved by discussion with a third reviewer (R.P.).

2.6. Risk of Bias Assessment

The quality of the included non-randomized studies was independently evaluated by two reviewers (L.D.B. and B.Z.) using the Methodological Index for Non-randomized Studies (MINORS) score. [20] The following domains were assessed; a clearly stated purpose, inclusion of consecutive subjects, prospective data collection, endpoints appropriate to the purpose of the study, unbiased assessment of the study endpoints, follow-up period appropriate for the study, loss to follow-up of less than 5%, prospective calculation of the study size, adequate control group, contemporary group, baseline group equivalence, and adequate statistical analysis. The last four items are specific to comparative studies. Each item was scored from 0 to 2 points, with a global ideal score of 16 points for non-comparative studies and 24 points for comparative studies.

2.7. Quantitative Analysis

Meta-analysis was carried out to investigate the effect of UKA on the return to sport activity either in comparison with TKA or in non-comparative studies. Furthermore, return to specific sport activities was pooled if at least three studies reported the same sport. Odds ratios (ORs) and raw, i.e. untransformed, proportions were used to report the pooled effect of UKA on the return to sport probabilities in comparative (vs. TKA) and non-comparative studies, respectively. Heterogeneity was evaluated using Q statistic, expressed as the p value for the χ test under the null hypothesis that the between-study variance (τ) equals 0, and I2 test. All the conducted meta-analyses evidenced the presence of significant heterogeneity, defined as a I2 > 55% and/or a Q statistic p value below 0.05. Accordingly, random effect models were applied. Finally, the likelihood of methodological bias among included studies was estimated with the visual inspection of the funnel plot. Analyses were conducted using metafor and meta packages in R 3.6.1 (R Foundation for Statistical Computing, Vienna, Austria).

3. Results

3.1. Research Results

Electronic search identified 447 papers, and of these 287 scientific products were screened for analysis. Full text of 49 papers was accurately analyzed and 28 were excluded for following reasons; absence of postoperative sport-related outcomes, cohort mean age lower than 65 years old, duplicated papers and no UKA patients. Finally, 10 [10,21–29] articles were included according PRISMA selection process (Figure 1).

3.2. Included and Excluded Studies

Among 10 studies, only 2 study were prospective [24,26], 6 evaluated the cohort retrospectively (LOE III) [21–23,27–29], and 2 were case series (LOE IV) [10,25]. Five studies out of 10 compared clinical outcome of UKA and TKA cohorts [22–24,28,29]. Six studies reported specific RTS outcome like preoperative and postoperative sport participation, RTS rate, time to RTS and pre and postoperative sport-specific participation [10,21,22,27–29]. Canetti et al. compared two different cohort of lateral UKA performed with and without robotic assistance [21].

3.3. Demographic Results

Overall number of patients analyzed in the present review was 5220 with 2930 UKA and 2447 TKA implanted. Mean age of UKA's was 66.3, whereas mean age of TKA cohort was 74 years old. Mean follow-up was 2.1 years. In three studies type of prosthesis was not specified [22,24,29] while 4 papers reported outcome of mobile bearing UKA [25–28]. Demographic parameters of included study are summarized in Table 1.

Table 1. Demographic studies details.

Author and Year	LOE	N.er of Patients	M	F	Type of Arthroplasty	Type of Implant	Bearing and Fixation	Mean Age at Surgery	Mean Follow-up (Months)	MINORS Score
Canetti et al. 2018	3	25 (28 knees)	9	21	Robotic UKA 11 / Conventional UKA 17	Resurfacing Uni Evolution, Tornier; BlueBelt Navio robotic surgical system.	Fixed bearing and cemented.	66.5 ± 6.8 / 59.5 ± 9.9	34.4 ± 10.5 / 39.3 ± 15.5	17
Harbourne et al. 2018	3	995	44 / 6	54 / 9	UKA 420 / TKA 575	n/a	n/a	67 ± 10 / 70 ± 9	12	16
Lygre et al. 2010	3	1344	152 / 282	220 / 690	UKA: 372 / TKA: 972	Genesis Uni (Smith & Nephew), Miller-Galante all poly Uni (Zimmer), Oxford III (Biomet). / AGC (Biomet), Genesis I (Smith & Nephew), LCS (DePuy) and NexGen (Zimmer).	Fixed/mobile and cemented. / Fixed bearing and cemented.	68.8 ± 8.8 / 76 ± 7.7	58.8 ± 27.6 / 84 ± 28.8	15
Matthews et al. 2013	2	68	10 / 14	24 / 20	UKA 34 / TKA 34	n/a	n/a	UKA 67.3 ± 9.1 / TKA 69.2 ± 7.7	12	15
Naal et al. 2007	4	83 (83)	45	38	UKA	Preservation prosthesis (DePuy).	Fixed bearing and cemented.	65.5 ± 9.1 years (47–83)	12	10
Pandit et al. 2011	4	818 (1000)	-	-	UKA	Phase 3 Oxford medial UKA (Biomet)	Mobile bearing and cemented.	66 (32–88)	67.2	11
Pandit et al. 2015	4	579 (520)	299	221	UKA	Phase 3 Oxford medial UKA (Biomet).	Mobile bearing and cementless	65.1 ± 10.3 (35–94)	40.8 ± 20.4	12
Pietschmann et al. 2012	3	131	57	74	UKA	Phase 3 Oxford medial UKA (Biomet).	Mobile bearing and cemented.	65.3 (44–90)	50.4 (12–120)	7
Walton et al. 2010	3	150 (183) / 120 (142)	76 / 61	74 / 59	UKA / TKA	Phase 3 Oxford medial UKA (Biomet). / n/a	Mobile bearing and cemented. / n/a	71.5 ± 9.85 / 71.53 ± 9.87	12	12
Wylde et al. 2008	3	966	48	52	UKA: 100 TKA: 866	n/a	n/a	66 (45–88) 69.6 (26–93)	24	16
			511	355						

UKA: Unicompartmental Knee Arthroplasty TKA: Total Knee Arthroplasty (TKA), LOE: Level: of Evidence, M: Males, F: Females.

3.4. Return to Sport Activity

Sport-specific return rates were analyzed in 50% of the studies included [10,21,22,27–29]. Mean RTS rate for UKA was 89.5%, ranging from 75% [22,29] to 100% [28]. Mean preoperative sport participation rate was 71.8% of the patients, ranging from 36% [29] to 100% [21], and mean postoperative sport participation rate was 70.2% of the patients, ranging from 27% [29] to 100% [21]. Mean time to RTS was 6.2 months. Results of the study published by Canetti et al. [21], showed for UKA robotic assisted group a statistically significant difference in terms of time to return to sport compared to conventional UKA with a similar RTS rate (100% vs. 94%). The cohort of medial UKA of Pietschmann et al. [27] had an 88% of RTS rate with 80.1% of patients that returned to preoperative activity level. Naal et al. [10] reported RTS rate of 95%; moreover, the activity frequency (session per week) was maintained in postoperative assessment (2.9 vs. 2.8) with a slight decrease in terms of session length (66 vs. 55 minutes). Overall, by meta-analyzing available studies, we evidenced a good proportional RTS (0.86 95% CI 0.78, 0.94), with sport-specific RTS favoring those sports with low-impact. Meta-analysis results were showed in Figures 2–8.

Study	Cases	Total	Proportion	95% C.I.
Canetti R. 2018	27	28	0.96	[0.82; 1.00]
Naal F. 2007	73	77	0.95	[0.87; 0.99]
Pietschmann M. 2012	69	78	0.88	[0.79; 0.95]
Harbourne et al. 2018	315	420	0.75	[0.71; 0.79]
Walton N. 2006	129	150	0.86	[0.79; 0.91]
Wylde V. 2008	27	36	0.75	[0.58; 0.88]
Random effects model		.	**0.86**	**[0.78; 0.94]**

Heterogeneity: $I^2 = 90\%$, $\tau^2 = 0.0086$, $p < 0.01$

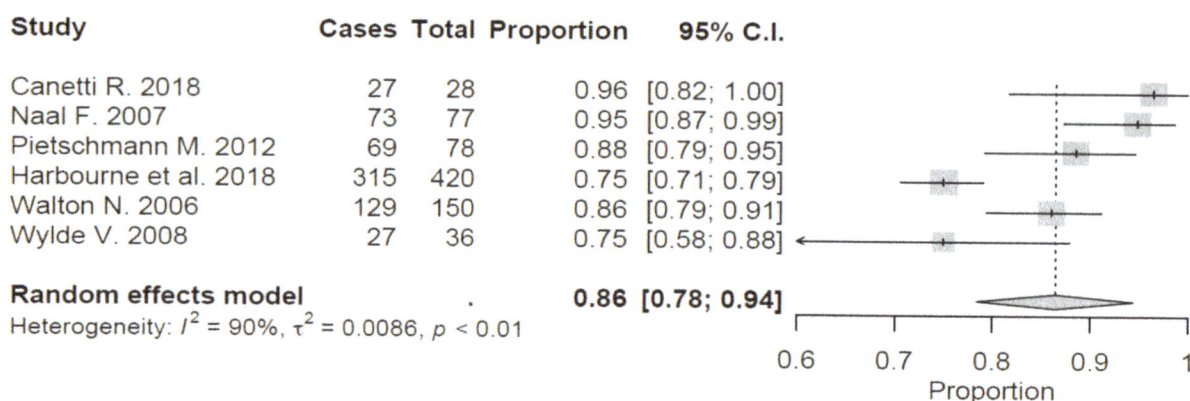

Figure 2. Overall return to sport after UKA (C.I.: Confidence Intervals).

Study	Cases	Total	Proportion	95% C.I.
Canetti R. 2018	23	25	0.92	[0.74; 0.99]
Naal F. 2007	43	56	0.77	[0.64; 0.87]
Pietschmann M. 2012	12	12	1.00	[0.74; 1.00]
Walton N. 2006	10	18	0.56	[0.31; 0.78]
Random effects model		.	**0.83**	**[0.68; 0.99]**

Heterogeneity: $I^2 = 83\%$, $\tau^2 = 0.0187$, $p < 0.01$

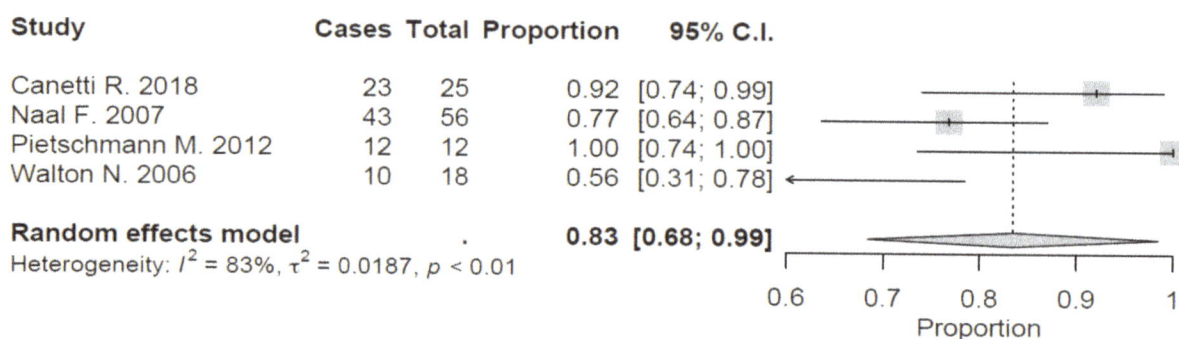

Figure 3. Return to hiking after UKA (C.I.: Confidence Intervals).

Study	Cases	Total	Proportion	95% C.I.
Canetti R. 2018	13	13	1.00	[0.75; 1.00]
Naal F. 2007	42	49	0.86	[0.73; 0.94]
Pietschmann M. 2012	44	45	0.98	[0.88; 1.00]
Walton N. 2006	19	19	1.00	[0.82; 1.00]
Random effects model		.	**0.97**	**[0.91; 1.00]**

Heterogeneity: $I^2 = 52\%$, $\tau^2 = 0.0015$, $p = 0.10$

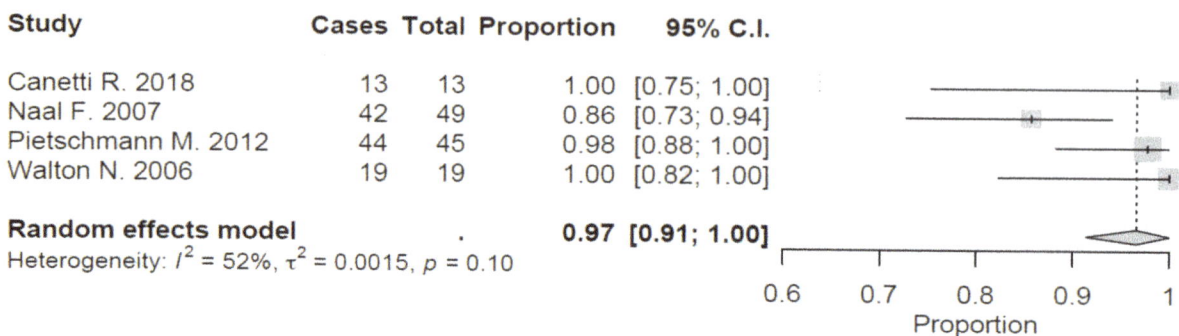

Figure 4. Return to cycling after UKA (C.I.: Confidence Intervals).

Study	Cases	Total	Proportion	95% C.I.
Canetti R. 2018	4	4	1.00	[0.40; 1.00]
Naal F. 2007	34	42	0.81	[0.66; 0.91]
Pietschmann M. 2012	13	17	0.76	[0.50; 0.93]
Walton N. 2006	23	23	1.00	[0.85; 1.00]
Random effects model		.	**0.90**	**[0.76; 1.00]**

Heterogeneity: $I^2 = 74\%$, $\tau^2 = 0.0128$, $p < 0.01$

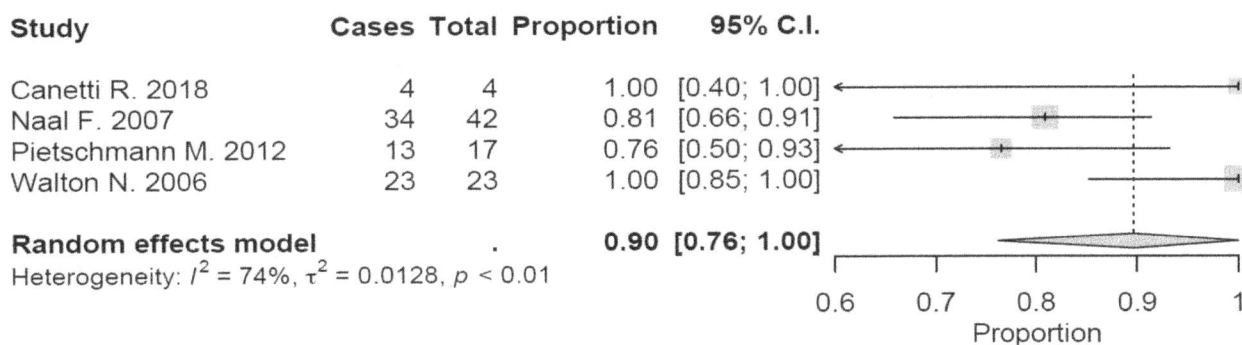

Figure 5. Return to swimming after UKA (C.I.: Confidence Intervals).

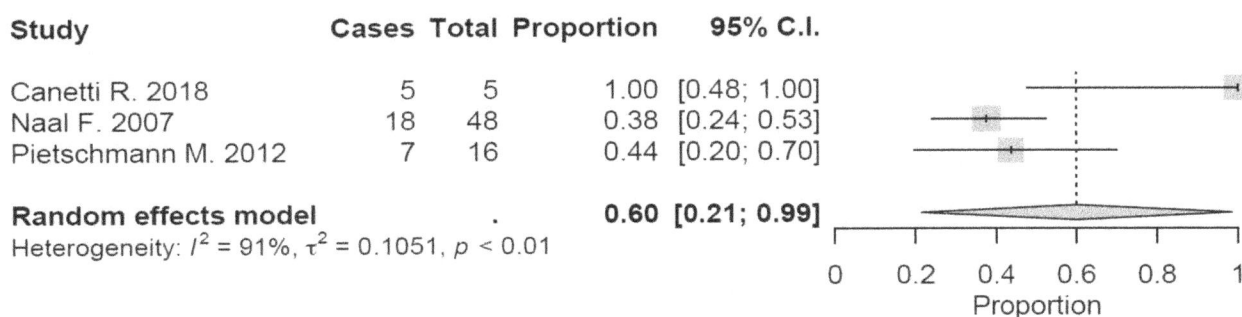

Study	Cases	Total	Proportion	95% C.I.
Canetti R. 2018	5	5	1.00	[0.48; 1.00]
Naal F. 2007	18	48	0.38	[0.24; 0.53]
Pietschmann M. 2012	7	16	0.44	[0.20; 0.70]
Random effects model		.	**0.60**	**[0.21; 0.99]**

Heterogeneity: $I^2 = 91\%$, $\tau^2 = 0.1051$, $p < 0.01$

Figure 6. Return to alpine ski after UKA (C.I.: Confidence Intervals).

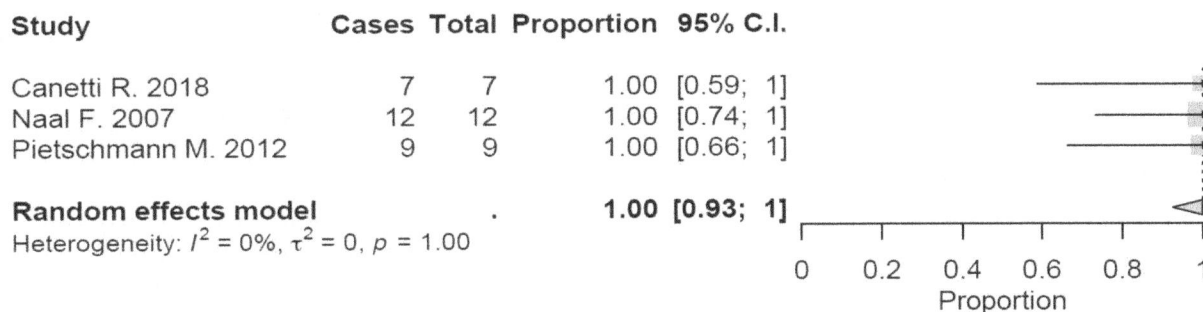

Study	Cases	Total	Proportion	95% C.I.
Canetti R. 2018	7	7	1.00	[0.59; 1]
Naal F. 2007	12	12	1.00	[0.74; 1]
Pietschmann M. 2012	9	9	1.00	[0.66; 1]
Random effects model		.	**1.00**	**[0.93; 1]**

Heterogeneity: $I^2 = 0\%$, $\tau^2 = 0$, $p = 1.00$

Figure 7. Return to fitness after UKA (C.I.: Confidence Intervals).

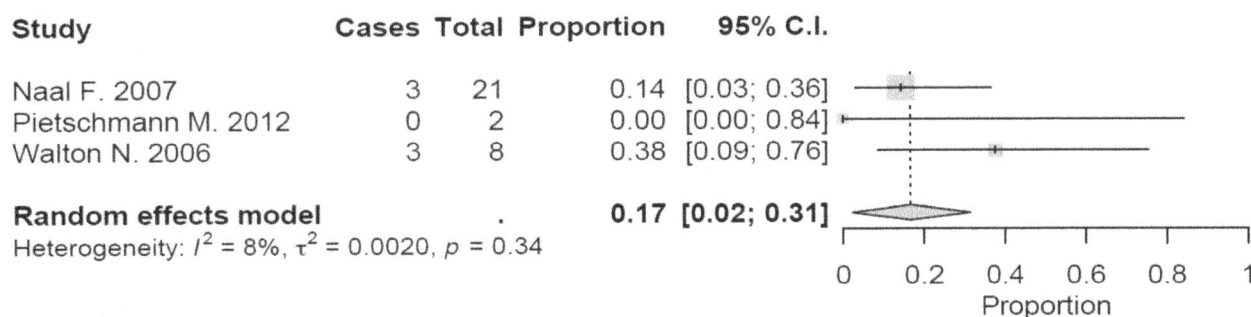

Study	Cases	Total	Proportion	95% C.I.
Naal F. 2007	3	21	0.14	[0.03; 0.36]
Pietschmann M. 2012	0	2	0.00	[0.00; 0.84]
Walton N. 2006	3	8	0.38	[0.09; 0.76]
Random effects model		.	**0.17**	**[0.02; 0.31]**

Heterogeneity: $I^2 = 8\%$, $\tau^2 = 0.0020$, $p = 0.34$

Figure 8. Return to tennis after UKA (C.I.: Confidence Intervals).

3.5. Comparison with TKA

Three papers compared RTS outcome of UKA and TKA patients' cohort [22,28,29]. Harbourne et al. [22] at 12 months of follow-up recorded a higher rate of return to activity in patients with UKA than TKA (75% vs. 59% $p < 0.001$). According to results of Walton et al. [28], the UKA group had a better percentage of patients that increased or maintained sport activity compared to the TKA group (P_.0003); moreover, TKA patients significantly reduced postoperative sport activity compared to UKA's (P_.0001). Wylde et al. [29] investigated return to sport after different type of implant (THA, Hip Resurfacing, TKA, UKA) and no significant difference differences were detected in postoperative sport participation between UKA and TKA (75% vs. 73.1%). Meta-analysis study pooling showed a better RTS in patients undergoing UKA (Odds Ratio 2.14 95% CI 1.29, 3.55). Results are shown in Figure 9.

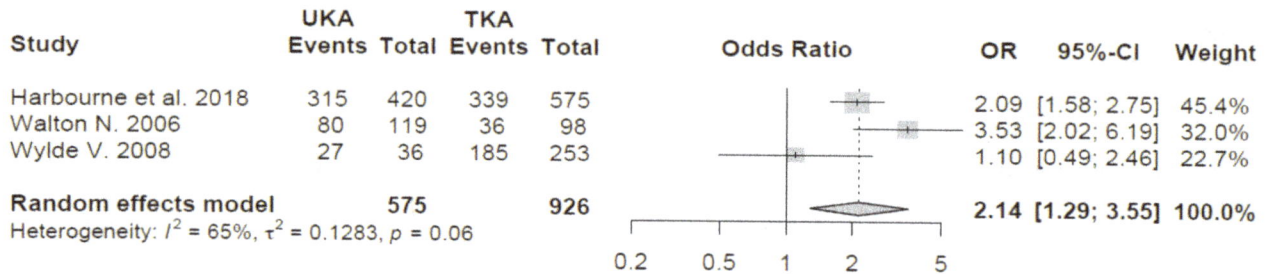

Study	UKA Events	Total	TKA Events	Total	Odds Ratio	OR	95%-CI	Weight
Harbourne et al. 2018	315	420	339	575		2.09	[1.58; 2.75]	45.4%
Walton N. 2006	80	119	36	98		3.53	[2.02; 6.19]	32.0%
Wylde V. 2008	27	36	185	253		1.10	[0.49; 2.46]	22.7%
Random effects model		575		926		2.14	[1.29; 3.55]	100.0%

Heterogeneity: $I^2 = 65\%$, $\tau^2 = 0.1283$, $p = 0.06$

0.2 0.5 1 2 5

Figure 9. Return to sport after UKA vs. TKA (C.I.: Confidence Intervals, O.R.: Odds Ratio).

3.6. Clinical Outcome Data

Several clinical outcome assessment measure and sport specific questionnaires were utilized. Oxford Knee score were used in six studies [22,24–28], Knee Society Score (KSS) in five studies [10,21,24–27], WOMAC in three studies [21,24,27,29], Forgotten Joint Score (FJS) and UCLA in two studies [21,24], Tegner Activity Score in two studies [25,26], KOOS [23] and Lysholm Knee Scale [21] in one study. Clinical results of Canetti et al. [21] showed a higher IKSS-Objective (97.2 ± 5.9 vs. 91.2 ± 6.5; $p < 0.05$) and a higher IKSS-Objective improvement (+ 30.9 ± 7.7 vs. + 22.8 ± 12.2; $p < 0.05$) compared to conventional group of lateral UKA. Naal et al. [10] obtained an improvement on KSS score in their postoperative assessment (from 129.9 ± 24.8, vs. to 186.9 ± 18.3) with a good result in terms of quality of life stated with SF-36. Pandit et al. [26] obtained a good postoperative results with the first 1000 cases of Oxford phase 3 medial UKA at 5 years: mean OKS was 41.3 (SD 7.2), mean AKS Objective Score 86.4 (SD 13.4), mean AKS Functional Score 86.1 (SD 16.6), and mean Tegner activity score 2.8 (SD 1.1). The same group, in 2015 [25], published results of cementless fixation for the same implant with similar postoperative clinical and functional results: OKS 43 (SD 7), AKSS (objective) 81 (SD 13), AKSS (functional) 86 (SD 17), and Tegner activity score of 3 (1–8). Pietschmann et al. [27] had a higher postoperative OKS, KSS, WOMAC and UCLA score. Active patients in sport preoperatively, except for KSS knee objective score, obtained statistically significant higher score than inactive patients group (OKS < 0.01, UCLA < 0.0001, KSS function < 0.01, KSS knee subjective < 0.01, KSS overall < 0.01, WOMAC < 0.05, WOMAC stiffness < 0.05, WOMAC ADL < 0.01, WOMAC overall < 0.01). Results are summarized in Table 2.

3.7. Clinical Outcome Data UKA vs. TKA

Four studies compared clinical outcome in patients aged more than 65 years old and underwent to UKA and TKA [23,24,28,29]. In the patients' cohort of Lygre et al. [23], UKA had a statistically significant superiority over TKA in terms of KOOS "Symptoms" (adjust mean diff 2.7 $p = 0.04$), KOOS "Function in Daily Living" (ADL) (adjust mean diff 4.1 $p = 0.01$) and KOOS "Function in Sport and Recreation" (adjust mean diff 5.4 $p = 0.006$). A prospective study designed by Matthews et al. [24] showed no statistical difference according to satisfaction (89 vs. 87 $p = 0.41$) and perception of knee normality (69 vs. 68 $p = 0.99$) scores between UKA and TKA; nevertheless, UKA reached a statistically significant higher WOMAC ($p = 0.003$), SF-36 (physical $p < 0.001$; mental $p = 0.25$), Oxford knee ($p < 0.001$), American Knee Society (clinical $p = 0.002$; function $p < 0.001$) and Total Knee Function Questionnaire scores (ADL $p = 0.002$; sport and exercise $p = 0.02$; movement and lifestyle $p = 0.02$). Walton et al. [28] compared in their study Mini-Incision Unicompartmental Knee Arthroplasty versus TKA and reported better results in terms of OKS ($p = 0.0426$) and mean modified Grimby score

(3.89 SD:1.27 vs. 2.76 (SD:1.12). In the last comparative study, performed by Wylde et al. [29], no clinical difference between UKA and TKA in terms of WOMAC pain (81.5 SD = 20.8 vs. 81.6 SD = 19.3) and function (76.3 SD = 21.4 vs. 79.1 SD = 20.5).

Table 2. Functional outcomes of included studies.

Author and Year	N.er of Patients	Preoperative		Postoperative		Outcome
		Mean	SD	Mean	SD	
Canetti R. 2018	28	66.3	8.9	97.2	5.9	KSS-Objective
		84.6	11.3	96.4	9.2	KSS-Functional
		6.4	1.6	6.6	1.4	UCLA
Naal F. 2007	83	n/a	n/a	96.4	8.3	Lysholm scale
		129.9	24.8	186.9	18.3	KSS total
		24.7	8.7	38.6	8.4	OKS
Pandit H. 2011	1000	2.3	1.1	2	8.4	Tegner activity score
		68.7	18	81.1	11.3	AKSS-F
		47.4	20	81.1	16	AKSS-O
		27	9	43	7	OKS
Pandit H. 2015	520	3	n/a	3	n/a	Tegner activity score
		71	17	86	16	AKSS-F
		52	20	92	12	AKSS-O
Pietschmann M. 2012	131	n/a	n/a	95.3	9.5	KSS-Objective
		n/a	n/a	86.7	13.8	KSS-Functional
		n/a	n/a	6	1	UCLA
		n/a	n/a	189	26.8	KSS total
		n/a	n/a	38.6	7.3	OKS
		n/a	n/a	90.6	9.7	WOMAC ADL

S.D.: Standard Deviation, N/A: Not Available, OKS: Oxford Knee Score, KOOS: Knee injury and Osteoarthritis Outcome Score, KSS: Knee Society Score, AKSS: American Knee Society Score, UCLA: University of California Los Angeles, WOMAC: Western Ontario McMaster universities osteoarthritis index.

3.8. Quality Assessment (MINORS)

The MINORS score ranged from 7 [27] to 12 [25] for non-comparative studies and from 12 [28] to 17 [21] for the comparative ones (Table 1). The mean value was 10 for non-comparative studies and 15 for comparative studies. The funnel plot of studies evaluating RTS after UKA showed a symmetrical distribution, while a rather poor precision of observations, suggesting an overall low-moderate risk of methodological bias (Figure 10).

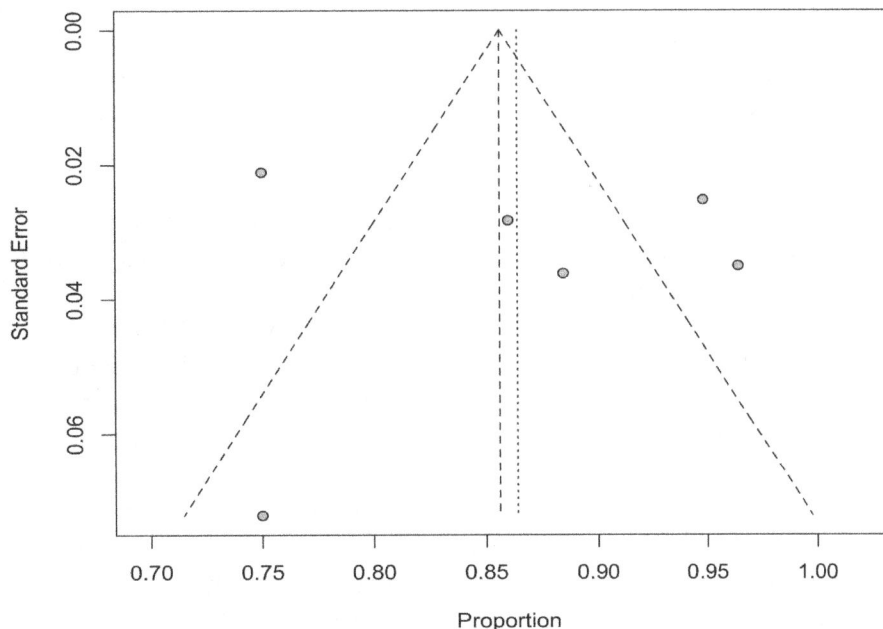

Figure 10. Funnel plot showing studies evaluating RTS after UKA.

4. Discussion

Elderly patients represent a selected population, which is changing in activity needs in recent years, according to general lifestyle modifications of the society. The main findings of the present investigation suggest a good proportional same level RTS in elderly patients after UKA (return proportion 0.86, 95%CI 0.78, 0.94), showing also better relative RTS and time to RTS of patients undergoing UKA, in comparison to those undergoing TKA. Moreover, patients undergoing TKA were more likely to reduce their activity level after the surgery [28]. Meta-analysis of the sport-specific RTS showed that higher return rates were observed for low-impact sports (e.g., swimming, fitness, hiking), whereas high-impact sports (e.g., tennis and alpine ski) prevented a full return to activities. The proportion of RTS for cohorts of patients undergoing UKA is in line with authors' experience and with literature-reported rates [10,21,30]. However, given the high heterogeneity of the studies concerning this outcome (90%), the result should be carefully interpreted. A first consideration concerns the average age of the cohorts, which was higher in those study reporting a lower RTS proportion. Furthermore, the differences in type of UKA implants could determine the activity level, with possible implications in polyethylene wearing [31]. Another major concern in general study heterogeneity is the absence, in almost all the studies, of a description of rehabilitation protocols and of surgical incision. In an era of wide differences in rehabilitation (i.e., fast-track, aquatic rehabilitation), understanding the post-operative protocols may be the key to evaluate the postoperative outcomes [32]. Moreover, the knee extension apparatus, thus the surgical approach plays a major role in return to activity and its timing.

Clinical outcomes reported in the included studies were filtered to collect those relative to sport participation and activity level. Although heterogeneous, an overall evaluation of the scores showed that either objective and subjective assessment improved significantly after UKA, suggesting that patient perception of the beneficial effects of the surgery reflects a standardized clinical examination and ROM assessment. Similarly, comparison of clinical outcomes after UKA with those after TKR favored the patients undergoing UKA. However, given the absence of control groups in most of the included studies, the meta-analysis evaluation was not possible, given the impossibility to calculate the standardized mean difference.

Concerning comparison of RTS and clinical outcomes between cohorts undergoing UKA and TKA, a potential confounding factor is age, as average age of UKA cohorts was 66.3 years, while mean age of TKA cohorts was 74 years. A 10-year difference is relevant by the observation that younger patients are more likely to continue in sport participation. This is especially true, given the higher and higher percentage of elderly population involved in sport activities in recent years [33]. Focusing on elderly population underlined some differences with available evidence on general population (non-elderly) [34,35]. First of all, as reported in previous literature reviews [11], the return to high-impact sport in patients that underwent either TKA and UKA was high, and not excessively different from those of low-impact sports [36,37]. Common experience leads the orthopedic surgeon to suggest caution in sport participation after joint arthroplasty, for the risk of component migration, loosening, and periprosthetic fractures. However, no specific evidence advices about long term results of sport involvement after UKA [30].

The UKA, a joint preserving arthroplasty, has been designed for those patients with localized osteoarthritis and was found especially beneficial in active individuals. However, the follow-up length reported in available literature is too short to assess failure and revision rates. It is opinion of the authors that until clear data will be available, the general attitude for patients and surgeon in regard to RTS will go toward a careful approach.

Another concern, in regards of the available literature, is the lack of information about reasons of not to return to sport activities. None of the articles included in this review reported the clinical and functional reasons that prevented the patients to return to activity, except a few reported surgical complications (i.e., common peroneal paralysis [21]). The issue of motivational causes that prevent RTS is relevant and only some studies in the gerontology field address the question [6,14]. An interesting point to improve future research would be to introduce motivational and depression scales next to functional patient reported outcome measures.

The overall LOE of included studies was low, as most of the evaluations were retrospective or were case series. This is reflected in the relatively high risk of bias which MINORS score showed. In particular, the worst item was the blinding of participants. However, given the type of therapeutic intervention considered, blinding was impossible.

The funnel plot evaluation was limited to those studies assessing the proportional RTS of patients after UKA. A balanced funnel was observed at visual inspection, but a relatively low precision was found for some studies, suggesting an overall low–moderate risk of methodological bias.

This is the first literature review and meta-analysis that selected age of the cohorts undergoing UKA, focusing the research questions on the elderly population. Meta-analysis had a two-fold aim: to investigate proportional RTS in UKA-only cohorts and to compare UKA and TKA patients. However, the study was not free from limitations. First of all, the limited number of studies reporting sport-specific outcomes after UKA and the low LOE prevented the authors to gather a sufficient evidence to finally answer to the research questions. Furthermore, the differences in study design, age of the cohorts and effect sizes yielded to high heterogeneity and prevented to draw a robust overall meta-analysis.

5. Conclusions

UKA is a valid and reliable option for elderly patients to satisfactorily resume their sport practice, especially for low impact activities. The rate of return to sports following UKA is higher than TKA. The most practiced sports after surgery are low contact activities such as swimming, fitness, and hiking. Unfortunately, there is a lack of consistent clinical data on the functional improvement before and after surgery in elderly patients, thus a standardized evaluation of patient after surgery is prevented. More, prospective, comparative studies are needed to determine the standardized functional improvement of elderly patients after UKA.

Author Contributions: Conceptualization, R.P. and B.Z.; methodology, A.D.V. and G.T.; formal analysis, A.D.V.; data curation, L.A.D.B. and B.Z.; writing—original draft preparation, G.T. and B.Z.; writing—review and editing, G.P. and S.V.; supervision, R.P. and V.D. All authors have read and agreed to the published version of the manuscript.

References

1. Dieppe, P.; Basler, H.; Chard, J.; Croft, P.; Dixon, J.; Hurley, M.; Lohmander, S.; Raspe, H. Knee replacement surgery for osteoarthritis: Effectiveness, practice variations, indications and possible determinants of utilization. *Rheumatology (Oxf. Engl.)* **1999**, *38*, 73–83. [CrossRef]
2. Felson, D.T.; Naimark, A.; Anderson, J.; Kazis, L.; Castelli, W.; Meenan, R.F. The prevalence of knee osteoarthritis in the elderly. The Framingham Osteoarthritis Study. *Arthritis Rheum. Off. J. Am. Coll. Rheumatol.* **1987**, *30*, 914–918. [CrossRef] [PubMed]
3. Hunter, D.J.; Bierma-zeinstra, S. Osteoarthritis. *Lancet* **2019**, *393*, 1745–1759. [CrossRef]
4. Dunlop, D.D.; Song, J.; Semanik, P.A.; Chang, R.W.; Sharma, L.; Bathon, J.M.; Eaton, C.B.; Hochberg, M.C.; Jackson, R.D.; Kwoh, C.K. Objective physical activity measurement in the osteoarthritis initiative: Are guidelines being met? *Arthritis Rheum.* **2011**, *63*, 3372–3382. [CrossRef] [PubMed]
5. Davis, M.; Ettinger, W.; Neuhaus, J.; Mallon, K. Knee osteoarthritis and physical functioning: Evidence from the NHANES I Epidemiologic Followup Study. *J. Rheumatol.* **1991**, *18*, 591–598. [PubMed]
6. Ettinger, W.H., Jr.; Fried, L.P.; Harris, T.; Shemanski, L.; Schulz, R.; Robbins, J.; Group, C.C.R. Self-reported causes of physical disability in older people: The Cardiovascular Health Study. *J. Am. Geriatr. Soc.* **1994**, *42*, 1035–1044. [CrossRef] [PubMed]

7. Ethgen, O.; Bruyère, O.; Richy, F.; Dardennes, C.; Reginster, J.-Y. Health-related quality of life in total hip and total knee arthroplasty: A qualitative and systematic review of the literature. *JBJS* **2004**, *86*, 963–974. [CrossRef] [PubMed]

8. Cartier, P.; Khefacha, A.; Sanouiller, J.-L.; Frederick, K. Unicondylar knee arthroplasty in middle-aged patients: A minimum 5-year follow-up. *Orthopedics* **2007**, *30*, 62.

9. Pandit, H.; Gulati, A.; Jenkins, C.; Barker, K.; Price, A.; Dodd, C.; Murray, D. Unicompartmental knee replacement for patients with partial thickness cartilage loss in the affected compartment. *Knee* **2011**, *18*, 168–171. [CrossRef]

10. Naal, F.D.; Fischer, M.; Preuss, A.; Goldhahn, J.; von Knoch, F.; Preiss, S.; Munzinger, U.; Drobny, T. Return to sports and recreational activity after unicompartmental knee arthroplasty. *Am. J. Sports Med.* **2007**, *35*, 1688–1695. [CrossRef]

11. Papalia, R.; Del Buono, A.; Zampogna, B.; Maffulli, N.; Denaro, V. Sport activity following joint arthroplasty: A systematic review. *Br. Med Bull.* **2012**, *101*, 81. [CrossRef] [PubMed]

12. Blair, S.; Sallis, R.; Hutber, A.; Archer, E. Exercise therapy–the public health message. *Scand. J. Med. Sci. Sports* **2012**, *22*, e24–e28. [CrossRef] [PubMed]

13. Kohl, H.W., 3rd; Craig, C.L.; Lambert, E.V.; Inoue, S.; Alkandari, J.R.; Leetongin, G.; Kahlmeier, S.; Group, L.P.A.S.W. The pandemic of physical inactivity: Global action for public health. *Lancet* **2012**, *380*, 294–305. [CrossRef]

14. Haskell, W.L.; Lee, I.-M.; Pate, R.R.; Powell, K.E.; Blair, S.N.; Franklin, B.A.; Macera, C.A.; Heath, G.W.; Thompson, P.D.; Bauman, A. Physical activity and public health: Updated recommendation for adults from the American College of Sports Medicine and the American Heart Association. *Med. Sci. Sports Exerc.* **2007**, *39*, 1423–1434. [CrossRef] [PubMed]

15. Seyler, T.M.; Mont, M.A.; Ragland, P.S.; Kachwala, M.M.; Delanois, R.E. Sports activity after total hip and knee arthroplasty. *Sports Med.* **2006**, *36*, 571–583. [CrossRef]

16. Chatterji, U.; Ashworth, M.J.; Lewis, P.L.; Dobson, P.J. Effect of total knee arthroplasty on recreational and sporting activity. *Anz J. Surg.* **2005**, *75*, 405–408. [CrossRef]

17. McGrory, B.J.; Stuart, M.J.; Sim, F.H. Participation in sports after hip and knee arthroplasty: Review of literature and survey of surgeon preferences. *Mayo Clin. Proc.* **1995**, *70*, 342–348. [CrossRef]

18. Swanson, E.A.; Schmalzried, T.P.; Dorey, F.J. Activity recommendations after total hip and knee arthroplasty: A survey of the American Association for Hip and Knee Surgeons. *J. Arthroplast.* **2009**, *24*, 120–126. [CrossRef]

19. Moher, D.; Liberati, A.; Tetzlaff, J.; Altman, D.G.; Group, P. Preferred reporting items for systematic reviews and meta-analyses: The PRISMA statement. *PLoS Med.* **2009**, *6*, e1000097. [CrossRef]

20. Slim, K.; Nini, E.; Forestier, D.; Kwiatkowski, F.; Panis, Y.; Chipponi, J. Methodological index for non-randomized studies (MINORS): Development and validation of a new instrument. *Anz J. Surg.* **2003**, *73*, 712–716. [CrossRef]

21. Canetti, R.; Batailler, C.; Bankhead, C.; Neyret, P.; Servien, E.; Lustig, S. Faster return to sport after robotic-assisted lateral unicompartmental knee arthroplasty: A comparative study. *Arch. Orthop. Trauma Surg.* **2018**, *138*, 1765–1771. [CrossRef]

22. Harbourne, A.D.; Sanchez-Santos, M.T.; Arden, N.K.; Filbay, S.R. Predictors of return to desired activity 12 months following unicompartmental and total knee arthroplasty. *Acta Orthop.* **2019**, *90*, 74–80. [CrossRef] [PubMed]

23. Lygre, S.H.L.; Espehaug, B.; Havelin, L.I.; Furnes, O.; Vollset, S.E. Pain and function in patients after primary unicompartmental and total knee arthroplasty. *JBJS* **2010**, *92*, 2890–2897. [CrossRef] [PubMed]

24. Matthews, D.J.; Hossain, F.S.; Patel, S.; Haddad, F.S. A cohort study predicts better functional outcomes and equivalent patient satisfaction following UKR compared with TKR. *HSS J.* **2013**, *9*, 21–24. [CrossRef] [PubMed]

25. Pandit, H.; Campi, S.; Hamilton, T.; Dada, O.; Pollalis, S.; Jenkins, C.; Dodd, C.; Murray, D. Five-year experience of cementless Oxford unicompartmental knee replacement. *Knee Surg. Sports Traumatol. Arthrosc.* **2017**, *25*, 694–702. [CrossRef] [PubMed]

26. Pandit, H.; Jenkins, C.; Gill, H.; Barker, K.; Dodd, C.; Murray, D. Minimally invasive Oxford phase 3 unicompartmental knee replacement: Results of 1000 cases. *J. Bone Jt. Surgery. Br. Vol.* **2011**, *93*, 198–204. [CrossRef] [PubMed]

27. Pietschmann, M.F.; Wohlleb, L.; Weber, P.; Schmidutz, F.; Ficklscherer, A.; Gülecyüz, M.F.; Safi, E.; Niethammer, T.R.; Jansson, V.; Müller, P.E. Sports activities after medial unicompartmental knee arthroplasty Oxford III—what can we expect? *Int. Orthop.* **2013**, *37*, 31–37. [CrossRef]

28. Walton, N.P.; Jahromi, I.; Lewis, P.L.; Dobson, P.J.; Angel, K.R.; Campbell, D.G. Patient-perceived outcomes and return to sport and work: TKA versus mini-incision unicompartmental knee arthroplasty. *J. Knee Surg.* **2006**, *19*, 112–116. [CrossRef]

29. Wylde, V.; Blom, A.; Dieppe, P.; Hewlett, S.; Learmonth, I. Return to sport after joint replacement. The Journal of bone and joint surgery. *Br. Vol.* **2008**, *90*, 920–923.

30. Witjes, S.; Gouttebarge, V.; Kuijer, P.P.F.; van Geenen, R.C.; Poolman, R.W.; Kerkhoffs, G.M. Return to sports and physical activity after total and unicondylar knee arthroplasty: A systematic review and meta-analysis. *Sports Med.* **2016**, *46*, 269–292. [CrossRef]

31. Kuster, M.S. Exercise recommendations after total joint replacement. *Sports Med.* **2002**, *32*, 433–445. [CrossRef] [PubMed]

32. Vasta, S.; Papalia, R.; Torre, G.; Vorini, F.; Papalia, G.; Zampogna, B.; Fossati, C.; Bravi, M.; Campi, S.; Denaro, V. The Influence of Preoperative Physical Activity on Postoperative Outcomes of Knee and Hip Arthroplasty Surgery in the Elderly: A Systematic Review. *J. Clin. Med.* **2020**, *9*, 969. [CrossRef] [PubMed]

33. Zampogna, B.; Papalia, R.; Papalia, G.F.; Campi, S.; Vasta, S.; Vorini, F.; Fossati, C.; Torre, G.; Denaro, V. The Role of Physical Activity as Conservative Treatment for Hip and Knee Osteoarthritis in Older People: A Systematic Review and Meta-Analysis. *J. Clin. Med.* **2020**, *9*, 1167. [CrossRef] [PubMed]

34. Ho, J.C.; Stitzlein, R.N.; Green, C.J.; Stoner, T.; Froimson, M.I. Return to sports activity following UKA and TKA. *J. Knee Surg.* **2016**, *29*, 254–259.

35. Kleeblad, L.J.; van der List, J.P.; Zuiderbaan, H.A.; Pearle, A.D. Larger range of motion and increased return to activity, but higher revision rates following unicompartmental versus total knee arthroplasty in patients under 65: A systematic review. *Knee Surg. Sports Traumatol. Arthrosc.* **2018**, *26*, 1811–1822. [CrossRef]

36. Mont, M.A.; Rajadhyaksha, A.D.; Marxen, J.L.; Silberstein, C.E.; Hungerford, D.S. Tennis after total knee arthroplasty. *Am. J. Sports Med.* **2002**, *30*, 163–166. [CrossRef]

37. Lefevre, N.; Rousseau, D.; Bohu, Y.; Klouche, S.; Herman, S. Return to judo after joint replacement. *Knee Surg. Sports Traumatol. Arthrosc.* **2013**, *21*, 2889–2894. [CrossRef]

13

Family Caregiver Strain and Challenges When Caring for Orthopedic Patients

Umile Giuseppe Longo [1,*], **Maria Matarese** [2], **Valeria Arcangeli** [2], **Viviana Alciati** [2], **Vincenzo Candela** [1], **Gabriella Facchinetti** [2], **Anna Marchetti** [2], **Maria Grazia De Marinis** [2] and **Vincenzo Denaro** [1]

[1]   Department of Orthopedic and Trauma Surgery, Campus Bio-Medico University, Via Alvaro del Portillo, 200, 00128 Trigoria, Rome, Italy; v.candela@unicampus.it (V.C.); denaro@unicampus.it (V.D.)

[2]   Research Unit Nursing Science, Campus Bio-Medico di Roma University, 00128 Rome, Italy; m.matarese@unicampus.it (M.M.); arcangeli.valeria@libero.it (V.A.); vivianaalciati@gmail.com (V.A.); g.facchinetti@unicampus.it (G.F.); a.marchetti@unicampus.it (A.M.); m.demarinis@unicampus.it (M.G.D.M.)

*   Correspondence: g.longo@unicampus.it

Abstract: Background: Caregivers represent the core of patients' care in hospital structures, in the process of care and self-care after discharge. We aim to identify the factors that affect the strain of caring for orthopedic patients and how these factors are related to the quality of life of caregivers. We also want to evaluate the role of caregivers in orthopedic disease, focusing attention on the patient–caregiver dyad. Methods: A comprehensive search on PubMed, Cochrane, CINAHL and Embase databases was conducted. This review was reported following PRISMA statement guidance. Studies were selected, according to inclusion and exclusion criteria, about patient–caregiver dyads. For quality assessment, we used the MINORS and the Cochrane Risk of BIAS assessment tool. Results: 28 studies were included in the systematic review; in these studies, 3034 dyads were analyzed. Caregivers were not always able to bear the difficulties of care. An improvement in strain was observed after behavioral interventions from health-care team members; Conclusions: The role of the caregiver can lead to a deterioration of physical, cognitive and mental conditions. The use of behavioral interventions increased quality of life, reducing the strain in caregivers of orthopedic patients. For this reason, it is important to consider the impact that orthopedic disease has on the strain of the caregiver and to address this topic.

Keywords: caregiver; orthopedic disease; caregiver strain; hip; knee; shoulder; caregiver stress; dyads

1. Introduction

Orthopedic surgery is one of the most commonly performed surgeries worldwide [1,2]. Patients undergoing orthopedic surgery can experience difficulties in the management of post-surgical symptoms and physical limitations [3]. Orthopedic patients may experience barriers such as difficulties with Activities of Daily Living (ADL) [4,5], and problems returning to post-surgical lives. For these reasons, the role of the caregiver is of paramount importance in supporting dependent people both in simple and complex activities [6]. Although they are often family members without formal training, they take part in the activities of daily care, offering emotional support to the patients and replacing, in whole or in part, the physically dependent patients in the ADLs. Additionally, they monitor the patient's care pathway, managing the symptoms and taking on the family responsibilities previously managed by the patients [7]. All these factors contribute to increasing the caregivers' workload and they could affect caregivers' quality of life, both pre to post the patients' orthopedic surgeries [8]. The poor physical conditions of patients are associated with a decrease in the quality of life of the caregiver and an increase in stressors, due to all the caregivers' responsibilities; the caregiver can also present physical problems due to the effort involved in helping the patient to move. It is therefore important to enhance the caregiver's safety to improve his/her physical condition [9]. Caregiving is emotionally and cognitively demanding, and literature indicates that caregivers' overall health is adversely altered [10].

The term "dyad" refers to the relationship between patient and caregiver, who are involved physically and emotionally. The dyad is an important foundation for problem identification and problem-solving included in the orthopedic patient process, from the pre-operative period to the post-operative period. Humor, reassurance, and empathy are also important factors in this dyad relationship. There is a need to enhance patient–caregiver dyad research, by studying the relationship from pre-operative to follow-up to evaluate the changes in the patient's outcomes, but also in the caregiver's psychological and cognitive sphere. There is a need to identify the type of supportive relationship that is established with informal caregivers to offer them an appropriate educational plan. Furthermore, it is necessary to evaluate if the degree of instruction received during the hospitalization period and the knowledge of informal caregivers about the disease, is sufficient for them to be able to face a functional recovery process in the postoperative period in order to maintain the role of caregiver after patients' surgery [11].

The present systematic review aims to identify, analyze and synthesize the studies on the role of informal caregivers' strain and difficulties when caring for orthopedic patients, focusing attention on the patient–caregiver dyad, during the pre-operative to post-operative period.

2. Materials and Methods

A literature review was performed and reported following PRISMA statement guidance [12]. Preliminary searches of main databases could not find any existing or ongoing systematic reviews on caregiver strain or difficulties of caring for orthopedic patients.

2.1. Eligibility Criteria and Search Strategy

Key words and combinations of key words were used to search the electronic databases and were organized according to the Population Intervention Comparison Outcome (PICO) model as follows.

Study: original studies with different study designs; English language; recent studies (from 2003 to 2020).

Participants: patient–caregiver dyads, orthopedic patients and informal caregivers.

Interventions: educational interventions, home-care rehabilitations, emotional and social supports.

Outcome measures: The primary outcome of the review is the caregivers' role in the orthopedic patients' functional recovery, the caregivers' knowledge to manage orthopedic disease symptoms, the caregivers' strain, and the dyads' quality of life; the secondary outcome is the impact that orthopedic disorders have on quality of life, on stress level and on the psychological and physical status of patients.

A comprehensive search of the databases PubMed, Medline, Cochrane, CINAHL, and Embase databases was conducted since the inception of the database to March 2020 with the English language constraint. To ensure a comprehensive search, facet analysis, necessary to identify the key terms to be used in the search strategy, was carried out. Keywords were combined using the Boolean operators "AND" and "OR". The search strategy was iterative and flexible within the limits of the search engines of the individual databases.

The following medical subject heading (MeSH) keywords and free terms were used for the search: caregiver, spouse, orthopedic disease, orthopedic, caregiver burden, hip, knee, shoulder, elbow, wrist, hand, humerus, femur, patella, spine, ankle, foot, caregiver stress, patient–caregiver dyads. Search strategies were checked by two reviewers (VC and GF). The exclusion criteria included: formal caregivers, reviews, books, patients and caregivers without a relation. Further details about search strategies are in Appendix A.

2.2. Study Selection and Data Collection

Two researchers (VAr and VAl) independently reviewed all studies (title, abstract and full text) that met the inclusion criteria and extracted relevant data. Disagreements were resolved by a discussion among the reviewers.

We included observational studies, prospective studies, cohort studies, mixed studies, pre–post quasi-experimental designs, randomized controlled trials, descriptive cross-sectional studies, prospective longitudinal cohort studies, non-randomized trials, qualitatively focused ethnographic approaches and retrospective analyses. The studies included articles published from 2003 to 2020. Disagreement regarding the exclusion and inclusion criteria were decided by the senior reviewer (VD).

2.3. Quality Assessment

Two reviewers independently evaluated (VAr/VAl) the potential risk of bias of the studies included using MINORS [13], a methodological index for non-randomized studies, and the Cochrane Risk of Bias Tool [14] for randomized controlled trials.

The MINORS items were scored as 0 if not reported, 1 when reported but inadequate, 2 when reported and adequate. The global ideal score was 16 for non-comparative studies and 24 for comparative studies.

The Cochrane Risk of Bias Tool assessed randomized controlled trials with the following criteria: selection, performance, detection, attrition, reporting and other biases. Each criterion was evaluated assigning zero for low risk, one point for unclear risk, and two points for high risk of bias. The potential total score range was 0–14, in which a low score indicated a higher quality level, and a high score indicated lower quality. Based on this score, an overall score of 0–1 shows high quality, an overall score of 2–3 shows moderate quality, and an overall score of >3 shows low quality [15].

2.4. Data Synthesis and Analysis

Data were extracted and synthesized through Microsoft Excel. Several data were extracted, and they concern outcome measures; authors and year; study design; orthopedic disease; aim of each study follow-up period; the relationship between patient and caregiver; number of patients and caregivers for each study; data findings; and study conclusion.

Data analysis was done using the description of the study and patient and intervention characteristics. Categorical variable data were reported as percentage frequencies. Continuous variable data were reported as mean values, with the range between the minimum and maximum values.

3. Results

The selection process is illustrated in Figure 1. The search strategy yielded 61 articles. After duplicate removal and title, abstract and full texts review, 28 studies were evaluated for methodological quality and were eligible for the review.

3.1. Study and Patient Characteristics

A total of 3034 patients–caregiver dyads were reviewed (Table 1).

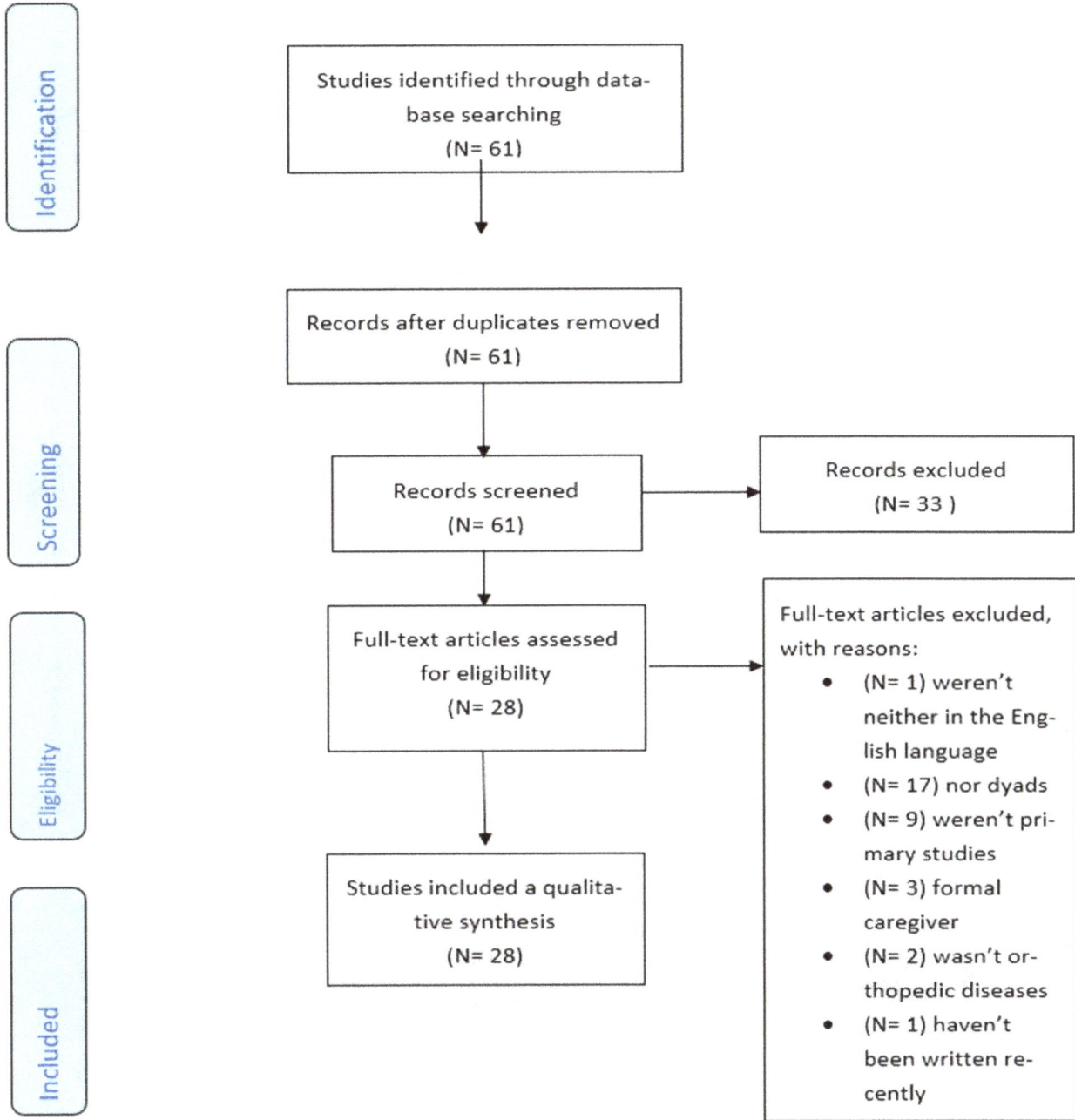

Figure 1. Study selection process and screening according to the PRISMA flow chart [12].

According to the aim of the review, the studies included analyzed the patient–caregiver dyad in the orthopedic disease context. It was found that the majority of the studies included (75%) analyzed dyad characteristics in hip disease (hip fracture, hip arthroplasty, hip deformity). To a lesser extent, 11% of the studies considered patients affected by knee orthopedic disease (knee fracture, knee arthroplasty, patella fracture) and 14.3% with backbone conditions (spinal arthrodesis, scoliosis, spine deformity, and cord injury) (Table 2).

Table 1. Characteristics of included studies: author and country; number of patients; number of caregivers; outcome measures; follow-up; data findings; conclusion; relationship with the patients.

Author and Country; Number of Patients; Number of Caregivers	Outcomes Measures *; Follow-up	Outcome Measures *; Follow-up	Relationship with the Patients
Shen, 2015, China [13]; 492; 539.	FES-I ($p < 0.001$); FRS ($p < 0.001$); VAS 24 months	75.4% of family caregiver and 70.7% of patients showed FOF; Regular follow-up examinations showed a lower family caregiver FES-I score and a higher patient FRS.	321 spouses (59.5%), 171 (31.7%) offsprings
Patrocinio Ariza-Vega, 2019, Spain [14]; 172; 172.	CSI ($p < 0.001$); 1 year	High level of caregiver difficulties at the hospital, at 1 and 3 months, and at 1 year after surgery; Support and training as strategies of treatment to reduce caregivers' difficulties.	Partner/spouse 39 (23%), son 15 (8%), daughter 94 (55%), others 24 (14%)
Margaret J. Bull, 2017, US [7]; 39; 39.	CAM (Sensitivity of 94–100%, Specificity of 90–95%) FAM-CAM (Sensitivity of 92.4%); Specificity of 87.5, 3 weeks pre-surgery; 2-weeks and 2 months post-hospitalization. Caregivers: 2-days post-surgery	The caregiver rating is high on the FAM-CAM 2 days after surgery; Recognizing presence or absence of delirium symptoms by caregivers.	Spouse 24 (62%), daughter 8 (21%), others 7 (17%)
Maria Crotty, 2003, Australia [15]; 32; 66.	MBI ($p = 0.738$); TUG ($p = 0.001$) Medical Outcomes; SF-36 ($p = 0.689$); CSI ($p = 0.140$); 4 months; 12 months	Caregiver difficulty reduction is achieved by home-based therapy and rehabilitation for patients; Functionally independent patients, return home earlier, with increased involvement of caregivers.	NS
Cuicui Li, 2018, China [16]; 87; 87.	ZBI (36.83 ± 13.30); GSE (21.67 ± 7.65); 0	Moderate or severe caregiver difficulties; Social support and self-efficacy might be helpful to reduce caregivers' difficulties.	Mothers 51 (58.6%), others 36 (41.4%)
Rachel L. Difazio, 2016, US [17]; 44; 44.	CP CHILD ($p < 0.001$); ACEND ($p = 0.26$); 1 year	Children's HRQOL improved over 12 months after spinal surgery; steady improvement over time after hip surgery, decrease at 6 weeks; Caregivers reported an improvement in HRQOL 1 year after orthopedic surgery.	NS
Mohammad Hossein Ebrahimzadeh, 2013, Iran [18]; 72; 72.	SF-36 ($p < 0.001$); 6 months	Wives worked full time at home. 88.9% of veterans had a paraplegic lesion; The SF-36 scores of the spouses were lower. The caregivers' challenges can impact the QOL of caregivers.	Spouse 72 (100%)
Jacobi Elliott, 2014, Canada [19]; 8; 11.	Questionnaire; 0	Facilitators and barriers included prior health care experience, trusting relationships, and the rural setting; Effective strategies to improve information sharing and care continuity may be involved.	Adult children 6 (54.5%), spouses 2 (18.1%)

Table 1. *Cont.*

Author and Country; Number of Patients; Number of Caregivers	Outcomes Measures; Follow-up	Outcome Measures *; Follow-up	Relationship with the Patients
Amit Jain, 2018, US [20]; 251; 251.	HRQOL ($p < 0.001$); 2 years post-surgery RNLI (33.3); CBI	HRQL: 74% of caregivers are a "lot better"; Caregiving in spinal surgery is ranked as the most beneficial intervention in the patients' lives. Caregiver burden is high at 18 and 24 months post-hip-fracture;	NS
Katherine S. McGilton, 2019, Canada [21]; 76; 76.	2 years post-hip fracture	There is a need for interventions for patients to enhance their RNLI and to support caregivers in decreasing their difficulties in caring.	Marital status, married or common-law partner 26 (34%)
Laura Churchill, 2018, GB [22]; 14; 14.	Questionaire; 6 months Questionnaire;	Concerns and challenges are mobility, pain, self-care and caregiver support; Outpatient THA can be implemented with pre-operative education, clarification of recovery processes and expectations. More details are needed from care providers to self-manage symptoms.	NS
Odom-Forren J, 2017, US [3]; 9; 10.	2 weeks after surgery	Nurses should be focused on preparing patients to manage sustained recovery issues at home.	Spouses 7 (70%), parents 2 (20%)
Jung-Ah Lee, 2014, US [11]; 30; 30.	Questionaire; At hospitalization	Patients and caregivers take daily injections of heparin. Patients with hip fracture and their caregivers may need further VTE preventive education.	child or son/daughter-in-law 19 (63.4%), 3 (10%) spouses
Pi-Chu Lin, 2007, Taiwan [23]; 95; 95.	OMFAQ; SERS; FOS; FFRS; FRS; CBI; 1 week and 1 month after discharge	1 week after hospital discharge the patients' physical functioning, self-efficacy, and social support contributed to variance in caregivers' difficulties; A health education and social support program should be designed to improve the primary caregiver's knowledge and to reduce the burden of care.	Apouses 30 (31.6%), sons 20 (21.1%), 18 (18.9%) daughters, 17 daughters-in-law (17.9%), grandchildren 7 (7.4%)
Hsin-Yun Liu, 2015, Taiwan [24]; 276; 276.	CBI; CMMSE; PS; MICROFET2; MNA; SF-36; 1-3-6-12 months after discharge	MCS levels were lower (22.4%), moderate (34.1%) and highest (43.5%); Health care providers could consider family caregivers' mental well-being while estimating recovery times and health outcomes of patients.	Spouse 70 (25.3%), son 61 (22.1%), daughter 57 (20.6%), daughter-in-law 71 (25.7%), other 17 (6.1%)

Table 1. *Cont.*

Author and Country; Number of Patients; Number of Caregivers	Outcomes Measures; Follow-up	Outcome Measures *; Follow-up	Relationship with the Patients
Asha Manohar, 2014, US [25]; 44; 44.	Questionnaire; ADL; Post-operative days; 0-3-7-30	Many patients needed more time to resume their ADL. Primary caregivers' disturbances were emotional and physical; Informal caregiving may be an unrecognized physical and psychological burden and may have a significant societal impact.	NS
Mariana Ortiz-Piña, 2019, Spain [26]; 70; 70.	FIM; Euro-Qol/EQ-5D; TUG; CBZI; SPPB; ADS; 4 weeks and 12 weeks after discharge	70 patients with a high pre-fracture functional level were allocated into a telerehabilitation group; Telerehabilitation is an option to promote recovery of the pre-fracture functional level.	NS
Mashfiqul A Siddiqui, 2010, Singapore [27]; 76; 76	CSI; 6 months	To 1 week of admission, and at 6 months, the caregivers were stressed. The stress factor was a financial strain. Adequate resources should be available to caregivers of patients with osteoporotic hip fractures.	NS
Benedict U. Nwachukwu, 2019, NS [28]; 95; 95.	UCLA Activity Score; HRQoL; Rehabilitation; 2 years post-surgery	Active adolescents assigned higher utility to achieve a stable return to the same function and lower utility to health states in which they were not fully participating in sport; These findings provide insight into the health-related quality of life impact for acute patella dislocations and their management.	NS
Joshua A. Parry, 2019, NS [29]; 29; 29.	CBI; DS; 6 months	Caregivers have negative effects on their finances, relationships, work hours, or intent to place the patient in a care facility. Caregivers with high caregiver burdens were more likely to consider the placement of the patient into a long-term care facility.	NS
Sara Elli, 2018, Italy [30]; 147; 147.	BRASS; At the beginning of the rehabilitation program	The caregivers assign lower scores than the doctor; Caregivers' altered perceptions can lead to a general lack of satisfaction with the outcome at the end of the rehabilitation process.	NS
Yea-Ing Lotus Shyu, 2012, Taiwan [31]; 135; 151.	PRS; MOS; SF-36; CBI; 1-3-6-12 months after discharge	Caregivers' mental health was lower at 12 and 1 month after discharge; The home care nurses should develop interventions early after discharge.	1/3 sons (32.66%), daughters-in-law (26.7%), spouses (20%), daughters (14.1%).

Table 1. *Cont.*

Author and Country; Number of Patients; Number of Caregivers	Outcomes Measures; Follow-up	Outcome Measures *; Follow-up	Relationship with the Patients
Åsa Johansson Stark, 2016, Finland [32]; 306; 306.	During recovery	If nurses gave information to partners, they experienced a greater quality of recovery; Spouses' emotional state is important in the patients' quality of recovery.	Spouses 306 (100%).
Justine Toscan, 2012, Canada [33]; 6; 6.	Questionnaire; During transition care	Four factors related to illness were confusion, unclear roles and responsibilities, diluted personal ownership over care, and role strain; Supports the notion of collaborative practice and includes an appropriate, informed role for patients and informal caregivers.	Children 5 (99%)
Cornelis L. P. van de Ree, 2017, Netherland [34]; 123; 123.	CarerQoL; 7D score; 1-3-6 months	The average amount of informal care provided per patient per week was 39.5 during the first six months; The Carer QoL was not associated with the intensity of the provided informal care.	Partners (44.7%), child (43.1%), sibling (5.7%), others (6.5%)
Li-Chu Wu, 2013, Taiwan [35]; 116; 116.	Questionnaire; 1 month after discharge	Impairments in physical functions were standing up/sitting down and dressing. The care needs were wound care, medical visits, cleaning, maintaining living; The physical function status was improved 1 week and after 1 month after discharge. The care needs and the difficulty of tasks for caregivers were negatively related to physical functional status.	Daughters or Sons (54.3%), Spouses (34.5%), Foreign workers (11.0%).
Jayson D. Zadzilka, 2018, US [36]; 150; 150.	CSI; KOOS; 4 weeks and 1 year after surgery	CSI scores at 1 year were lower; The caregivers' difficulties were high in the early post-operative period. It was close to zero by one year post-operation.	NS

ACEND: Assessment of Caregiver Experience with Neuromuscular Disease; BRASS: Blaylock Risk Assessment Screening Score; BSS: Bakas Satisfaction Scale; Carer QoL 7D Score: Carer Quality of Life 7D Score; CAM: Confusion Assessment Method; CBI: Chinese Barthel Index; CBS: Caregiver Burden Rating Scale; CBZI: Caregiver Burden Zarit Intervention; CMMSE: Chinese Mini Mental Status Examination; CP CHILD: Cerebral Plasty Child; CSI: Caregiver Strain Index; DS: Depression Scale; EQoL-5D: Euro Quality of Life 5D; FAM-CAM: Family Confusion Assessment Method; FES-I: Falls Efficacy Scale-International; FFRS: Family Function Rating Scale; FIM: Functional Independence Measure; FOS: Filial Obligation Scale; GSE: General Self-Efficacy Scale; HADS: The Hospital Anxiety and Depression Scale; HRQoL: Health Related Quality of Life; HSS-Pedi-FABS: Hospital for Special Surgery Pediatric Functional Activity Brief Scale; IFS: International Fitness Scale; IADL: Instrumental Activities of Dayly Living; KEso: Knowledge Expectations of Significant Other; KOOS: Knee Injury and Osteoarthritis Outcome Score; MBI: Maslach Burnout Inventory; MCI: Mild Cognitive Impairment; MICRO FET2: Micro Force Evaluation Testing 2; MNA: Mini Nutritional Assesment; MOS: Medical Outcome Study; MOS SF-36: Medical Outcome Study Short Form-36; OMFAQ: Multidimensional Functional Assessment Questionnaire; PRS: Performance Related Scale; PS: Pain Scale; QoL: Quality of Life; RKso: Received Knowledge of Significant Other; RNLI: Reintegration to Normal Living Index; SERS: Self Efficacy Rating Scale; SFES-I: Short Falls Efficacy Scale-International; SF-36: Short Form 36; SPPB: Short Physical Performance Battery; TUG: Timed Up and Go Test; UCLA: University of California, Los Angeles Loneliness Scale; VAS: Visual Analog Scale; VTE: Venous Thromboembolism; ZBI: Zarit Burden Interview.

Table 2. Characteristics of orthopedic diseases in included studies.

JOINTS		TOT *	%
Hip	Hip fracture	19	
	Hip arthroplasty	1	21	75%
	Hip deformity	1		
Backbone	Spinal arthrodesis	1		
	Scoliosis	1	4	14.3%
	Spine deformity	1		
	Cord injury	1		
Knee	Knee fracture	1		
	Knee artrhroplasty	1	3	10.7%
	Patella fracture	1		

* TOT: Total.

The topics of the studies included in the systematic review make it possible to evaluate the caregiver's role in the orthopedic patients' functional recovery, dealing with knowledge to manage symptoms and orthopedic disease in 8 studies, caregiver strain in 15 studies and dyads' quality of life in 5 studies.

In the studies evaluating the quality of life of the dyad, 7.14% of the studies affirmed that the patient's quality of life was improved due to the assistance provided by the informal caregiver. Despite the improvement in patients' quality of life, their quality of functional recovery does not improve, and the 14.2% of studies state that it is influenced by caregivers' psychological factors.

Regarding the caregivers' quality of life, 7.14% of the studies say the decrease in caregivers' quality of life is related to the increasing intensity of care and caregiver strain [14].

The studies analyzing caregiver strain report that the factors affecting caregiver difficulties are increased recovery time (21.4%), complication and symptom management (14.2%), financial resources (10.7%), functional level reduction (10.7%), bad healthcare experiences (7%), any trusting relationships (7%), patients' and caregivers' age (7%), poor social support (7%), poor self-efficacy (7%), transport (3.5%), and rural environment (3.5%). Two studies identified a significant correlation between caregiver strain and caregiver characteristics such as age [16,17] and gender [17].

The studies included in the review used some different follow-up periods: the pre-operative period (12.5%) and 2 weeks (4.6%), 1 month (18.2%), 3 months (20.4%), 6 months (23.3%), and 1 year (21%) after surgery. The follow-up period analysis was useful for analyzing the caregivers' strain duration. In studies that analyzed the duration of caregiver strain, fourteen percent of studies reported that caregiver strain lasted for one year, 10.7% for six months, 7.1% for one month and 3.5% for two years.

Regarding the studies that analyzed knowledge to manage symptoms, they reported that pre-operative education was fundamental to improve the management of symptoms. Pre-operative education and postoperative social support reduced caregiver strain in 46.5% of studies.

To understand the relationship between the informal caregivers and the patients that form the dyads, studies reported that the major of informal caregivers were patients' relatives. The most common relationships between the primary caregiver and the care recipient in this review included spouses (22.1%), daughters (8.7%), sons (6.7%), daughters-in-law (5.2%), and others, including partners, mothers, grandchildren and siblings (9.2%) (Table 3).

Table 3. Caregivers' demographic characteristics (relationship with patients).

Relationship with Patients	N	%
SPOUSE	726	23.9%
CHILDREN (DAUGHTERS AND SONS)	468	15.4%
OTHERS	162	5.3%
DAUGHTER IN LAW	160	5.2%
MOTHERS	51	1.7%
GRANDCHILDREN	25	0.8%
SIBLING	7	0.2%
TOTAL	1599	52.7%
N/A	**1435**	**47.2%**

3.2. Intervention Characteristics

The most common outcome measures observed in original studies according with the aim of this review were Caregiver Strain Index (CSI), utilized in 32% of the studies recruited [18–25]; Zarit Burden Interview (ZBI), in 7.14% [26,27]; Mini-Mental Test (M-MT) in 7.14% [22,27]; and Health-Related Quality of Life score (HRQL) in 14.2% of the studies [27–30].

Participants' knowledge of the intervention and post-surgical management was tested via Knowledge Expectations of significant others (KEso) and Received Knowledge of significant others (RKso) [16]; confusion assessment method (CAM) and family version (FAM-CAM) [7] were used to measure empowering by knowledge.

Measures for general health status included the Short Form 36 Health Survey (SF-36) [18,22,31,32], the Functional Independence Measure Score (FIM) [27]; the Short Physical Performance Battery (SPPB) [27]; Time Up and Go Test (TUG) [18,19,27]; International Fitness Scale (FIS) [27]; The University of California, Los Angeles Activity Scale (UCLA) [29]; The Blaylock Risk Assessment Screening Score (BRASS) [37]; and the italics Self-Efficacy Scale (GSE) [21,26].

ADLs for patients and caregivers were assessed using the Barthel index [18,22,32]; the Reintegration to Normal Living Index (RNLI) [20]; and the Family Function Rating Scale [21]. The Visual Analogue Scale for Pain (VAS) [27,33] was the scale most often used to evaluate symptoms, as well as depression scales [24,27].

3.3. Quality Assessment

Most of studies included in this review (N = 27; 96.4%) were evaluated with MINORS. Of these, one study (3.57%) had low risk of bias and 26 (92.8%) had high risk of bias. The only RCT (Crotty, 2003) in this review had moderate quality due to insufficient details about the double-blinding procedure.

4. Discussion

This review aimed to synthesize the studies on the role of informal caregiver strain and difficulties when caring for orthopedic patients, focusing attention on the patient–caregiver dyad, from the pre-operative period to the post-operative period. Family caregivers are a relatively unused resource as a way to identify early symptoms and complications in orthopedic patients and to improve health outcomes for orthopedic patients. When pre-operative education is performed, family caregivers can apply their knowledge by acting on early recognition of symptoms [3,7].

Learning about diseases drives caregivers to satisfaction and to learn strategies to help patients, also with emotional support. Extensive efforts have been made to understand the strain felt by caregivers of patients with orthopedic disease. Orthopedic caregivers without enough information had less security in dealing with the patients' disease than those who received an appropriate education from health care team members: this is a finding that was consistent with the stress and coping model of caregiving [29].

Caregiving and poor quality of life can relate bidirectionally. In the dyad, concerns are about mobility, pain, self-care, support from the caregiver and discharge on the same day regarding recovery expectations, and drugs and their effect on postoperative recovery [34]. Orthopedic patients feel more pain and greater difficulties with physical activity; this leads to an increase in the caregiver's workload, and several studies underestimate this result [35]. The impact of the orthopedic disease on dyads is crucial for patients' outcomes and caregiver strain. The physical outcomes of patients and their functional recovery, and also the impact of caregiver assistance on care transition, have been studied more frequently [36].

In this context, the formal rehabilitation program has a key role in restoring patient autonomy and also involving the caregiver to reduce and improve rehabilitation times [38,39]. When the patients' formal post-surgery rehabilitation program is insufficient, the supply of a family caregiver is fundamental. For example, it could be necessary to improve the information and caregivers' education about the management of symptoms. A focus on the orthopedic patient and caregiver education regarding the clinical post-operative problems, potential risks involved, and patient and caregiver roles to improve the caring process is necessary.

In many of the studies recruited, caregiver strain is one of the main topics. The difficulty of assistance is often not recognized, and it can lead to mental and physical problems, but can also have a strong impact on social life [35]. Caregiver stress increases in the immediate postoperative period, while decreasing a lot after a year after surgery [25]. Especially in patients undergoing hip replacement, the caregiver strain is very high, which is why it is important to ease caregiver stress and increase the quality of care throughout the functional recovery period, including the periodic follow-up [24]. In most of the studies analyzed, the follow-up period of the dyad is approximately one year. This means that it cannot be said that the interventions implemented on the dyad provide long-term benefits and that the outcomes are valid.

Concerning the strain of care [30], we have found that caregivers showed disorders in the cognitive and physical spheres of their daily lives during the treatment period, from the pre-operative to post-operative period, leading to a reduction in their quality of life.

This review showed the importance of information and education before and after orthopedic surgery, to limit the functional restriction of patients by scared caregivers and to analyze its influence on functional recovery. The patient's functional level, quality of life, physical performance, pain, caregiver strain, and their the emotional and cognitive state should be evaluated, and perception of physical state should be assessed [40]. A study conducted in 2010 aimed to investigate the causes of stress attributed to the caregivers of patients with orthopedic disease [23]. The caregiver tension can result from changes in the patient's physical and cognitive states, and the sustained role during the patient's daily life activities. Several factors can contribute to caregiver stress, including financial strain, which is one of the most significant causes of caregiver stress. The financial problems arise from the need to incur medical expenses, rehabilitation, and transportation. This can be added to the physical and mental stress of the caregiver.

Post-operative recovery of patients was associated with the mental state of their family members. When a caregiver's mental state is "poor", the patient is more likely to relapse, which could lead a prolongation of recovery. Agreeing with this hypothesis, it is recommended to consider the mental well-being of the informal carers by evaluating patient recovery time [22].

The patient–caregiver dyad has also been studied in the traumatological and chronic fields. It has been well documented in hip injuries, while less attention is paid to other orthopedic conditions. Quantitatively, 19 studies deal with hip fractures, four studies deal with knee injuries, five studies with spine injuries, and two studies with general orthopedic pathologies. All revised studies refer to the caregiver strain and the amount of care for the patient with the orthopedic condition, which will reduce the quality of life of the caregiver due to the resulting growing stress. Many studies focus on patient outcomes related to care by a caregiver. The aim is to improve care but also to reduce the strain and stress factors attributable to this type of relationship established with the patient.

The present results should be interpreted in the context of the strengths and weaknesses of the studies composing the orthopedic caregiver. For example, most studies of orthopedic caregivers have used self-report questionnaires rather than assess the level of quality of life or have used rating scales that emphasize increasing caregiver strain.

Self-reported quality of life was greater than objective measures of quality of life, so it is possible that the actual caregivers' stress level was even worse than that estimated by the present systematic review. Repeating objective measures for all the caregivers would yield more accurate estimates of the real caregiver strain when caring for orthopedic patients.

Caregivers could be important to patients' healthcare, particularly according to the duration of caregiving, workload and stress level: these are also the factors that increase caregiver difficulties. Patients demonstrated the greatest increase in quality of recovery thanks to communication with their caregiver and thanks to the help they received from caregivers in maintaining social interaction. Besides, caregivers could improve orthopedic patients' life with behavioral interventions such as emotional comfort and support, both during pre-operative and post-operative periods.

Limitations

There were several limitations to this study. Further research is needed to examine how the intervention described would be successful with a larger sample. The study lacked a control group: future research is needed using a design that randomly assigns participants to intervention and control groups. Despite these limitations, the interventions were successful in increasing knowledge of caregivers' importance in orthopedic disease.

5. Conclusions

Despite the challenges in studying the role of caregivers in orthopedic diseases and family caregiver strain and challenges when caring for orthopedic patients, the literature indicates that not only the increase in caregivers' stress levels but also the decrease in quality of life was less severe in caregivers who received appropriate behavioral interventions including health care advice, such as medication advice or psychological tips. To improve the quality of health care, stressors should be considered for caregivers due to the high strain, especially in the post-discharge period.

Clinicians should consider the importance of caregiver interventions, not only for the orthopedic patient but also for the spouse, child, or friend who will be providing care for that individual. Further studies should focus on the important physical and mental role of the informal caregiver for patients who receive orthopedic surgery and the importance of psychological sphere for the patient–caregiver dyad. Focusing on caregivers' welfare rather than only on patient well-being could radically improve both caregivers' performance and patients' recovery.

Author Contributions: Conceptualization, M.M. and U.G.L.; methodology, V.A. (Valeria Arcangeli); software, V.A. (Viviana Alciati); validation, V.C., and M.M.; formal analysis, G.F.; investigation, A.M.; resources, M.G.D.M.; data curation, V.C.; writing—original draft preparation, writing—review and editing, A.M.; visualization, M.M.; supervision, V.D.; project administration, U.G.L. All authors have read and agreed to the published version of the manuscript.

Acknowledgments: This research did not receive any specific grant from funding agencies in the public, commercial, or not-for-profit sectors.

Appendix A. List of Search Terms Used for Systematic Review

Search terms for Medline Complete (via EBSCO Host): 1971 to 27 January 2019

1.   MH "Chronic Disease"
2.   chronic disease*
3.   chronic illness*
4.   chronically Ill
5.   1 or 2 or 3 or 4
6.   MH "Aged+"
7.   Aged
8.   Elderly
9.   older adults
10. 6 or 7 or 8 or 9
11. MH "Continuity of Patient Care+"
12. continuity of patient care
13. patient care continuity
14. continuum of care
15. continuity of care
16. care continuity
17. 11 or 12 or 13 or 14 or 15 or 16
18. MH "Patient Readmission"
19. re-admission*
20. readmission*
21. patient readmission*
22. hospital readmission*
23. post discharge*
24. postdischarge*
25. re-hospitalization
26. rehospitalization
27. re-admit*
28. 18 or 19 or 20 or 21 or 22 or 23 or 24 or 25 or 26 or 27
29. 5 and 10 and 17 and 28

269. records found

Search terms for PubMed: 1971 to 27 January 2019

1.   Chronic Disease [Mesh]
2.   chronic disease*
3.   chronic illness*
4.   chronically ill
5.   1 or 2 or 3 or 4
6.   Aged [Mesh]
7.   aged
8.   elderly
9.   older adult
10. 6 or 7 or 8 or 9
11. Continuity of Patient Care"[Mesh]
12. patient care continuity

13. continuum of care
14. care continuity
15. 11 or 12 or 13 or 14
16. Patient Readmission"[Mesh]
17. re-admission*
18. readmission*
19. patient readmission*
20. hospital readmission*
21. post discharge*
22. postdischarge*
23. re-hospitalization
24. rehospitalization
25. re-admit*
26. readmit*
27. 16 or 17 or 18 or 19 or 20 or 21 or 22 or 23 or 24 or 25 or 26
28. 5 and 10 and 15 and 27

233. records found

Search terms for CINHAL (via EBSCO Host): 1995 to 27 January 2019

1. MH "Chronic Disease"
2. chronic disease*
3. chronic illness*
4. chronically Ill
5. 1 or 2 or 3 or 4
6. MH "Aged"
7. aged
8. older adult*
9. 6 or 7 or 8 or 9
10. MH "Continuity of Patient Care"
11. patient care continuity
12. continuum of care
13. continuity of care
14. care continuity
15. 10 or 11 or 12 or 13 or 14
16. MH "Readmission"
17. re-admission*
18. readmission*
19. patient readmission*
20. hospital readmission*
21. post discharge*
22. postdischarge*
23. re-hospitalization
24. rehospitalization

25. re-admit*
26. readmit*
27. 16 or 17 or 18 or 19 or 20 or 21 or 22 or 23 or 24 or 25 or 26
28. 5 and 9 and 15 and 27

169. records found

Search terms for Embase: 1971 to 27 January 2019

1.   'chronic disease'/exp
2.   'chronic disease'
3.   'chronic illness'/exp
4.   'chronic illness'
5.   1 or 2 or 3 or 4
6.   AND 'aged'/exp
7.   'aged'
8.   'aged patient'/exp
9.   'aged patient'
10. 'aged people'/exp
11. 'aged people'
12. 'aged person'/exp
13. 'aged person'
14. 'aged subject'/exp
15. 'aged subject'
16. 'elderly'/exp
17. 'elderly'
18. 'elderly patient'/exp
19. 'elderly patient'
20. 'elderly people'/exp
21. 'elderly people'
22. 'elderly person'/exp
23. 'elderly person'
24. 'elderly subject'/exp
25. 'elderly subject'
26. 'senior citizen'/exp
27. 'senior citizen'
28. 'senium'/exp
29. 'senium'
30. 6 or 7 or 8 or 9 or 10 or 11 or 12 or 13 or 14 or 15 or 16 or 17 or 18 or 19 or 20 or 21 or 22 or 23 or 24 or 25 or 26 or 27 or 28 or 29
31. 'advance care planning'/exp
32. 'advance care planning'
33. 'care, continuity of'/exp
34. 'care, continuity of'
35. 'continuity of patient care'/exp
36. 'continuity of patient care'
37. 'episode of care'/exp

38. 'episode of care'
39. 'night care'/exp
40. 'night care'
41. 'patient care'/exp
42. 'patient care'
43. 'patient care management'/exp
44. 'patient care management'
45. 'patient care team'/exp
46. 'patient care team'
47. 'patient centered care'/exp
48. 'patient centered care'
49. 'patient helper'/exp
50. 'patient helper'
51. 'patient isolation'/exp
52. 'patient isolation'
53. 'patient management'/exp
54. 'patient management'
55. 'patient navigation'/exp
56. 'patient navigation'
57. 'patient-centered care'/exp
58. 'patient-centered care'
59. 'continuity of care'/exp
60. 'continuity of care'
61. 'continuum of care'
62. 'care continuity'
63. 30 or 31 or 32 or 33 or 34 or 35 or 36 or 37 or 38 or 39 or 40 or 41 or 42 or 43 or 44 or 45 or 46 or 47 or 48 or 49 or 50 or 51 or 52 or 53 or 54 or 55 or 56 or 57 or 58 or 59 or 60 or 61 or 62
64. 'hospital readmission'/exp
65. 'hospital readmission'
66. 'patient readmission'/exp
67. 'patient readmission'
68. 'readmission'/exp
69. 'readmission'
70. 'readmission rate'/exp
71. 'readmission rate'
72. 'readmissions'/exp
73. 'readmissions'
74. 'rehospitalization'/exp
75. 'rehospitalization'
76. 'post discharge'
77. 62 or 63 or 64 or 65 or 66 or 67 or 68 or 69 or 70 or 71 or 72 or 73 or 74
78. 5 and 29 and 61 and 75

135. records found

References

1.   Longo, U.G.; Salvatore, G.; Rizzello, G.; Berton, A.; Ciuffreda, M.; Candela, V.; Denaro, V. The burden of rotator cuff surgery in Italy: A nationwide registry study. *Arch. Orthop. Trauma Surg.* **2017**, *137*, 217–224. [CrossRef]

2.   Salvatore, G.; Longo, U.G.; Candela, V.; Berton, A.; Migliorini, F.; Petrillo, S.; Ambrogioni, L.R.; Denaro, V. Epidemiology of rotator cuff surgery in Italy: Regional variation in access to health care. Results from a 14-year nationwide registry. *Musculoskelet. Surg.* **2019**. [CrossRef]

3.   Odom-Forren, J.; Reed, D.B.; Rush, C. Postoperative Distress of Orthopedic Ambulatory Surgery Patients. *AORN J.* **2017**, *105*, 464–477. [CrossRef]

4.   Oliva, F.; Ronga, M.; Longo, U.G.; Testa, V.; Capasso, G.; Maffulli, N. The 3-in-1 procedure for recurrent dislocation of the patella in skeletally immature children and adolescents. *Am. J. Sports Med.* **2009**, *37*, 1814–1820. [CrossRef]

5.   Longo, U.G.; Loppini, M.; Romeo, G.; Maffulli, N.; Denaro, V. Evidence-based surgical management of spondylolisthesis: Reduction or arthrodesis in situ. *J. Bone Joint Surg. Am.* **2014**, *96*, 53–58. [CrossRef]

6.   Holzer, J.; Bradford, A. Caregivers of Orthopedic Trauma Patients: Perspectives on Participating in Caregiver-Related Research. *IRB* **2014**, *36*, 8–12.

7.   Bull, M.J.; Boaz, L.; Maadooliat, M.; Hagle, M.E.; Gettrust, L.; Greene, M.T.; Holmes, S.B.; Saczynski, J.S. Preparing Family Caregivers to Recognize Delirium Symptoms in Older Adults After Elective Hip or Knee Arthroplasty. *J. Am. Geriatr. Soc.* **2017**, *65*, e13–e17. [CrossRef] [PubMed]

8.   Malley, A.M.; Bourbonniere, M.; Naylor, M. A qualitative study of older adults' and family caregivers' perspectives regarding their preoperative care transitions. *J. Clin. Nurs.* **2018**, *27*, 2953–2962. [CrossRef] [PubMed]

9.   Lee, S.Y.; Kim, S.C.; Lee, M.H.; Lee, Y.I. Comparison of shoulder and back muscle activation in caregivers according to various handle heights. *J. Phys. Ther. Sci.* **2013**, *25*, 1231–1233. [CrossRef] [PubMed]

10. Pinquart, M.; Sorensen, S. Differences between caregivers and noncaregivers in psychological health and physical health: A meta-analysis. *Psychol. Aging* **2003**, *18*, 250–267. [CrossRef] [PubMed]

11. Lee, J.A.; Donaldson, J.; Drake, D.; Johnson, L.; van Servellen, G.; Reed, P.L.; Mulnard, R.A. Venous thromboembolism knowledge among older post-hip fracture patients and their caregivers. *Geriatr. Nurs.* **2014**, *35*, 374–380. [CrossRef] [PubMed]

12. Liberati, A.; Altman, D.G.; Tetzlaff, J.; Mulrow, C.; Gotzsche, P.C.; Ioannidis, J.P.; Clarke, M.; Devereaux, P.J.; Kleijnen, J.; Moher, D. The PRISMA statement for reporting systematic reviews and meta-analyses of studies that evaluate health care interventions: Explanation and elaboration. *PLoS Med.* **2009**, *6*, e1000100. [CrossRef] [PubMed]

13. Slim, K.; Nini, E.; Forestier, D.; Kwiatkowski, F.; Panis, Y.; Chipponi, J. Methodological index for non-randomized studies (minors): Development and validation of a new instrument. *ANZ J. Surg.* **2003**, *73*, 712–716. [CrossRef] [PubMed]

14. Higgins, J.P.; Altman, D.G.; Gøtzsche, P.C.; Jüni, P.; Moher, D.; Oxman, A.D.; Savovic, J.; Schulz, K.F.; Weeks, L.; Sterne, J.A.; et al. The Cochrane Collaboration's tool for assessing risk of bias in randomised trials. *BMJ* **2011**, *343*, d5928. [CrossRef] [PubMed]

15. Facchinetti, G.; D'Angelo, D.; Piredda, M.; Petitti, T.; Matarese, M.; Oliveti, A.; De Marinis, M.G. Continuity of care interventions for preventing hospital readmission of older people with chronic diseases: A meta-analysis. *Int. J. Nurs. Stud.* **2020**, *101*, 103396. [CrossRef] [PubMed]

16. Stark, A.J.; Salantera, S.; Sigurdardottir, A.K.; Valkeapaa, K.; Bachrach-Lindstrom, M. Spouse-related factors associated with quality of recovery of patients after hip or knee replacement—A Nordic perspective. *Int. J. Orthop. Trauma Nurs.* **2016**, *23*, 32–46. [CrossRef] [PubMed]

17. Wu, L.C.; Chou, M.Y.; Liang, C.K.; Lin, Y.T.; Ku, Y.C.; Wang, R.H. Association of home care needs and functional recovery among community-dwelling elderly hip fracture patients. *Arch. Gerontol. Geriatr.* **2013**, *57*, 383–388. [CrossRef]

18. Crotty, M.; Whitehead, C.; Miller, M.; Gray, S. Patient and caregiver outcomes 12 months after home-based therapy for hip fracture: A randomized controlled trial. *Arch. Phys. Med. Rehabil.* **2003**, *84*, 1237–1239. [CrossRef]

19. Ariza-Vega, P.; Ortiz-Pina, M.; Kristensen, M.T.; Castellote-Caballero, Y.; Jimenez-Moleon, J.J. High perceived caregiver burden for relatives of patients following hip fracture surgery. *Disabil. Rehabil.* **2019**, *41*, 311–318. [CrossRef]

20. McGilton, K.S.; Omar, A.; Stewart, S.S.; Chu, C.H.; Blodgett, M.B.; Bethell, J.; Davis, A.M. Factors That Influence the Reintegration to Normal Living for Older Adults 2 Years Post Hip Fracture. *J. Appl. Gerontol.* **2019**, 733464819885718. [CrossRef]

21. Lin, P.C.; Lu, C.M. Psychosocial factors affecting hip fracture elder's burden of care in Taiwan. *Orthop. Nurs.* **2007**, *26*, 155–161. [CrossRef] [PubMed]

22. Liu, H.Y.; Yang, C.T.; Cheng, H.S.; Wu, C.C.; Chen, C.Y.; Shyu, Y.I. Family caregivers' mental health is associated with postoperative recovery of elderly patients with hip fracture: A sample in Taiwan. *J. Psychosom. Res.* **2015**, *78*, 452–458. [CrossRef] [PubMed]

23. Siddiqui, M.Q.; Sim, L.; Koh, J.; Fook-Chong, S.; Tan, C.; Howe, T.S. Stress levels amongst caregivers of patients with osteoporotic hip fractures—A prospective cohort study. *Ann. Acad. Med. Singap.* **2010**, *39*, 38–42. [PubMed]

24. Parry, J.A.; Langford, J.R.; Koval, K.J. Caregivers of hip fracture patients: The forgotten victims? *Injury* **2019**, *50*, 2259–2262. [CrossRef] [PubMed]

25. Zadzilka, J.D.; Klika, A.K.; Calvo, C.; Suarez, J.C.; Patel, P.D.; Krebs, V.E.; Barsoum, W.K.; Higuera, C.A. Caregiver Burden for Patients With Severe Osteoarthritis Significantly Decreases by One Year After Total Knee Arthroplasty. *J. Arthroplast.* **2018**, *33*, 3660–3665. [CrossRef] [PubMed]

26. Li, C.; Miao, J.; Gao, X.; Zheng, L.; Su, X.; Hui, H.; Hu, J. Factors Associated with Caregiver Burden in Primary Caregivers of Patients with Adolescent Scoliosis: A Descriptive Cross-Sectional Study. *Med. Sci. Monit.* **2018**, *24*, 6472–6479. [CrossRef]

27. Ortiz-Pina, M.; Salas-Farina, Z.; Mora-Traverso, M.; Martin-Martin, L.; Galiano-Castillo, N.; Garcia-Montes, I.; Cantarero-Villanueva, I.; Fernandez-Lao, C.; Arroyo-Morales, M.; Mesa-Ruiz, A.; et al. A home-based tele-rehabilitation protocol for patients with hip fracture called @ctivehip. *Res. Nurs. Health* **2019**, *42*, 29–38. [CrossRef]

28. Jain, A.; Sullivan, B.T.; Shah, S.A.; Samdani, A.F.; Yaszay, B.; Marks, M.C.; Sponseller, P.D. Caregiver Perceptions and Health-Related Quality-of-Life Changes in Cerebral Palsy Patients After Spinal Arthrodesis. *Spine (Phila Pa 1976)* **2018**, *43*, 1052–1056. [CrossRef]

29. Nwachukwu, B.U.; So, C.; Zhang, Y.; Shubin-Stein, B.E.; Strickland, S.M.; Green, D.W.; Dodwell, E.R. Adolescent and Caregiver-derived Utilities for Traumatic Patella Dislocation Health States. *J. Pediatr. Orthop.* **2019**, *39*, e755–e760. [CrossRef]

30. Van de Ree, C.L.P.; Ploegsma, K.; Kanters, T.A.; Roukema, J.A.; De Jongh, M.A.C.; Gosens, T. Care-related Quality of Life of informal caregivers of the elderly after a hip fracture. *J. Patient Rep. Outcomes* **2017**, *2*, 23. [CrossRef]

31. Ebrahimzadeh, M.H.; Shojaei, B.S.; Golhasani-Keshtan, F.; Soltani-Moghaddas, S.H.; Fattahi, A.S.; Mazloumi, S.M. Quality of life and the related factors in spouses of veterans with chronic spinal cord injury. *Health Qual. Life Outcomes* **2013**, *11*, 48. [CrossRef] [PubMed]

32. Shyu, Y.I.; Chen, M.C.; Liang, J.; Tseng, M.Y. Trends in health outcomes for family caregivers of hip-fractured elders during the first 12 months after discharge. *J. Adv. Nurs.* **2012**, *68*, 658–666. [CrossRef] [PubMed]

33. Shen, J.; Hu, F.; Liu, F.; Tong, P. Functional Restriction for the Fear of Falling in Family Caregivers. *Medicine (Baltimore)* **2015**, *94*, e1090. [CrossRef] [PubMed]

34. Churchill, L.; Pollock, M.; Lebedeva, Y.; Pasic, N.; Bryant, D.; Howard, J.; Lanting, B.; Laliberte Rudman, D. Optimizing outpatient total hip arthroplasty: Perspectives of key stakeholders. *Can. J. Surg.* **2018**, *61*, 370–376. [CrossRef]

35. Manohar, A.; Cheung, K.; Wu, C.L.; Stierer, T.S. Burden incurred by patients and their caregivers after outpatient surgery: A prospective observational study. *Clin. Orthop. Relat. Res.* **2014**, *472*, 1416–1426. [CrossRef]

36. Toscan, J.; Mairs, K.; Hinton, S.; Stolee, P.; InfoRehab Research, T. Integrated transitional care: Patient, informal caregiver and health care provider perspectives on care transitions for older persons with hip fracture. *Int. J. Integr. Care* **2012**, *12*, e13. [CrossRef]

37. Elli, S.; Contro, D.; Castaldi, S.; Fornili, M.; Ardoino, I.; Caserta, A.V.; Panella, L. Caregivers' misperception of the severity of hip fractures. *Patient Prefer. Adherence* **2018**, *12*, 1889–1895. [CrossRef]

38. Lima, C.A.; Sherrington, C.; Guaraldo, A.; Moraes, S.A.; Varanda, R.D.; Melo, J.A.; Kojima, K.E.; Perracini, M. Effectiveness of a physical exercise intervention program in improving functional mobility in older adults after hip fracture in later stage rehabilitation: Protocol of a randomized clinical trial (REATIVE Study). *BMC Geriatr.* **2016**, *16*, 198. [CrossRef]

39. Longo, U.G.; Facchinetti, G.; Marchetti, A.; Candela, V.; Risi Ambrogioni, L.; Faldetta, A.; De Marinis, M.G.; Denaro, V. Sleep Disturbance and Rotator Cuff Tears: A Systematic Review. *Medicina (Kaunas)* **2019**, *55*, 453. [CrossRef]

40. Longo, U.G.; Risi Ambrogioni, L.; Berton, A.; Candela, V.; Carnevale, A.; Schena, E.; Gugliemelli, E.; Denaro, V. Physical therapy and precision rehabilitation in shoulder rotator cuff disease. *Int. Orthop.* **2020**. [CrossRef]

14

Physical Activity for the Treatment of Chronic Low Back Pain in Elderly Patients

Gianluca Vadalà, Fabrizio Russo *, Sergio De Salvatore, Gabriele Cortina, Erika Albo, Rocco Papalia and Vincenzo Denaro

Department of Orthopaedic and Trauma Surgery, University Campus Bio-Medico of Rome, 00128 Rome, Italy; g.vadala@unicampus.it (G.V.); s.desalvatore@unicampus.it (S.D.S.); g.cortina@unicampus.it (G.C.); e.albo@unicampus.it (E.A.); r.papalia@unicampus.it (R.P.); denaro@unicampus.it (V.D.)
* Correspondence: fabrizio.russo@unicampus.it

Abstract: Chronic low back pain (CLBP) affects nearly 20–25% of the population older than 65 years, and it is currently the main cause of disability both in the developed and developing countries. It is crucial to reach an optimal management of this condition in older patients to improve their quality of life. This review evaluates the effectiveness of physical activity (PA) to improve disability and pain in older people with non-specific CLBP. The Preferred Reporting Items for Systematic reviews and Meta-Analyses (PRISMA) guidelines were used to improve the reporting of the review. Individual risk of bias of single studies was assessed using Rob 2 tool and ROBINS-I tool. The quality of evidence assessment was performed using GRADE analysis only in articles that presents full data. The articles were searched in different web portals (Medline, Scopus, CINAHL, EMBASE, and CENTRAL). All the articles reported respect the following inclusion criteria: patients > 65 years old who underwent physical activities for the treatment of CLBP. A total of 12 studies were included: 7 randomized controlled trials (RCT), 3 non-randomized controlled trials (NRCT), 1 pre and post intervention study (PPIS), and 1 case series (CS). The studies showed high heterogeneity in terms of study design, interventions, and outcome variables. In general, post-treatment data showed a trend in the improvement for disability and pain. However, considering the low quality of evidence of the studies, the high risk of bias, the languages limitations, the lack of significant results of some studies, and the lack of literature on this argument, further studies are necessary to improve the evidences on the topic.

Keywords: chronic low back pain; elderly; old aged patients; physical therapy; physical activity; walking; global postural rehabilitation; cycling; hydrotherapy; yoga

1. Introduction

Low back pain (LBP) is a common symptom that can improve spontaneously within a few weeks. However, about 2–7% [1] of cases may evolve into chronic low back pain (CLBP) that may lead to significant disability. Age is a well-known risk factor for CLBP in association to [2,3], psychological distress, inactivity, social environment, comorbidity, gender, genetic, and prior work exposure. CLBP affects approximately 20–25% of the elderly population (older than 65 years) [4], and it currently is the main cause of disability both in the developing and developed countries [5,6]. It increases linearly from the third decade of life affecting more women than men [7]. After a single episode of LBP, there is a higher risk to become recurrent [8]. CLBP, that is one of the most important conditions that leads to work-related disability, has dramatic consequences on the costs for the health system [9]. It is defined by the location of pain between the lower rib margins and the buttock that lasts for more than 12 weeks [10,11] and it can be often accompanied by neurological symptoms in the lower limbs (i.e., sciatica). Causes of CLBP can be distinguished into specific (degenerative process to the spinal segments of the lumbar spine such as lumbar spinal stenosis, spondylolisthesis, or disc herniation) [12] or non-specific, apparently when there is no underlying source of pain [13]. Among patients affected by LBP in primary care, patients affected by CLBP represent the greatest part (over 85%) [14]. CLBP in older adults has multifactorial causes, including both biological (insufficient muscle function around the spine [15]), and psychosocial factors [16] and, especially in the older adults it can lead to a severe reduction of independence and performance of normal daily activities [17].

Thus, it is crucial to reach an optimal management of this condition in older patients in order to improve their quality of life. However, limited evidence is available about the effectiveness of commonly recommended treatments for the older patient with CLBP. Paeck et al. showed that only a few clinical trials published in the literature were focused on older people. In fact, most studies include people younger than 65 years [18]. However, not all treatment options normally indicated for young people can also be pursued in the elderly population, since there may be other comorbidities, such as osteoporosis, that can limit their applicability.

Clinical practice guidelines for CLBP recommend physical activity (PA) as one of the most used interventions based on its biological rationale [19] and since it is easily applicable and low cost [20–22]. PA improves functions, mobility, quality of life, and some psychological distress that can be often found in older adults. Moreover, PA can improve social and work participation, coping strategies, and reduces fear-related beliefs regarding CLBP [23]. In the same way, physical inactivity is significantly correlated with the worsening of several chronic conditions including type 2 diabetes mellitus, congestive heart failure, and cognitive disorders such as depression and neurodegenerative diseases [24]. Therefore, PA can be useful and have positive effects on older patients with CLBP and other chronic conditions [25].

In the current review, PA is defined as a supervised activity program including general physical fitness programs, total body cardiovascular exercises, back schools, and specific techniques aimed at increasing single muscle strength or stretching such as Pilates, McKenzie, Feldenkrais, Tai Chi, or aquatic physiotherapy/hydrotherapy. The aim of this systematic review is to evaluate the effectiveness of PA in improving disability and pain in elderly patients with non-specific CLBP, comparing the results with groups of patients treated through manual therapy and other therapies that include non-physical intervention (advice to keep active) and untreated groups.

2. Materials and Methods

We focused our research on studies concerning PA as a treatment for CLBP in elderly patients. The Preferred Reporting Items for Systematic reviews and Meta-Analyses (PRISMA) guidelines were used to improve the reporting of the review. The Grading of Recommendations Assessment Development and Evaluation (GRADE) [26] approach was used to assess the quality of evidence of the articles that include full data.

2.1. Eligibility Criteria

2.1.1. Study Inclusion Criteria

- Peer-reviewed studies of each level of evidence according to Oxford Classification. We included randomized clinical trials (RCT) and non-randomized controlled studies (NRCT) designs such as observational studies (OS), pre-post interventional studies (PPIS), and case-series studies (CS). We excluded case reports, technical notes, letters to editors, instructional courses, in vitro studies, cadaver investigation, systematic reviews, and meta-analyses.
- Studies including elderly patients (mean age > 65 years) suffering by CLBP (at least > 3 months).

- Clinical outcomes (disability and pain) of patients treated with PA (cardiovascular or aerobic) or exercise programs that included loaded (against gravity or resistance) as a component. To define a study as eligible, it had to include at least one pain assessment or one disability assessment. The disability outcome needed to be evaluated by one or more of the following scales: 36-Item Short Form Health Survey (SF-36) Version 1.0 and 2.0 (SF-36); Roland Morris Disability Questionnaire (RMDQ); Oswestry Disability Index (ODI); and Back function (FFBH-R) [27]. The pain outcome had to be evaluated by one or more of the following scales: Numerical pain rating scale (NRS); Global Rating Change (GRC); Patient Pain Questionnaire (PPQ); and Visual rating scale (VRS).
- Only articles written in English and Italian languages were included.

2.1.2. Study Exclusion Criteria

- Studies with a mean age of patients < 65 years old;
- Studies in which PA was a part of a multidisciplinary program;
- Studies including participants who had physical problems that did not allow them to perform PA (diabetes untreated, muscle-skeletal problems, postural problems, neurological diseases, cardiovascular conditions).

2.2. Search Protocol

The following articles were screened from inception to March 2019: Medline, Scopus, CINAHL, EMBASE, and CENTRAL. For the search strategy we decided to use the following keywords: "low back pain" OR "chronic low back pain" AND "physical activity" OR "physical therapy" AND "elderly" OR "old aged" OR "older age" AND "Meziere" AND "Souchard" AND "global postural rehabilitation" "Feldenkrais" AND "McKenzie" AND "back school program" AND "Tai-Chi" AND "Pilates" AND "water therapy" OR "hydrotherapy" OR "balneotherapy" OR "hydrokinesis." We used the keywords isolated or combined. We searched for more studies among the reference lists of the selected papers and systematic reviews.

2.3. Study Selection

We accepted only English and Italian publications. The initial search of the article was conducted by two reviewers (D.S.S. and C.G). They used the protocol of search previously described to identify literature. In case of disagreements, the consensus of a third reviewer (R.F.) was asked. The researchers used the following research order. Titles were screened first, then abstracts and full papers. A paper was considered potentially relevant and its full text reviewed if, following discussion between the two independent reviewers, it could not be unequivocally excluded on the basis of its title and abstract. The full text of all papers not excluded on the basis of abstract or title was evaluated. The number of articles excluded or included were registered and reported in a PRISMA flowchart (Figure 1). For designing the PRISMA we followed the rules by Moher et al. [28].

2.4. Data Extraction

Data were extracted on: author, n of participants, year of study, content of intervention and control group, follow-up, outcomes (disability and pain), and mean age.

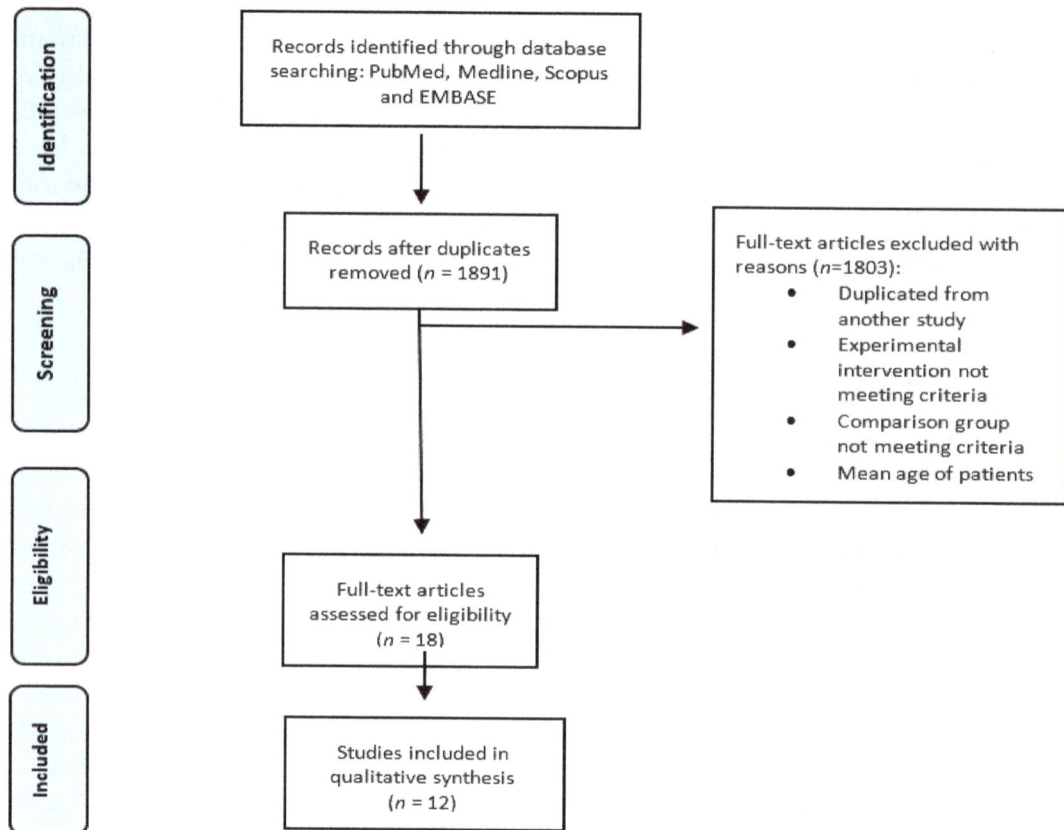

Figure 1. Preferred Reporting Items for Systematic reviews and Meta-Analyses (PRISMA) flow diagram.

2.5. Quality of Evidence

To estimate the potential bias that were most relevant for the study, we used the following tools: the Cochrane tool for assessing risk of bias in randomized trials (RoB 2 tool) [29] (Table 1) and the Risk Of Bias In Non-randomized Studies of Interventions (ROBINS-I) [30] (Table 2). In order to avoid imprecisions, the elected papers were rated independently by two reviewers (E.A. and S.D.S.) and verified by a third (G.V.). We used the GRADE approach (Tables 3 and 4) to rate the overall quality of evidence. However, only six articles [31–36] showed full post-treatment data, therefore it was not possible to assess all the studies included using GRADE approach. The GRADE approach classifies the quality of evidence for each outcome grading the following domains: study design, risk of bias, inconsistency, indirectness, imprecision, publication bias, magnitude of the effect (not assessed in this study), dose-response gradient (not assessed in this study), and influence of all plausible residual confounding (not assessed in this study). The quality of evidence was then classified as follow:

- High Quality of Evidence: among 75% of articles included are considered with low risk bias. Further researches are useful to change either the estimate or confidence in results.
- Moderate Quality of Evidence: one of the GRADE domains is not met. Further studies are required to improve the quality of the study and the evidence.
- Low Quality of Evidence: two of the GRADE domains are not met. Further research is very important.
- Very Low Quality of Evidence: three of the GRADE domains are not met. The results of the study are very uncertain. In the case of studies with a sample size inferior to 300 subjects the quality of the study is considered very low if there was also a high risk of bias (assessed with different tools. In our study we used Rob2 and ROBINS-I).

Table 1. Cochrane tool for assessing risk of bias in randomized trials (RoB 2 tool).

Unique ID	Randomization process	Deviations From Intended Interventions	Missing Outcome Data	Measurement of the Outcome	Selection of the Reported Result	Overall
Vincent et al. 2014	?	+	+	+	?	?
Vincent et al. 2014 II study	+	+	?	+	+	?
Tsatsako et al. 2016	+	+	+	−	?	−
Costantino et al. 2014	?	+	+	−	?	?
Ferrel et al. 1996	−	+	+	+	?	−
Teut et al. 2016	+	+	+	+	+	+
Holmes et al. 1996	+	+	−	−	?	−

+ : low risk; ? : some concern; − : high risk.

Table 2. Risk of bias in non-randomized studies of interventions (ROBINS-I).

Unique ID	D1	D2	D3	D4	D5	D6	D7	Overall
Iversen et al.	X	-	+	-	X	-	-	X
Beissner et al.	!	X	-	-	X	X	X	!
Khalil et al.	!	X	+	-	-	+	-	-
Mailloux et al.	X	-	-	+	-	-	-	-
Hicks et al.	-	-	+	+	-	-	-	-

! : Critical; X : Serious; - : Moderate; + : Low.

Table 3. GRADE evidence profile.

№ of Studies	Study Design	Certainty Assessment					№ of Patients		Effect	Certainty	Comments
		Risk of Bias	Inconsistency	Indirectness	Imprecision	Other Considerations	Physical Activity	NO Intervention	Absolute (95% C.I.)		
Disability RCTs (assessed with: ODI; Scale from: 0% to 100%)											
2 [33,35]	randomized trials	not serious	serious	not serious	serious	none	52	46	MD 1.24% lower (1.94 lower to 0.54 lower), (p = 0.0005 *)	⊕⊕◯◯ LOW	PA group shows a lower ODI mean value after treatment. It represents a possible positive influence of PA in improving disability
Disability RCTs (assessed with: SF-36; Scale from: 0 to 100)											
2 [31,32]	randomised trials	not serious	serious	not serious	serious	none	77	67	MD 2.88 point higher (−3.30 lower to 9.6 higher), (p = 0.36)	⊕⊕◯◯ LOW	PA group shows a higher SF-36 mean value after treatment. It represents a possible positive influence of PA in improving disability
Pain RCT (assessed with: NRS; Scale from: 0 to 10)											
1 [36]	randomized trials	not serious	not serious	not serious	serious	none	35	17	MD 1.73 points lower (3.11 lower to 0.35 lower), (p = 0.01 *)	⊕⊕⊕◯ MODERATE	PA group shows a lower mean NRS after treatment. It represents a possible positive influence of PA in improving pain
Pain NRCT (assessed with: Global Rating Change; Scale from: 1 to 10)											
1 [34]	observational studies	serious	not serious	not serious	serious	none	238	154	MD 1 points lower (1.53 lower to 0.47 lower), (p < 0.001 *)	⊕⊕◯◯ LOW	PA group shows a lower mean pain value after treatment. It represents a possible positive influence of PA in improving pain

C.I.: confidence interval; MD: mean difference; *: statistically significant; NRCT: non-randomized controlled trials; RCT: randomized controlled trials; PA: physical activity; SF-36: 36-Item Short Form Health Survey; ODI: Oswestry Disability Index; NRS: Numerical pain rating scale.

Table 4. GRADE summary of findings table.

Outcomes	Anticipated Absolute Effects * (95% C.I.) Risk with PA	№ of Participants (Studies)	Certainty of the Evidence (GRADE)
Disability RCTs assessed with: ODI Scale from: 0% to 100%	MD 1.24% lower (1.94 lower to 0.54 lower), ($p = 0.0005$ *)	98 (2 RCTs) [33,35]	⊕⊕〇〇 LOW
Disability RCTs assessed with: SF-36 Scale from: 0 to 100	MD 2.88 point higher (−3.30 lower to 9.6 higher), ($p = 0.36$)	144 (2 RCTs) [31,32]	⊕⊕〇〇 LOW
Pain RCT assessed with: NRS Scale from: 0 to 10	MD 1.73 points lower (3.11 lower to 0.35 lower), ($p = 0.01$*)	52 (1 RCT) [36]	⊕⊕⊕〇 MODERATE
Pain NRCT assessed with: Global Rating Change Scale from: 1 to 10	MD 1 points lower (1.53 lower to 0.47 lower), ($p < 0.001$ *)	392 (1 observational study) [34]	⊕⊕〇〇 LOW

MD: mean difference, *: statically significant; C.I.: confidence interval.

The outcomes assessed were improvement in pain and disability, both evaluated at the end of the treatment. Follow-up were different and ranged from 1 month to 48 months. Furthermore, the outcomes were subgrouped into RCTs, NRCTs, and other studies (pre-post intervention and case series).

3. Results

3.1. Study Selection

We created a flow-chart diagram according to the PRISMA protocol that shows the selection process of the studies (Figure 1). We found a total of 2173 studies (no additional studies were found in gray literature). We obtained 1891 studies when the duplicates were removed. Of the 1891 studies, 1709 articles were excluded from our study through the title screening. We assessed the abstracts of 182 articles and we excluded 94. Then, 88 full-text articles were screened. Out of these studies, 76 were excluded for the following reasons: mean age of patients < 65 years old ($n = 64$); experimental intervention not meeting the inclusion criteria ($n = 8$), and comparison group not meeting the inclusion criteria ($n = 4$). After this process, we included 12 articles in our study. No unpublished studies were retrieved.

3.2. Study Characteristics

A description of the characteristics of the studies that was considered eligible for this review is reported in Table 5. A total of 12 articles were selected for this systematic review. We included 7 RCT of I level of evidence (LOE), 3 NRCT (3 OS of II LOE), 1 PPS of III LOE, and 1 CS of IV LOE. Studies were published between 1992 [37] and 2016 [31].

Table 5. Characteristics of the included studies.

Study	Type of Study (LOE)	n. of Patients/Mean Age (y)	Exclusion	Inclusion	Type of Intervention	Control Group	Frequency	Outcome Summary	Outcome Measure/Difference Between Groups	Conclusions
Mailloux et al. [38] 2006	CS (IV)	126/76/48	Compression fracture within the last 6 months; and lack of cognitive or language skills necessary to complete paper-and-pencil measures.	CLBP	Stretching and endurance	No	6 weeks 2 session/week 2 hour/session	Disability Pain	ODI T0–T1 value Physical activity group: 28 (17) to 16 (13) (p = 0.01) Control: 38 (17) to 25 (17) (p = 0.01)	The exercise behaviours of older adults with CLBP can increase after an exercise-oriented spine physical therapy.
Beissner et al. [39] 2012	OS (II)	59/75.57/2	Not reported	Patients >60 years old; ability to speak English or Spanish; LBP in the past three month, cognitively intact.	Overall fitness: warmup, stretching, endurance exercises, walking, and a cool down	No	9 weeks 2 session/week	Disability	RMDQ T0–T1 values Physical activity group: 3.12 (0.72) to 7.83 (0.77), (p < 0.001)	The race/ethnicity could have a role in the improvement of CLBP with a conservative treatment
Iversen et al. [40] 2003	PPIS (III)	26/72/3	Pain with lumbar flexion; low back surgery in the last year; epidural steroid injection during the last 6 months; currently receiving physical therapy or participating in an exercise training program; other medical problems that limited their function more than LBP	Patients >65 years old; low back, buttock, and/or leg pain exacerbated by passive lumbar extension in standing; and symptoms that last for at least 6 months.	Indoor cycling	No	3 months 3 session/week	Disability	SF-36 T0–T1 Physical activity group: 7.2 (p = 0.6)	The bicycle program was safe and effective for improving functional status and well-being.
Costantino et al. [41] 2014	RCT (I)	56/73.46/3	Musculoskeletal disorders, cardiac diseases; fever or infectious disease; previous spinal surgery, trauma; previous physical therapies in the last three months	Patients >65 and <80 years old; Diagnosis of chronic non-specific low back pain; Chronic low back pain recurrence in the last three months.	Back school Program	Yes: Hydrotherapy	3 months 2 session/week 1 hour/session	Disability	RMDQ T0–T1 difference Back school: 3.26 ± 1.02, (p < 0.001); Hydrotherapy: 4.96 ± 0.71 (p < 0.001) SF-36 (Version 2.0) T0–T1 difference Back school: 13.30 ± 1.44 (p < 0.001); Hydrotherapy: 14.19 ± 1.98 (p < 0.001)	Back School program and Hydrotherapy could be valid treatment options in the rehabilitation of non-specific CLBP in older people.

Table 5. *Cont.*

Study	Type of Study (LOE)	n. of Patients/Mean Age (y)	Exclusion	Inclusion	Type of Intervention	Control Group	Frequency	Outcome Summary	Outcome Measure/Difference Between Groups	Conclusions
Ferrel et al. [32] 1997	RCT (I)	33/73/1.5	Unstable cardiovascular or pulmonary diseases, inflammatory arthritis or nerve root compression; psychiatric disease, or alcohol abuse	Age >65 years CLBP, use of analgesic medication; ability to walk independently and able to understand and read English.	Three groups: Group 1: low intensity walking.Group 2: pain education program. Group 3: usual care	Yes: Education programme (one 90-minute session + weekly telephone reinforcement)	6 weeks 4 session/week 1 hour/session	Pain Disability	SF-36 (Version 1.0) T0–T1 difference Intervention: 58.5 (27.7), ($p < 0.001$) Control: 43 (16.7), ($p < 0.001$) PPQ T0–T1 difference Intervention: 28.9 (18.5), ($p < 0.001$) Control: 57.8 (24,9), ($p < 0.001$)	Patient education and fitness walking can improve overall pain management and related functional limitations
Hicks et al. [34] 2012	OS (II)	392/66.8/12	Unstable angina, hypertension, pulmonary disease, dementia, aphasia, back pain attributable to organic causes, back, presence of 2 or more of the following sign: lower-extremity strength, sensation, or reflexes	LBP > 4 months, capability to rise from a chair and walk, capability to travel to the exercise facility, and limited participation in physical activity at the initiation of the exercise program	Strengthening; abdominal strengthening, thoracolumbar, and scapula retraction in lying or standing position or sitting Stretching: hamstring and calf Endurance: 5–10 minutes walking	No	12 months 2 session/week 1 hour/session–20–30 steps	Pain Adherence to exercise Performance	GRC T0–T1 difference Physical activity group: 4.6 (2.5) Control: 4.9 (2.7) ($p = 0.246$)	Patients were able to safely participate in exercise program and back pain improved 12 months later.
Holmes et al. [42] 1996	RCT (I)	38/68.3/3	Not reported	CLBP	Flexion and extension cycles of isotonic resistance exercises	Yes: No exercises	4 weeks, 2 session/week	Pain	VRS T0–T1 values Physical activity group: from 5.3 to 2.1 ($p < 0.05$) Control: data not reported ($p > 0.05$)	In many patients lumbar exercises and resistance exercises could improve CLBP
Khalil et al. [37] 1992	OS (II)	59/68/1	Not reported	In the active restoration program: Low back pain and a diagnosis of myofascial pain syndrome. In the passive restoration program: weakness of quadriceps and/or tibialis anterior.	Mixed isotonic and isokinetic progressive resistive exercise of muscles	No control group The passive approach was based on the use of functional electric stimulation (FES) as an adjunct treatment to strengthen lower extremity muscles weakened by disuse	4 weeks 1 session/day	Pain	Pain level 1–10 T0–T1 values Physical activity group: 5.5 to 3.3 ($p < 0.01$) Control: data not reported	Physical activity can improve symptoms and functional ability of older people that suffer of low back pain. Moreover, FES could be a helpful device in the rehabilitation of weak muscles

Table 5. *Cont.*

Study	Type of Study (LOE)	n. of Patients/Mean Age (y)	Exclusion	Inclusion	Type of Intervention	Control Group	Frequency	Outcome Summary	Outcome Measure/Difference Between Groups	Conclusions
Teut et al. [31] 2016	RCT (I)	176/73/3	Acute neurological symptoms within the last 3 months, severe organic or psychiatric disease, metastatic bone disease	Adults ≥65 years old, chronic low back pain for at least 6 months	Yoga group:Viniyoga methodQuijong group: "Dantian" and Nei Yang Gong exercises from the Training System Liu Ya Fei	Yes: No intervention group	Yoga group: 3 months 24 classes 45 minutes/class Quijong group: 3 months 12 classes 90 minutes/class	Disability	SF-36 T0-T1 value Yoga: 36.3 ± 8.7 to 59.47 (C.I. 54.73; 64.21) Qijong: 37.5 ± 7.8 to 61.01 (C.I. 55.88; 66.14) Control: 36.5 ± 9.3 to 61.17 (C.I. 56.32; 66.02), (p = 0.50) FFBH-R T0-T1 value Yoga: 68.7 ± 15.4 to 66.55 (C.I. 62.89; 70.21) Qijong: 70.4 ± 18.7 to 69.23 (C.I. 65.9)	High satisfaction of patients with the yoga and qigong classes, but participation in a 3- or 6-month period of yoga or qigong program did not improve chronic back pain, back function and quality of life.
Tsatsakos [35] et al. 2014	RCT (I)	80/67.7/1	Back surgery, Cauda equina syndrome, spondylolisthesis, rheumatoid conditions	Patients >60 years old, of both sexes and with pain in the lumbar region for a period over 12 weeks	10.000 steps/day performed on a treadmill and during the common life.	Yes: recommendation relaxation, and ergonomic	1 month 8000 steps/day	Disability	ODI T0-T1 value Physical activity group: 7.56 (3.22) to 8.06 (4.94) Control: 11.77 (5.27) to 10.00 (5.03), p = 0.46	Walking shows that it has no effect in the functional status of the elderly with CLBP.
Vincent et al. [33] 2014	RCT (I)	49/67.5/4	Being wheelchair bound	In men and women, BMI ≥30 kg/m² LBP for ≥6 months	Resistance exercise intervention (TOTRX) Lumbar extension intervention (LEXT)	Yes: No intervention	TOTRX: 4 months, 3 session/week 15 exercise/session LEXT: 4 months, 3 session/week 2 sets of lumbar	Disability	ODI T0-T1 values TOTRX: 29.4 (11.2) to 18.0 (12.6) LEXT: 28.6 (15.2) to 22.6 (14.2) Control: 24.4 (12.1) to 22.9 (12.4), (p = 0.015) RMDQ	Resistance exercise show improvement in patients walking endurance. Lumbar extension strength in obese older adults with CLBP
Vincent et al. [36] 2014	RCT (I)	49/68.5/4	Wheelchair bound, ability to participate in resistance exercise, acute back pain back surgery within the previous two years	CLBP> 6 months and abdominal obesity and free of abnormal cardiovascular responses during electrocardiogram (ECG) screening tests	TOTRX LEXT	Yes: Behavioural advices: strengthening exercise and nutritional choices	TOTRX: 4 months, 3 session/week 15 sets/exercise/session LEXT: 4 months, 3 session/week 2 sets of lumbar exercises- 15 reps/exercise/session	Pain	NRS T1 value TOTXR: 4.3 (1.8) to 2.0 (1.7) LEXTR: 5.0 (1.8) to 3.7 (2.6) Control: 5.2 (2.4) to 4.6 (2.4), (p <0.006)	Total body resistance exercise (including lumbar extension exercise) was more effective than lumbar extension exercise alone in reducing self-reported disability scores due to back pain

CLBP: chronic low back pain, LBPL low back pain; CS: case-series; LOE: level of evidence; LEXT: lumbar extension intervention; TOTRX: resistance exercise intervention; ODI; Oswestry disability index OS; observational studies; NRS: numerical pain rating scale (NRS); PPIS: pre-post interventional study; PPQ: patient pain questionnaire; RCT: randomized clinical trial, RMDQ: Roland Morris Disability Questionnaire; VRS: Visual rating scale; SF-36: 36-Item short form health survey; FES: functional electric stimulation; T0: baseline values; T1: last follow up values; C.I.: confidence interval; numbers reported in brackets refer to standard deviations.

Based on the data of the included studies, a total of 1581 patients were treated for CLBP. The mean age of patients at the time of treatment was 71.88 ± 3.01 and ranged between 67.5 [36] and 76.0 [42].

The outcome measures used in these studies included: (3 studies) 36-Item Short Form Health Survey (SF-36) Version 2.0 (SF-36); (3 studies) Roland Morris Disability Questionnaire (RMDQ); (3 studies) Oswestry Disability Index (ODI); (2 studies) Numerical pain rating scale (NRS); (1 study) SF-36 Version 1.0; (1 study) Patient Pain Questionnaire (PPQ); (1 study) Global Rating Change (GCR); (1 study) Visual rating scale (VRS); and (1 study) Back function (FFBH-R) [27].

The studies cited in this review show high heterogeneity in terms of study design, interventions, and outcome variables. The results are presented descriptively, focusing on disability and pain and further issues of potential interest. In general, post-treatment data showed a moderate range of improvement for disability and pain. Otherwise, these results need to be evaluated carefully due to the high risk of bias and the high heterogeneity of the studies included.

3.3. Methodological Quality

The Rob2 tool for RCT and ROBINS-I tool for NRCT, pre-post intervention and case-series were used to assess the methodological quality of each study. For RCT we found three studies with an overall risk identified as "some concerns," 3 as "high risk," and 1 as "low risk". Concerning the NRCT we found 1 study with an overall risk of bias identified as "critical" [38] and 2 studies as "moderate" [34,37]. We assessed the pre-post intervention study with an overall risk of bias identified as "serious" [41]; instead the case series was identified as "moderate" [42].

The quality of evidence of the studies included in GRADE ranges from low to moderate. All the studies, except one [34], have a small sample (n < 300). Methodological quality assessments of each study are summarized in Tables 1 and 2. The quality of evidence of full data trials was performed using GRADE approach (Tables 3 and 4). The analysis of the data of the study was reported using the mean difference between studies. RevMan5 (version 5.3) was used to calculate the mean difference of the included studies. Because of the lack of post treatment results in some studies, we decided to perform a systematic review and not a meta-analysis. We report the outcomes of each study in Table 5.

3.4. Results of Individual Studies

The intervention methods are usually well described in all the included studies. High heterogeneity in the type of PA was reported in all the studies. We included all types of PA (walking [32,35], back school and hydrotherapy [39], isotonic resistance exercises [40] yoga and qijong [31], TOTXR [33] and LEXTR). The authors divided the description of intervention per outcome (pain and disability) in three subgroups (randomized controlled trials, non-randomized controlled trials, and other studies, including pre-post intervention and case series).

3.4.1. Randomized Controlled Trials (RCTs)

Seven RCTs were included. They were divided per outcome: 2 studies [36,40] examined the improvement in pain (measured by NRS and VRS); 5 studies [31–33,35,39] assessed the disability outcome (measured by ODI, RMDQ, PPQ, FRI, FFBH-R, and SF-36). Single studies were assessed for risk of bias using Rob2 tool. Two studies were classified as "high risk," three as "some concerns," and one as "low risk." It was possible to include only 5 articles in GRADE analysis [31–33,35,36]. The overall quality of evidence in these studies ranges from "low" to "moderate" according to GRADE. The quantitative effect estimate was reported as mean difference between and within studies (when possible). This heterogeneity among studies and the low quality of evidence could lead to an overestimation of the results. The results of the outcome of the other studies are reported in Table 5.

Outcome: Pain

Two RCTs studies [36,40] presented data on pain at the end of the treatment. The authors used NRS and VRS to evaluate the improvements in pain. Follow-up was 3 months in the study carried out by Holmes et al. [42] and 4 months in the study by Vincent et al. [36]. At the end of the treatment, they both reported a reduction of pain in the group treated by PA (isotonic resistance exercises in Holmes et al. [42] group and TOTXR and LEXTR in Vincent [36] group). The study by Holmes et al. was classified as "high risk," and the risk of bias of the study by Vincent et al. was assessed as "some concern" using Rob2 tool. The study by Vincent et al. [36] was assessed as "moderate" quality using GRADE analysis. It was not possible to evaluate the overall quality of the other study according to GRADE [26] because of the lack of data. Otherwise, in both articles it was reported an improvement in pain evaluated by NRS and VRS. Vincent et al. [36] reported a better NRS in the intervention group compared to the control group at the end of the treatment (MD −1.73, 95% C.I. −3.11 to −0.35, $p = 0.01$). Holmes et al. [42] reported a difference from 5.3 to 2.1 points in VRS from the beginning to the end of the treatment (no full data were reported concerning to control group results). Otherwise, the authors reported an improvement in pain between the intervention and the control group, but this was not statistically significant ($p > 0.05$). The results of the outcome of the other studies are reported in Table 5.

Outcome: Disability

Five RCT studies [31–33,35,39] presented data on disability at the end of the treatment. The authors used ODI, RMDQ, SF-36, PPQ, FRI, and FFBH-R to assess the improvements in disability. Follow-up was heterogenous: 1 month for Tsatsakos et al. [35]; 1.5 months for Ferrel et al. [32]; 3 months for Teut et al. [31] and Costantino et al. [41]; and 4 months for Vincent et al. [33]. At the end of the treatment, all studies reported an overall improvement in disability. The PA program was different between studies (walking [32,35], back school and hydrotherapy [39], yoga and Qijong [31] and TOTXR [33]). In the study by Ferrel et al. [32] the control group was constituted by the hydrotherapy group and not by a no-intervention group as in the other studies. Also, in this study they reported an overall increase in disability in both groups. The studies by Tsatsakos et al. and Ferrel et al. were classified as "high risk," Teut et al. as "low risk," Costantino et al. and Vincent et al. as "some concern" using Rob2 tool. It was not possible to assess the quality of evidence of the study by Costantino et al. [41] because of the absence of a "no-intervention" control group. The overall quality of the other 4 studies [31–33,35] was evaluated as "low" according to GRADE [26]. In specific, the authors divided the studies into two subgroups: RCTs measured by ODI and RCTs measured by SF-36. We used only these scales since they were reported in all studies. We found a reduction of disability evaluated by ODI (MD −1.24, 95% C.I. −1.94 to −0.54; $p = 0.0005$ *). Moreover, an improvement of SF-36 in patients treated by PA was reported (MD 2.88, 95% C.I. −3.30 to 9.06, $p = 0.36$). Costantino et al. [41] observed a highly significant statistical difference of SF-36 (13.30 ± 1.44, $p < 0.001$ *), measured in both intervention groups (back school and hydrotherapy) at the end of the treatment. The results of outcome of the other studies are reported in Table 5.

3.4.2. Non-Randomized Controlled Trials (NRCT)

We included in our review three NRCT [34,37,38] studies. They were divided per outcome: 2 studies [34,37] examined the improvement in pain (measured by GRS and PPQ); 1 study [38] assessed the disability outcome (measured by RMDQ). The latter study did not have a control group. Single studies were assessed for risk of bias using ROBINS-I tool [30]. Two studies [34,37] were classified as "moderate" overall risk and one [38] as "critical." Because of the lack of data, it was possible to assess the quality of evidence, according to GRADE, only of the study by Hicks et al. [34] classifying as "low." The quantitative effect estimate of this study was reported as mean difference between groups. The high heterogeneity among studies and the low quality of evidence could lead to an overestimation of the results. The results of outcome of the other studies were reported in Table 5.

Outcome: Pain

Two NRCT studies [34,37] presented data on pain at the end of the treatment. The authors used GRS and PPS to evaluate improvements in pain. Follow-up was 1 month in the study by Khalil et al. [37] and 12 months in the study by Hicks et al. [34]. At the end of the treatment they both reported a reduction of pain in the group treated by PA (strengthening and stretching programs [34] and isotonic and isokinetic progressive resistive exercise [37]). The overall quality of the study by Hicks et al. [34] was evaluated as "low" according to GRADE [26]. The study by Khalil et al. [37] was classified as "moderate" risk of bias using ROBINS-I tool. In specific, Hicks et al. [34] reported an improvement in pain after the treatment in the intervention group compared to controls measured by GRC (MD-1.00, 95% C.I. −1.53 to −0.47, $p = 0.006$ *). Khalil et al. [37] also reported a reduction of pain measured by pain scale (1–10) from 5.5 to 3.3 ($p < 0.01$ *), but no data concerning to control group were found.

Outcome: Disability

One NRCT study [38] presented data on disability at the end of the treatment. The authors used RMDQ to evaluate improvements in disability. Follow-up was 2 months. One important limitation in the study was the lack of a control group. However, at the end of the treatment the authors concluded by reporting an improvement in disability in the group treated by PA (stretching and resistance exercises [38]). The risk of bias of this study was evaluated using ROBINS-I and it was classified as "serious." Beissner et al. [39] reported a reduction of disability measured by RMDQ scale in patients treated by PA (−5.29 points, $p < 0.001$ *).

3.4.3. Other Studies (Pre-Post Intervention and Case Series)

One pre-post intervention study [41] and one case series [42] presented data on disability at the end of the treatment. The authors used respectively SF-36 and ODI to evaluate improvements in disability. One important limitation of these studies was the lack of a control group. Because of the lack of a control group it was not possible to classify the evidence of these studies according to GRADE. Otherwise, the study by Mailloux et al. [38] was classified as "moderate" risk and Iversen et al. [40] as "serious" according to the ROBINS-I tool.

Outcome: Disability

Two studies [41,42] presented data on disability at the end of the treatment. They reported an improvement in disability in the groups treated by PA (cycling [41], stretching, resistance training, and endurance activities [42]). Follow-up was respectively 48 months in the study by Mailloux et al. [38] and 3 months in the study by Iversen et al. [40]. Iversen et al. [40] reported a non-statistically significant improvement in physical function measured by SF-36 of 7.2 points ($p = 0.6$). Mailloux et al. [38] reported a reduction of ODI from 28% ± 17 to 16% ± 13 ($p = 0.001$ *) in the intervention group after 48 months of follow-up. On the other hand, it was reported only a reduction of ODI from 38 ± 17 to 25 ± 17 ($p = 0.001$ *) in the control group.

4. Discussion

CLBP currently affects approximately one-fifth of the global population [43,44]. Cayea et al. reported that 36% of older adults aged 65 years or more are affected by at least one episode of this condition per year, of which 21% reported moderate or intense pain representing an important priority for the health system. In the literature, as confirmed by Paeck et al. [16], there is a lack of studies on CLBP in the elderly. In fact, most of the studies on CLBP treatment options are focused on the so-called "working age" and this calls into question the reliability of several treatment options in the older population, especially because in the older age we can often find several comorbidities that may limit the rehabilitation.

In our systematic review, we screened the recent literature (1992–2018) with the aim to assess the effectiveness of PA to improve disability and pain in the elderly population affected by non-specific CLBP comparing it to no treatment and other conservative treatments. Indeed, 12 studies were included at the end of the search process. Among these, only 5 RCTs with an overall quality of evidence that ranges from "low" to "moderate" and 1 NRCT of "low" quality could be assessed according to GRADE approach. The quality of the other studies was evaluated by Rob2 for RCT and ROBINS-I for the other study types. The lack of data in some articles, and the poor literature among this topic could lead to low quality of evidence. Our research highlighted that older patients with CLBP treated with PA showed an overall pain and disability improvement in the majority of the studies. Otherwise, these conclusions need to be taken carefully, considering the high risk of bias, the low quality of evidence of the literature, and the languages limitations of this study (only English and Italian articles were included). Because of these limitations and the absence of high-quality literature, we decided to perform only a systematic review of the literature and not a meta-analysis.

However, the extreme variability of type, duration, intensity, and execution modality of the proposed PA, the different body district on which PA were focused on in each different program and the compliance of the patients, are important variables that make it impossible to recommend a specific protocol in the elderly population. This lack of standardization was also confirmed by Airaksinen et al. [18] that found a considerable variety of PA, such as stretching, aerobic exercises, or muscle reconditioning.

In this systematic review, we analyzed different PA protocols, based on walking [35], cycling [41], back school exercises [39], hydrotherapy [39], Yoga and Quigong [31], endurance, resistance, stretching and strengthening exercises [33,37]. Regarding the trained muscle groups, we found that most of the included studies were focused on abdominus muscles [40], iliopsoas, hamstring, gastrocnemius, quadriceps, hip flexors, abductor/adductor muscles of the hip and erector spinae muscles [37].

Regarding the 4 studies evaluating pain (2 RCTs and 2 NRCTs), they showed that both lumbar isotonic resistance exercise cycles and abdominal, thoracolumbar and upper limb isotonic and isokinetic strengthening exercises, improve pain in elderly patients with CLBP. In their RCT, Vincent et al. [32] also reported, at a 4-months follow-up, an improvement in walking speed and endurance. This finding confirms that the physical treatment of CLBP might be focused not only on the lumbar muscles but also on the lower limbs and thorax (exercises for breathing muscle districts [39]). Otherwise, one study [40] reported an improvement in pain, but not statistically significant if compared with the control group ($p > 0.05$).

The studies which assessed disability (5 RCTs, 1 NRCT, 1 pre-post intervention and 1 case series) confirmed that walking, back school exercise, hydrotherapy, yoga and Qijong, bicycle program, strengthening and stretching program, and combined PA and cognitive-behavioral program improve the functional performances of elderly people with CLBP. However, because of the high heterogeneity of the studies, we found a significant reduction of disability evaluated by ODI ($p = 0.000\,5*$), but the improvement of SF-36 in patients treated by PA was not significant ($p = 0.36$). Moreover, we also found an improvement in patients treated by different types of PA such as back school and hydrotherapy [39] ($p < 0.001\,*$) at the end of the treatment.

Other important concerns are compliance and motivation of the patient that may represent decisive parameters during CLBP treatment in the elderly. Beissner et al. [39] emphasized an interesting treatment option represented by the cognitive-behavioral therapy (CBT) in association with PA to reduce symptoms in patients with CLBP. This novel treatment is becoming increasingly important. In a recent systematic review, Vitoula et al. [45] highlighted that CBT was effective in patients with CLBP, especially in reducing pain perception and helping them to improve their functionality. Furthermore, the review showed that better outcomes can be achieved when treatments are personalized. This represents a remarkable issue. In fact, several studies included in our research [34,38,39] showed that patients that maintain a prolonged compliance to the rehabilitation protocols and were highly motivated had better outcomes in pain relief and function outcomes.

It is crucial to focus on the biological effects of PA [46,47]. One major limit to perform PA in old-aged patients is the sarcopenia, defined as a loss of muscle mass (lean body mass) with a reduction of muscle function [48]. This process represents a specific condition of normal energy balance in the elderly, with an increase in body fat percentage. Limb surgery postoperative period, disuse, endocrine diseases (such as diabetes type II), and uncontrolled nutrients intake lead to sarcopenia [49]. This condition could lead to a frailty status, with a reduction of PA [50]. Landi et al. [51] conducted a review of the literature reporting that PA has an important role in the reduction of sarcopenia in old-aged people. PA could also increase irisin [52] and osteocalcin [53]. The former is a hormone-like myokine produced by skeletal muscle during PA [54]. Irisin can induce thermogenesis from brown adipocytes. This protein has also an effect in the control of bone mass, with positive effects on cortical mineral density. It is also demonstrated that irisin plays a crucial role in the reduction of sarcopenia in old people [55,56]. Osteocalcin is a bone-derived hormone-like protein. It could favor physiological functions increasing the bone formation [57], regulating the muscle decrease related to age [58], and reducing the risk of diabetes type II [4,59]. Chahla et al. [60] reported in their study that osteocalcin is higher in patients who perform regular PA, with an increase in bone mineralization, muscle function, and reduction of risk of diabetes type II.

Moreover, several studies [61–63] report that PA could also reduce the level of osteoporosis, resulting in a valid therapeutical approach for this disease in elderly people.

Limitations

The results of this study should be considered with caution, as there was a high heterogeneity in terms of follow-up, type of intervention, and standardization of physical protocols. In fact, the follow-up varies from a minimum of 1 month to a maximum of 48 months, as well as the number of patients (49 to 392). The small sample size and the high heterogeneity among trials as well as the absence of a control group in three studies [38,41,42], make the estimate of the effect of intervention extremely challenging. Moreover, the low quality of the studies (from "low" to "moderate"), and the high risk of bias of some studies included, decrease the power of our conclusions. Nevertheless, some studies reported an improvement of outcomes in patients treated by PA, even if their results were not statistically significant. These data could lead the authors to overestimate the results considered. Another important limitation of this systematic review is the decision of the authors to include only English and Italian articles. This limitation could lead to an exclusion of relevant studies related to this specific topic. Therefore, further high quality evidences that take into account the standardized methods and a similar cohort of patients are desirable. At the same time, this review should promote future investigations, also including other languages, to better understand which type of PA is preferred to treat older patients with CLBP and help our clinical practice.

5. Conclusions

In the available literature PA seems to have a trend of improvement in pain and disability in elderly patients with non-specific CLBP. However, because of the limited and low-quality literature it is not possible to state this positive effect as a definitive conclusion. In order to avoid the overestimated effectiveness of PA on CLBP from high risk of bias studies, new high-quality evidence is needed.

Author Contributions: Conceptualization, G.V., R.P., and V.D.; methodology, F.R.; writing—original draft preparation, S.D.S., G.C., and E.A.; writing—review and editing, F.R., S.D.S., G.C., and E.A.; supervision G.V., R.P., and V.D.; funding acquisition, G.V. All authors have read and agreed to the published version of the manuscript.

References

1. Burton, A.K.; Balagué, F.; Cardon, G.; Eriksen, H.R.; Henrotin, Y.; Lahad, A.; Leclerc, A.; Müller, G.; van der Beek, A.J. Chapter 2 European guidelines for prevention in low back pain. *Eur. Spine J.* **2006**, *15*, s136–s168. [CrossRef] [PubMed]

2. Wong, A.Y.; Karppinen, J.; Samartzis, D. Low back pain in older adults: Risk factors, management options and future directions. *Scoliosis Spinal Disord.* **2017**, *12*, 14. [CrossRef] [PubMed]

3. Dunn, K.M.; Hestbaek, L.; Cassidy, J.D. Low back pain across the life course. *Best Pract. Res. Clin. Rheumatol.* **2013**, *27*, 591–600. [CrossRef] [PubMed]

4. Cannata, F.; Vadalà, G.; Ambrosio, L.; Fallucca, S.; Napoli, N.; Papalia, R.; Pozzilli, P.; Denaro, V. Intervertebral disc degeneration: A focus on obesity and type 2 diabetes. *Diabetes Metab. Res. Rev.* **2020**, *36*, e3224. [CrossRef]

5. Hoy, D.; Bain, C.; Williams, G.; March, L.; Brooks, P.; Blyth, F.; Woolf, A.; Vos, T.; Buchbinder, R.A. Systematic review of the global prevalence of low back pain. *Arthritis Rheum.* **2012**, *64*, 2028–2037. [CrossRef]

6. Hartvigsen, J.; Hancock, M.J.; Kongsted, A.; Louw, Q.; Ferreira, M.L.; Genevay, S.; Hoy, D.; Karppinen, J.; Pransky, G.; Sieper, J.; et al. What low back pain is and why we need to pay attention. *Lancet* **2018**, *391*, 2356–2367. [CrossRef]

7. Meucci, R.D.; Fassa, A.G.; Faria, N.M.X. Prevalence of chronic low back pain: Systematic review. *Rev. Saúde Pública* **2015**, *49*, 73. [CrossRef]

8. Vadalà, G.; Russo, F.; Battisti, S.; Stellato, L.; Martina, F.; Del Vescovo, R.; Giacalone, A.; Borthakur, A.; Zobel, B.B.; Denaro, V. Early intervertebral disc degeneration changes in asymptomatic weightlifters assessed by t1ρ-magnetic resonance imaging. *Spine* **2014**, *39*, 1881–1886. [CrossRef]

9. Gallagher, R.M. Low back pain, health status, and quality of life in older adults: Challenge and opportunity. *Pain. Med.* **2003**, *4*, 305–307. [CrossRef]

10. Deyo, R.A.; Weinstein, J.N. Low back pain. *N. Engl. J. Med.* **2001**, *344*, 363–370. [CrossRef]

11. Vadalà, G.; Russo, F.; Musumeci, M.; D'Este, M.; Cattani, C.; Catanzaro, G.; Tirindelli, M.C.; Lazzari, L.; Alini, M.; Giordano, R.; et al. Clinically relevant hydrogel-based on hyaluronic acid and platelet rich plasma as a carrier for mesenchymal stem cells: Rheological and biological characterization. *J. Orthop. Res.* **2017**, *35*, 2109–2116. [CrossRef] [PubMed]

12. Hubert, M.G.; Vadala, G.; Sowa, G.; Studer, R.K.; Kang, J.D. Gene therapy for the treatment of degenerative disk disease. *J. Am. Acad. Orthop. Surg.* **2008**, *16*, 312–319. [CrossRef] [PubMed]

13. Maher, C.; Underwood, M.; Buchbinder, R. Non-specific low back pain. *Lancet* **2017**, *389*, 736–747. [CrossRef]

14. Cayea, D.; Perera, S.; Weiner, D.K. Chronic low back pain in older adults: What physicians know, what they think they know, and what they should be taught. *J. Am. Geriatr. Soc.* **2006**, *54*, 1772–1777. [CrossRef]

15. Macedo, L.G.; Maher, C.G.; Latimer, J.; McAuley, J.H. Motor control exercise for persistent, nonspecific low back pain: A systematic review. *Phys. Ther.* **2009**, *89*, 9–25. [CrossRef]

16. Scheele, J.; Enthoven, W.T.M.; Bierma-Zeinstra, S.M.A.; Peul, W.C.; van Tulder, M.W.; Bohnen, A.M.; Berger, M.Y.; Koes, B.W.; Luijsterburg, P.A.J. Course and prognosis of older back pain patients in general practice: A prospective cohort study. *Pain* **2013**, *154*, 951–957. [CrossRef]

17. Weiner, D.K.; Rudy, T.E.; Kim, Y.S.; Golla, S. Do medical factors predict disability in older adults with persistent low back pain? *Pain* **2004**, *112*, 214–220. [CrossRef]

18. Paeck, T.; Ferreira, M.L.; Sun, C.; Lin, C.W.C.; Tiedemann, A.; Maher, C.G. Are older adults missing from low back pain clinical trials? A systematic review and meta-analysis. *Arthritis Care Res.* **2014**, *66*, 1220–1226. [CrossRef]

19. Richardson, C.A.; Jull, G.A. Muscle control-pain control. What exercises would you prescribe? *Man. Ther.* **1995**, *1*, 2–10.

20. Airaksinen, O.; Brox, J.I.; Cedraschi, C.; Hildebrandt, J.; Klaber-Moffett, J.; Kovacs, F.; Mannion, A.F.; Reis, S.; Staal, J.B.; Ursin, H.; et al. European guidelines for the management of chronic nonspecific low back pain. *Eur. Spine J.* **2006**, *15*, S192–S300. [CrossRef]

21. Chou, R.; Qaseem, A.; Snow, V.; Casey, D.; Cross, J.T.; Shekelle, P.; Owens, D.K.; Clinical Efficacy Assessment Subcommittee of the American College of Physicians; American College of Physicians; American Pain Society Low Back Pain Guidelines Panel. Diagnosis and treatment of low back pain: A joint clinical practice guideline from the American College of Physicians and the American Pain Society. *Ann. Intern. Med.* **2007**, *147*, 478–491. [PubMed]

22. Hayden, J.A.; van Tulder, M.W.; Malmivaara, A.V.; Koes, B.W. Meta-analysis: Exercise therapy for nonspecific low back pain. *Ann. Intern. Med.* **2005**, *142*, 765–775. [CrossRef] [PubMed]

23. Henschke, N.; Ostelo, R.W.; van Tulder, M.W.; Vlaeyen, J.W.; Morley, S.; Assendelft, W.J.; Main, C.J. Behavioural treatment for chronic low-back pain. *Cochrane Database Syst. Rev.* **2010**, CD002014. [CrossRef] [PubMed]

24. Ruegsegger, G.N.; Booth, F.W. Health Benefits of Exercise. *Cold Spring Harb. Perspect. Med.* **2018**, *8*, a029694. [CrossRef]

25. van Middelkoop, M.; Rubinstein, S.M.; Verhagen, A.P.; Ostelo, R.W.; Koes, B.W.; van Tulder, M.W. Exercise therapy for chronic nonspecific low-back pain. *Best Pract. Res. Clin. Rheumatol.* **2010**, *24*, 193–204. [CrossRef]

26. Ryan, R.; Hill, S. How to GRADE the quality of the evidence. *Cochrane Consum. Commun. Gr* **2019**, 1–24. [CrossRef]

27. Longo, U.G.; Loppini, M.; Denaro, L.; Maffulli, N.; Denaro, V. Rating scales for low back pain. *Br. Med. Bull.* **2010**, *94*, 81–144. [CrossRef]

28. Moher, D.; Liberati, A.; Tetzlaff, J.; Altman, D.G. Preferred Reporting Items for Systematic Reviews and Meta-Analyses: The PRISMA Statement. *PLoS Med.* **2009**, *6*, e1000097. [CrossRef]

29. Sterne, J.A.C.; Savović, J.; Page, M.J.; Elbers, R.G.; Blencowe, N.S.; Boutron, I.; Cates, C.J.; Cheng, H.Y.; Corbett, M.S.; Eldridge, S.M.; et al. RoB 2: A revised tool for assessing risk of bias in randomised trials. *BMJ* **2019**, *366*. [CrossRef]

30. Sterne, J.A.; Hernán, M.A.; Reeves, B.C.; Savović, J.; Berkman, N.D.; Viswanathan, M.; Henry, D.; Altman, D.G.; Ansari, M.T.; Boutron, I.; et al. ROBINS-I: A tool for assessing risk of bias in non-randomised studies of interventions. *BMJ* **2016**, *355*. [CrossRef]

31. Teut, M.; Knilli, J.; Daus, D.; Roll, S.; Witt, C.M. Qigong or Yoga Versus No Intervention in Older Adults with Chronic Low Back Pain—A Randomized Controlled Trial. *J. Pain* **2016**, *17*, 796–805. [CrossRef] [PubMed]

32. Ferrell, B.A.; Josephson, K.R.; Pollan, A.M.; Loy, S.; Ferrell, B.R. A randomized trial of walking versus physical methods for chronic pain management. *Aging Clin. Exp. Res.* **1997**, *9*, 99–105. [CrossRef] [PubMed]

33. Vincent, H.K.; George, S.Z.; Seay, A.N.; Vincent, K.R.; Hurley, R.W. Resistance Exercise, Disability, and Pain Catastrophizing in Obese Adults with Back Pain. *Med. Sci. Sports Exerc.* **2014**, *46*, 1693–1701. [CrossRef] [PubMed]

34. Hicks, G.E.; Benvenuti, F.; Fiaschi, V.; Lombardi, B.; Segenni, L.; Stuart, M.; Pretzer-Aboff, I.; Gianfranco, G.; Macchi, C. Adherence to a community-based exercise program is a strong predictor of improved back pain status in older adults: An observational study. *Clin. J. Pain* **2012**, *28*, 195–203. [CrossRef] [PubMed]

35. Tsatsakos, G.; Kouli, O.; Michalopoulou, M.; Malliou, P.; Godolias, G. Effect of Physical Activity on Functional Status in Elderly with Chronic Low Back Pain. *J. Yoga Phys. Ther.* **2014**, *4*, 2.

36. Vincent, H.K.; Vincent, K.R.; Seay, A.N.; Conrad, B.P.; Hurley, R.W.; George, S.Z. Back strength predicts walking improvement in obese, older adults with chronic low back pain. *PMR* **2014**, *6*, 418–426. [CrossRef]

37. Khalil, T.M.; Abdel-Moty, E.; Diaz, E.L.; Steele-Rosomoff, R.; Rosomoff, H.L. Efficacy of physical restoration in the elderly. *Exp. Aging Res.* **1994**, *20*, 189–199. [CrossRef]

38. Mailloux, J.; Finno, M.; Rainville, J. Long-term exercise adherence in the elderly with chronic low back pain. *Am. J. Phys. Med. Rehabil.* **2006**, *85*, 120–126. [CrossRef]

39. Beissner, K.; Parker, S.; Henderson, C.R., Jr.; Pal, A.; Papaleontiou, M.; Reid, M.C. Implementing a Combined Cognitive-Behavioral + Exercise Therapy Protocol for Use by Older Adults with Chronic Back Pain: Evidence for a Possible Race/Ethnicity Effect. *J. Aging Phys. Act.* **2012**, *16*, 246–265. [CrossRef]

40. Iversen, M.D.; Fossel, A.H.; Katz, J.N. Enhancing function in older adults with chronic low back pain: A pilot study of endurance training. *Arch. Phys. Med. Rehabil.* **2003**, *84*, 1324–1331. [CrossRef]

41. Costantino, C.; Romiti, D. Effectiveness of Back School program versus hydrotherapy in elderly patients with chronic non-specific low back pain: A randomized clinical trial. *Acta Biomedica* **2014**, *85*, 52–61. [PubMed]

42. Holmes, B.; Leggett, S.; Mooney, V.; Nichols, J.; Negri, S.; Hoeyberghs, A. Comparison of female geriatric lumbar-extension strength: Asymptotic versus chronic low back pain patients and their response to active rehabilitation. *J. Spinal Disord.* **1996**, *9*, 17–22. [CrossRef] [PubMed]

43. Di Martino, A.; Russo, F.; Denaro, L.; Denaro, V. How to treat lumbar disc herniation in pregnancy? A systematic review on current standards. *Eur. Spine J.* **2017**, *26*, 496–504. [CrossRef] [PubMed]

44. Di Martino, A.; Papapietro, N.; Lanotte, A.; Russo, F.; Vadalà, G.; Denaro, V. Spondylodiscitis: Standards of current treatment. *Curr. Med. Res. Opin.* **2012**, *28*, 689–699. [CrossRef]

45. Vitoula, K.; Venneri, A.; Varrassi, G.; Paladini, A.; Sykioti, P.; Adewusi, J.; Zis, P. Behavioral Therapy Approaches for the Management of Low Back Pain: An Up-To-Date Systematic Review. *Pain Ther.* **2018**, *7*, 1–12. [CrossRef]

46. Vadalà, G.; Russo, F.; Ambrosio, L.; Papalia, R.; Denaro, V. Mesenchymal stem cells for intervertebral disc regeneration. *J. Biol. Regul. Homeost. Agents* **2016**, *30*, 173–179.

47. Russo, F.; Hartman, R.A.; Bell, K.M.; Vo, N.; Sowa, G.A.; Kang, J.D.; Vadalà, G.; Denaro, V. Biomechanical Evaluation of Transpedicular Nucleotomy With Intact Annulus Fibrosus. *Spine* **2017**, *42*, E193–E201. [CrossRef]

48. Papalia, R.; Zampogna, B.; Torre, G.; Lanotte, A.; Vasta, S.; Albo, E.; Tecame, A.; Denaro, V. Sarcopenia and its relationship with osteoarthritis: Risk factor or direct consequence? *Musculoskelet. Surg.* **2014**, *98*, 9–14. [CrossRef]

49. Bijlsma, A.Y.; Meskers, C.G.M.; van den Eshof, N.; Westendorp, R.G.; Sipilä, S.; Stenroth, L.; Sillanpää, E.; McPhee, J.S.; Jones, D.A.; Narici, M.V.; et al. Diagnostic criteria for sarcopenia and physical performance. *Age* **2014**, *36*, 275–285. [CrossRef]

50. Morley, J.E. Frailty and sarcopenia in elderly. *Wien. Klin. Wochenschr.* **2016**, *128*, 439–445. [CrossRef]

51. Landi, F.; Marzetti, E.; Martone, A.M.; Bernabei, R.; Onder, G. Exercise as a remedy for sarcopenia. *Curr. Opin. Clin. Nutr. Metab. Care* **2014**, *17*, 25–31. [CrossRef] [PubMed]

52. Colaianni, G.; Cinti, S.; Colucci, S.; Grano, M. Irisin and musculoskeletal health. *Ann. NY Acad. Sci.* **2017**, *1402*, 5–9. [CrossRef] [PubMed]

53. Greenhill, C. Exercise: Osteocalcin in the adaptation to exercise. *Nat. Rev. Endocrinol.* **2016**, *12*, 434. [CrossRef] [PubMed]

54. Briganti, S.I.; Gaspa, G.; Tabacco, G.; Naciu, A.M.; Cesareo, R.; Manfrini, S.; Palermo, A. Irisin as a regulator of bone and glucose metabolism. *Minerva Endocrinol.* **2018**, *43*, 489–500.

55. Korta, P.; Pocheć, E.; Mazur-Biały, A. Irisin as a Multifunctional Protein: Implications for Health and Certain Diseases. *Medicina* **2019**, *55*, 485. [CrossRef]

56. Diaz-Franco, M.C.; Franco-Diaz de Leon, R.; Villafan-Bernal, J.R. Osteocalcin-GPRC6A: An update of its clinical and biological multi-organic interactions (Review). *Mol. Med. Rep.* **2019**, *19*, 15–22. [CrossRef]

57. Karsenty, G. Update on the biology of osteocalcin. *Endocr. Pract.* **2017**, *23*, 1270–1274. [CrossRef]

58. Mera, P.; Laue, K.; Ferron, M.; Confavreux, C.; Wei, J.; Galán-Díez, M.; Lacampagne, A.; Mitchell, S.J.; Mattison, J.A.; Chen, Y.; et al. Osteocalcin Signaling in Myofibers Is Necessary and Sufficient for Optimum Adaptation to Exercise. *Cell Metab.* **2016**, *23*, 1078–1092. [CrossRef]

59. Russo, F.; Ambrosio, L.; Ngo, K.; Vadalà, G.; Denaro, V.; Fan, Y.; Sowa, G.; Kang, J.D.; Vo, N. The Role of Type I Diabetes in Intervertebral Disc Degeneration. *Spine* **2019**, *44*, 1177–1185. [CrossRef]

60. Chahla, S.E.; Frohnert, B.I.; Thomas, W.; Kelly, A.S.; Nathan, B.M.; Polgreen, L.E. Higher daily physical activity is associated with higher osteocalcin levels in adolescents. *Prev. Med. Rep.* **2015**, *2*, 568–571. [CrossRef]

61. Castrogiovanni, P.; Trovato, F.M.; Szychlinska, M.A.; Nsir, H.; Imbesi, R.; Musumeci, G. The importance of physical activity in osteoporosis. From the molecular pathways to the clinical evidence. *Histol. Histopathol.* **2016**, *31*, 1183–1194. [PubMed]

62. McMillan, L.B.; Zengin, A.; Ebeling, P.R.; Scott, D. Prescribing Physical Activity for the Prevention and Treatment of Osteoporosis in Older Adults. *Healthcare* **2017**, *5*, 85. [CrossRef] [PubMed]

63. Warburton, D.E.R.; Nicol, C.W.; Bredin, S.S.D. Health benefits of physical activity: The evidence. *Can. Med. Assoc. J.* **2006**, *174*, 801–809. [CrossRef] [PubMed]

Permissions

List of Contributors

Pia Simonsen Lentz and Anna Havelund Rasmussen
Department of Physiotherapy and Occupational Therapy, North Denmark Regional Hospital, Bispensgade 37, DK-9800 Hjoerring, Denmark

Aysun Yurtsever
Department of Rheumatology, North Denmark Regional Hospital, Bispensgade 37, DK-9800 Hjørring, Denmark

Dorte Melgaard
Centre for Clinical Research, North Denmark Regional Hospital, DK-9800 Hjoerring, Denmark
Department of Clinical Medicine, Aalborg University, DK-9000 Aalborg, Denmark

Shao-Wei Huang
Graduate School of Design, National Yunlin University of Science and Technology, Yunlin 640, Taiwan

Tsen-Yao Chang
Department of Creative Design, National Yunlin University of Science and Technology, Yunlin 640, Taiwan

Maria Graça
Research Centre for Physical Activity, Health and Leisure, Faculty of Sport, University of Porto, 4200-450 Porto, Portugal
School of Health Sciences, University of Aveiro, 3810-193 Aveiro, Portugal
Porto Biomechanics Laboratory (LABIOMEP-UP), University of Porto, 4200-450 Porto, Portugal

José Alvarelhão and Rui Costa
School of Health Sciences, University of Aveiro, 3810-193 Aveiro, Portugal

Ricardo J. Fernandes and João Paulo Vilas-Boas
Porto Biomechanics Laboratory (LABIOMEP-UP), University of Porto, 4200-450 Porto, Portugal
Centre of Research, Education, Innovation and Intervention in Sport, Faculty of Sport, University of Porto, 4200-450 Porto, Portugal

Andrea Ribeiro
Porto Biomechanics Laboratory (LABIOMEP-UP), University of Porto, 4200-450 Porto, Portugal
School of Health, Fernando Pessoa University, 4200-253 Porto, Portugal

Daniel Daly
Department of Movement Sciences, KU Leuven, 3001 Leuven, Belgium

Sebastiano Vasta, Rocco Papalia, Guglielmo Torre, Ferruccio Vorini, Giuseppe Papalia, Biagio Zampogna, Stefano Campi and Vincenzo Denaro
Department of Orthopaedic and Trauma Surgery, Campus Bio-Medico University of Rome, 00128 Rome, Italy

Chiara Fossati
Department of Movement, Human and Health Sciences, University of Rome "Foro Italico", 00100 Rome, Italy

Marco Bravi
Department of Physical Medicine and Rehabilitation, Campus Bio-Medico University of Rome, 00128 Rome, Italy

Lorenzo Alirio Diaz Balzani and Anna Maria Alifano
Department of Orthopaedic and Trauma Surgery, Campus Bio-Medico University of Rome, 00128 Rome, Italy

Riccardo Borzuola, Arrigo Giombini, Paolo Borrione and Andrea Macaluso
Department of Movement, Human and Health Sciences, University of Rome "Foro Italico", 00135 Rome, Italy

Erika Albo
Department of Orthopaedic and Trauma Surgery, Campus Bio-Medico University of Rome, 00128 Rome, Italy

Marco Alessandro Minetto, Alessandro Giannini, Rebecca McConnell, Chiara Busso and Giuseppe Massazza
Division of Physical Medicine and Rehabilitation, Department of Surgical Sciences, University of Turin, 10126 Turin, Italy

Mauro Ciuffreda and Chiara De Andreis
Department of Orthopaedic and Trauma Surgery, Campus Bio-Medico University of Rome, 00128 Rome, Italy

Federica Fagnani, Attilio Parisi and Fabio Pigozzi
Department of Movement, Human and Health Sciences, University of Rome "Foro Italico", 00135 Rome, Italy

Matteo Turchetta
Department of Orthopaedics, Policlinico Casilino, 00169 Rome, Italy

Maurizio Casasco
Italian Federation of Sports Medicine, 00196 Rome, Italy

Antonio De Vincentis
Deaprtment of Orthopaedic and Trauma Surgery, Campus Bio-Medico University of Rome, Via A. Del Portillo, 21, 00128 Rome, Italy
Department of Internal Medicine and Gerontology, Campus Bio-Medico University of Rome, Via A. Del Portillo, 21, 00128 Rome, Italy

Umile Giuseppe Longo and Vincenzo Candela
Department of Orthopedic and Trauma Surgery, Campus Bio-Medico University, Via Alvaro del Portillo, 200, 00128 Trigoria, Rome, Italy

Maria Matarese, Valeria Arcangeli, Viviana Alciati, Gabriella Facchinetti, Anna Marchetti, Maria Grazia De Marinis
Research Unit Nursing Science, Campus Bio-Medico di Roma University, 00128 Rome, Italy

Gianluca Vadalà, Fabrizio Russo, Sergio De Salvatore and Gabriele Cortina
Department of Orthopaedic and Trauma Surgery, University Campus Bio-Medico of Rome, 00128 Rome, Italy

Index